**Wisconsin Publications in the
History of Science and Medicine
Number 8**

General Editors

†William Coleman
David C. Lindberg
Ronald L. Numbers

T0110833

The Middle English Gilbertus Anglicus, London, Wellcome MS 537, f. 275ᵛ.

HEALING AND SOCIETY
IN MEDIEVAL ENGLAND

A Middle English Translation of the Pharmaceutical Writings of

Gilbertus Anglicus

Edited with an Introduction and Notes by

Faye Marie Getz

The University of Wisconsin Press

The University of Wisconsin Press
1930 Monroe Street, 3rd floor
Madison, Wisconsin 53711-2059
uwpress.wisc.edu

3 Henrietta Street
London WC2E 8LU, England
eurospanbookstore.com

Printed in the United States of America

Library of Congress Cataloging-in-Publication Data
Getz, Faye Marie, 1952–
Healing and society in Medieval England: a Middle English translation of the
pharmaceutical writings of Gilbertus Anglicus / edited by Faye Marie Getz.
456 pp.   cm. — (Wisconsin publications in the history of science
and medicine ; no. 8)
Originally presented as the author's thesis (doctoral—University
of Toronto), 1981.
Includes bibliographical references.
1. Gilbertus, Anglicus. Compendium medicinae. English (Middle
English) 2. Medicine, Medieval—England. I. Series.
[DNLM: 1. Gilbertus, Anglicus. 2. History of Medicine, Medieval—
England. 3. Pharmacy—history—England. W1 WI805 no. 8 /
WZ 294
G466cG]
R487.G55313G48   1991
610'.942'0902—dc20   90-50643
ISBN 0-299-12930-6   CIP

ISBN-13: 978-0-299-12934-7 (pbk.: alk. paper)

For Hal

Contents

Preface

The Middle English Gilbertus Anglicus is a fifteenth century translation of the Latin practice of medicine found in *Compendium medicinae*, written before about 1250 by Gilbertus Anglicus, England's first notable medical writer. The fact that a scholastic medical text was translated from its original Latin into the English vernacular demonstrates an audience for learned medicine outside the walls of the university. Over a dozen witnesses to the text have been located. All are datable within about fifty years of each other and none contain any attribution to the author. Before my identification, no such translation was known to exist. This edition presents the entire text for the first time.

I am pleased to acknowledge the assistance of Mr. Eric Freeman, Librarian and Deputy Director of the Wellcome Institute; Mr. Robin Price, Deputy Librarian; Dr. Richard Palmer, Keeper of Western Manuscripts, Wellcome Library; Dr. W. F. Bynum, Head of the Wellcome Unit, London; Mr. Stephen Emberton, Administrator, Wellcome Institute; and the staff of the Library of the Wellcome Institute for the History of Medicine and of the Institute of Historical Research, London, without whose help this study would not have been possible. I would also like to express my gratitude to Prof. A. Rupert Hall, Dr. Marie Boas Hall, Dr. Charles Talbot, and Dr. Vivian Nutton, who advised and assisted me while I worked in London.

This book is based on my doctoral dissertation, presented at the Centre for Medieval Studies, University of Toronto, in 1981. Many people contributed to its completion, none more than Prof. George Rigg. I am also happy to thank Prof. Jeffrey Heath, Prof. John Munro, and the staff of both the Centre for Medieval Studies and the Pontifical Institute of Mediaeval Studies, who have acted variously as supportive friends and valued colleagues. Countless errors and omissions were remedied at various stages of this edition by gifts of time and expertise from the following readers: Prof. Martha Carlin, Prof. Harold J. Cook, Dr. Karis

Crawford, Mr. Eric Freeman, Mr. Peter Murray Jones, Dr. Vivian Nutton, Prof. George Rigg, the late Prof. Rossell Hope Robbins, Prof. Linda Voigts, and an anonymous reader. This edition was brought to completion with the help of my husband, Prof. Harold J. Cook, who prepared the photoready copy, and whose expertise with computers and patience with the complexities of book production were freely given in generous amounts. Finally, I would like to thank Professors Ronald L. Numbers, David C. Lindberg, and the late William Coleman, the editors of the series in which this book appears.

The following libraries have been of assistance in the preparation of this edition: the British Library, Glasgow University Library, Library of the Society of Antiquaries, Library of Trinity College, Cambridge, and the Wellcome Institute Library. The research for this book was funded by the Hannah Institute for the History of Medicine in Toronto, Canada, and by the Wellcome Trust in London, England. The final stages of the preparation of the manuscript were supported by a grant from the National Library of Medicine. Material from Wellcome manuscripts as well as extracts from manuscripts in the British Library are published with the permission of the Keeper of Western Manuscripts of the Wellcome Library and the Keeper of Manuscripts of the British Library. Parts of the introduction to this edition appeared in an article entitled "Gilbertus Anglicus Anglicized," *Medical History* 26 (1982): 436-42, and are reprinted here with the permission of the editors. The text is available on floppy disk from the author.

The following sigla and abbreviations have been established for use in this edition.

Sigla for manuscripts containing the Middle English Gilbertus Anglicus:

> Add 25589: London, British Library, Additional MS 25589.
> Add 30338: London, British Library, Additional MS 30338.
> H: San Marino, California, Huntington MS 19079.
> Har 2375: London, British Library, Harley MS 2375.
> Har 3407: London, British Library, Harley MS 3407.
> Hu U.7.1: Glasgow, Hunterian MS U.7.ll.
> Hu V.8.12: Glasgow, Hunterian MS V.8.12.
> Sl 5: London, British Library, Sloane MS 5.
> Sl 442: London, British Library, Sloane MS 442.
> Sl 2394: London, British Library, Sloane MS 2394.
> Sl 3486: London, British Library, Sloane MS 3486.
> Sl 3553: London, British Library, Sloane MS 3553.
> SoA: London, Society of Antiquaries MS 338.
> TCC: Cambridge, Trinity College MS O. 9. 37.
> W: the Middle English Gilbertus translation found in London, Wellcome MS 537.

Abbreviations:
EETS: Early English Text Society.
L: Gilbertus Anglicus, *Compendium medicine*. Lyons: J. Saccon for V. de Portonariis, 1510.
Seymour: *On the Properties of Things: John Trevisa's Translation of Bartholomaeus Anglicus* De proprietatibus rerum*: A Critical Text*. Edited by M. C. Seymour et al. 3 vols. Oxford: Clarendon Press, 1975-88.
Talbot and Hammond: Talbot, C. H., and Hammond, E. A. *The Medical Practitioners in Medieval England: A Biographical Register*. London: Wellcome Institute, 1965.
TK: *A Catalogue of Incipits of Mediaeval Scientific Writings in Latin*. Edited by Lynn Thorndike and Pearl Kibre. Revised and augmented. New York: Mediaeval Academy of America, 1963.

Middle English letters that do not survive in modern English are:
þ: thorn, a *th* sound; ex. *þat* = that.
3: yogh, a *g* or *y* sound; ex. *3eer* = year, *a3enst* = against.

Citations to W made in the Introduction and Glossary are by folio number. Scribal errors in ordering the material in the text have made it necessary to rearrange those folios in the following order: 48-152, 153-157ᵛ, 158ᵛ-168ᵛ, 170-170ᵛ, 169-169ᵛ, 172-172ᵛ, 171-171ᵛ, 173-194, 221-275ᵛ, 194-202, 203, 202ᵛ, 203ᵛ-221, 275ᵛ-310ᵛ.

Faye M. Getz

Madison, Wisconsin
January 14, 1991

Introduction

The Middle English Gilbertus Anglicus consists for the most part of medicinal recipes, grouped according to the diseases for which they were useful. These recipes in turn were arranged roughly from the head downward, with the text divided into chapters that are introduced by simple guides for diagnosis. The text also defined for its readers many Latin medical terms. The Gilbertus translation shares material with other Middle English recipe collections, although it is not clear whether the Middle English or Latin version of the *Compendium* was the source of this shared material.

The recipes found in the Middle English Gilbertus derive almost exclusively from the Latin exemplar, and thus cannot be said to be characteristic of "folk" medicine. Nor can those Middle English recipe collections that share material with the Middle English Gilbertus (as many seem to) be labeled as such. Instead, the Middle English Gilbertus and those collections that share material with it would seem to represent a popularization and simplification of Latin medical learning.[1] Not every recipe from every collection had a learned origin: these collections are

---

[1] Major sources for information about the scope and development of the Middle English medical text are as follows: Linda Ehrsam Voigts, "Medical Prose," in *Middle English Prose*: *A Critical Guide to Major Authors and Genres*, ed. A. S. G. Edwards (New Brunswick: Rutgers University Press, 1984), pp. 315-35; H. S. Bennett, "Medicine," in *English Books and Readers, 1475-1557*, 2d ed. (Cambridge: Cambridge University Press, 1970), pp. 97-109; Rossell Hope Robbins, "Medical Manuscripts in Middle English," *Speculum* 45 (1970): 393-415; Voigts, "Scientific and Medical Books," in *Book Production and Publishing in Britain, 1375-1475*," ed. Jeremy Griffiths and Derek Pearsall (Cambridge: Cambridge University Press, 1989), pp. 345-402.

themselves compendia from a variety of sources, especially from other recipe collections. But the Middle English Gilbertus must be regarded as representative of a larger trend in late medieval English vernacular literature as a whole: the production in manuscript form of a body of useful knowledge for popular consumption. It is, in short, a very early example of the "self-help" manual, derived from learned Latin sources.[2]

The Wellcome version of the Gilbertus translation is of special interest for several reasons. It provides excellent evidence of how a medieval manuscript was rearranged, divided, and corrected. It is unique among manuscripts of the Gilbertus text in that it contains numerous illuminated initials, and, more important, it demonstrates how the scribe edited his more complete exemplar to remove most references to the diseases of women and children, to travel, and to the use of animals and animal parts in medicinal preparations. The type of binding, the illumination, and the scribal editing indicate that the Wellcome Gilbertus, unlike other witnesses, was probably produced in a monastic house.[3]

This edition places one witness to the Middle English Gilbertus in its historical and textual context. It demonstrates that the Middle English Gilbertus is a translation of a Latin exemplar. It also shows how one manuscript was prepared, how this manuscript relates to others containing the same text, and how the translation was incorporated into various compendia. It also shows how Middle English recipe collections share material with the Gilbertus translation, and how that shared material can be traced to earlier Latin sources. Finally, it places the

---

[2] The increase in availability of information in the vernacular that took place in England from the beginning of the fifteenth century suggests that the printing press, rather than marking the onset of demand for such material, instead accelerated an already existing demand: Faye Marie Getz, "Gilbertus Anglicus Anglicized," *Medical History* 26 (1982): 436-42. On the nature of this demand, see Getz, "Charity, Translation, and the Language of Medical Learning in Medieval England," *Bull. Hist. Medicine* 64 (1990): 1-17. German scholarship into the production of useful knowledge in the vernacular is quite developed. See Volker Zimmermann, *Rezeption und Rolle der Heilkunde in landessprachigen handschriftlichen Kompendien des Spätmittelalters* (Stuttgart: Franz Steiner Verlag, 1986). See also Jerry Stannard, "Rezeptliteratur as Fachliteratur," in *Studies on Medieval Fachliteratur*, ed. William Eamon, *Scripta* 6 (Brussels, 1982): 59-63. More general are Bennett, "Translations and Translators," and "Trial List of Translations into English Printed between 1475-1569," in *English Books and Readers, 1474-1557*, pp. 152-77, 277-319. For the early modern period, see Paul Slack, "Mirrors of Health and Treasures of Poor Men: The Uses of the Vernacular Medical Literature of Tudor England," in *Health, Medicine and Mortality in the Sixteenth Century*, ed. Charles Webster (Cambridge: Cambridge University Press, 1979), pp. 237-73.

[3] See below p. lvi. I am grateful to Dr. Charles Talbot for his advice on the nature of the binding of the Wellcome manuscript.

recipe collection in a historical context, suggesting that the level of learning such collections represent deserves further exploration in the light of Latin textual traditions.

The function texts such as the Middle English Gilbertus were intended to serve is still very much an open issue. One way of approaching this question is to ask about the persons who owned or commissioned such texts. Middle English medical manuscripts often belonged to the less formally educated among medical practitioners. A fifteenth-century compendium of short texts belonged to Essex bailiff and leech John Crophill, and is preserved in British Library, Harley MS 1735. London barber-surgeon Richard Dod owned British Library, Sloane MS 5, and London barber-surgeon Thomas Plawdon had a medical compendium translated for him found in Cambridge, Gonville and Caius MS 176/97.[4]

More formally educated medical practitioners may have produced vernacular recipes, possibly for their students or patrons. Oxford physician John Cokkys (died ca. 1475) is credited with several Middle English recipes in Oxford, Bodley, Ashmole MS 1432 (late 15th-early 16th c.), a learned medical compendium in Middle English and Latin.[5] These recipes include preparations "for the pallesy in a mannes handis," "a goode drynke for the dropesie," "for the ye sight," and one to "breke the stone, made be Magister John Cokkes and proved uppon hymselffe." Other vernacular recipes included in the collection were associated with learned persons, including one for the stone said to have been used by George Neville, archbishop of York.[6]

Most medical manuscripts containing recipes are like Ashmole 1432. They have texts in more than one language: Middle English, Latin, and sometimes Norman French. Although in general one may say that Latin was the language of the university-educated physician, while English was easier to understand for those outside the university, be they lay person or medical practitioner, the division was not clear-cut. In a multilingual society like that of late medieval England, language alone must be regarded an exceedingly inexact indicator of ownership.

Closely related to the issue of ownership is that of intended usage. What little is known about the use of pharmaceuticals by medical practitioners points to the conclusion that recipes like those found in the

---

[4] For Crophill, see James K. Mustain, "A Rural Medical Practitioner in Fifteenth-Century England," *Bull. Hist. Medicine* 46 (1972): 469-76. Dod's manuscript contains a version of the Gilbertus translation and is discussed below, p. lxx and following. For Plawdon see Linda E. Voigts and Michael R. McVaugh, "A Latin Technical Phlebotomy and its Middle English Translation," *Trans. American Philos. Soc.* 74, 2 (1984), esp. pp. 15, 24-25.

[5] Talbot and Hammond, pp. 134-36.

[6] Ashmole MS 1432, pp. 11, 17, 18, 5, 4. Neville died in 1476, having followed Gilbert Kymer, MD, as chancellor of Oxford University. He was at Balliol with humanist physician John Free (*Dictionary of National Biography*, Vol. 14, pp. 252-57).

Middle English Gilbertus were more than exercises in "slavish copying": there is evidence of the actual use of these pharmaceuticals. For example, Oxford physician William Goldwyn recommended for his patron Lady Stonor syrup of roses, liverwort, endive seed, plantain, vinegar, and wormwood in a prescription filled by Goldwyn's apothecary John Byrrel in 1480.[7] All of these ingredients are common enough in many Middle English recipe collections, including the Gilbertus translation. The type of documentation provided by the Stonor letters is rare, but as will be shown below, there is evidence that the pharmaceuticals described in medieval English recipe collections were encountered on many levels of medieval English society.

These recipe collections were more complex in their origins and meaning than has generally been supposed, and they admit no easy generalizations about language, intended use, or ownership. Many gaps in our understanding of these documents can be supplied only by returning the recipe collection to its historical context, and by examining the place of pharmaceutical practice in medieval English culture.

I. HISTORICAL BACKGROUND

A. Theoretical Justifications for Pharmaceutical Practices

The notion that nothing in nature was without power underlies much of medieval pharmaceutical practice, and accounts in part for the enormous variety of substances medieval people employed in their medicines.[8]   The Gilbertus translation named nearly four hundred

---

[7] *The Stonor Letters and Papers, 1290-1483*, ed. C. L. Kingsford, 2 vols. Camden 3d ser. 29-30 (1919), vol. 2, pp. 107-8. Another patron of apothecaries was Queen Isabella, wife of Edward II, who was said to have died in 1358 from the "effect of too powerful a medicine, administered at her own desire":   Leslie G. Matthews, *The Royal Apothecaries* (London: Wellcome Institute, 1967), p. 25. Whether these distinguished persons can be regarded as representative of any widespread trend in medieval society can only be surmised. See Robbins and Slack, who attempt to infer from the growth in numbers of vernacular medical texts a marked increase in popular readership.

[8] A favorite scriptural citation in support of the utility of all of God's creation to humanity came from the Book of Ecclesiasticus: "The Lord has created medicines from the earth, and a sensible man will not disparage them" (37:4). A popular representative of this viewpoint was Hildegard of Bingen.   On her knowledge of medicinal plants, see Irmgard Müller, *Die pflanzlichen Heilmittel bei Hildegard von Bingen* (Salzburg: Otto Müller Verlag, 1982).

therapeutic substances, from gutted puppies to gold filings, and its Latin exemplar suggested many more. Theoretical justifications for the usage of these substances ranged from the merely empirical to what might be called the symbolic, and it is often impossible to tell just by examining the ingredients of a recipe in isolation precisely which levels of meaning were operating.

For instance, the cartilage found in a stag's heart was often recommended for strengthening the human heart.[9] A modern pharmacologist probably would find the cartilage medically inert. But for the medieval medical writer, the connection between the stag's heart and the human heart, from which flowed the body's heat and life, was powerfully symbolic and affirmed the writer's view of Creation. God put animals on the earth under human dominion.[10] The stag was an animal whose long life was legendary, and whose heart, when eaten, stimulated the body's natural heat, thus prolonging a person's life to its fullest extent.[11] The cartilage was rare, of course, a proof of its value, as rare as were gold, coral, pearls, precious spices, and gems, other commonly recommended medicines for the heart.[12]

It is tempting to assume that prescriptions containing rare and exotic ingredients were never intended for use, but were instead copied *pro forma*, in the same way as were literary or scriptural texts. Historical documentation suggests otherwise. Just as the "nobility" of the heart required rare and noble medicines, the same could be said for the nobility of the individual. A rich person was better served by costly medicines, while the poor needed only humble remedies.[13] A historical case in point involved apothecary Richard de Montpellier, spicer to Edward I. In collaboration with Oxford physician Nicholas Tyngewick, Richard sent the king, who was suffering from dysentery and an ailment of the feet and legs, an impressive array of medicaments. They included an electuary containing ambergris, musk, pearls, gold, and silver; rose sugar with ground pearls; pomegranate wine; and a plaster for his neck containing ambergris and rare gums. The value of Richard's prescription was over £134, a debt Edward died leaving unpaid.[14]

---

[9] See W, f. 189v.

[10] See Genesis 1:27-30.

[11] An anecdote about a stag which, when captured, bore a collar put round its neck at the time of Julius Caesar, is related in a text attributed to Roger Bacon: "Summaria expositio epistole fratris Rogeri Bacon de retardatione accidentium senectutis," in *De retardatione accidentium senectutis cum aliis opusculis de rebus medicinalibus*, ed. A. G. Little and E. Withington, Brit. Soc. Franciscan Studies 14 (1928), pp. 87-8.

[12] See W, f. 189v.

[13] See W, ff. 198v-199.

[14] A. Way, "Bill of Medicines Furnished for the Use of Edward I. 34 and 35 Edw. I., 1306-7," *Archaeological Journal* 14 (1857): 267-71. Compare these expensive drugs with those listed in a recipe for pills of diacastor in W, ff. 76-77.

Not all medicinal ingredients found in medieval recipe collections operated according to these symbolic justifications. Most received their theoretical underpinning from the humoral or dietetic medicine of the ancient Greeks as transmitted to the Latin West via Islam.[15] Very simply put, the humoral theory taught that the body was composed of four humors: blood, choler, phlegm, and melancholy. Each of these four had two qualities. Blood was hot and moist, choler hot and dry, phlegm cold and moist, and melancholy cold and dry. Health was the perfect balance of these humors and their qualities, disease their imbalance. The purpose of therapy was to restore this equilibrium.

According to the Middle English Gilbertus, all diseases were either hot, cold, moist, or dry. A hot headache was accompanied by a red forehead, a fast pulse, red urine, and an aversion to hot things.[16] Hot headaches were treated by cold remedies, and by the avoidance of too much thinking, staying awake, bathing, and sexual excitement.[17] Most diseases described in the Middle English text were treated by exactly the same method as was the hot headache: by drugs or regimen having the opposite effect to that of the disease.[18]

Where the Middle English Gilbertus parted company with other recipe books is in its technical explanations for the actions of drugs. Sensory qualities such as "cold," "sharp," and "biting" often appear. But more descriptive terms, usually based on the imagery of burning, freezing, and melting, were also employed. Dissolutives were "hot medicines that can dissolve the matter of the sickness just as the heat of the sun dissolves ice or snow into water" (W, f. 78v). Stupefactives such as opium should be used to deliver a medication to the kidneys because they are too cold to be dissolved along the way:

> Because medicines pass many ways before they
> come to the kidneys, it is therefore better for
> them to contain something to carry them to the
> kidneys that will not be consumed or wasted
> away too soon, such as opium. But remember
> that just as opium quenches a person's natural
> heat, so myrrh and balm tend a person's
> natural heat, just as oil tends and feeds fire.
> Therefore mix them together. (F. 278v)

The Middle English Gilbertus also defined the actions of confortatives, repercussives, mitigatives, corrosives, strictories, laxatives,

---

[15] See especially Jerry Stannard, "Botanical Data and Late Mediaeval 'Rezeptliteratur,'" in *Fachprosa-Studien: Beiträge zur mittelalterlichen Wissenschafts- und Geistesgeschichte*, ed. Gundolf Keil et al. (Berlin: Erich Schmidt Verlag, 1982), pp. 371-95, esp. pp. 388-95.

[16] Add 30338, f. 11v, printed in the Commentary, n. 1/ .

[17] W, f. 48.

[18] An excellent example of humoral diagnosis and therapy appears in W's chapter on mania (ff. 58-61).

subtilitives, diuretics, and maturatives.   In addition, media for
administering medications were described: pills, fumigations, enemas,
electuaries, and suppositories.   The care with which the translation
explained these terms makes it an invaluable tool for understanding the
language of medieval English pharmacy.

All medication was directed toward stimulating the power of the
body to heal itself. The practitioner was cautioned to mitigate the action
of harsh drugs with comforting ones,

> for unless the member is strong enough to
> function on its own, the strength of the
> medicine will do little good: The medicine is
> only a helper, and the principal actor is the
> part that is sick. (F. 79)

Yet another level of pharmaceutical speculation, beginning in
the Latin West about 1200, was all but absent from the Middle English
Gilbertus and from other Middle English recipe collections.   When
translations of Arabic pharmaceutical texts began to be read at Western
universities, scholars attempted to elaborate on Islamic applications of
quantification to the compounding of pharmaceutical substances.
Questions were asked about the relationship between the "degree" or
intensity of the qualities of hot, cold, moist, and dry and quantity of a
drug.   Mathematical formulas were then offered to illustrate how to
compound pharmaceuticals to achieve the desired effects.[19]   Gilbertus
Anglicus himself knew about recently made translations of Islamic
physicians (he cited Avicenna frequently).   But the basis for his
pharmaceutical system remained that propounded by the School of
Salerno, the oldest medical university in the West.[20]   The Gilbertus
translation reflects what might be called the twelfth-century character of
Gilbertus' pharmaceutical system, a simple one free of attempts at
quantification and taking advantage of a large number of medicinal

---

[19] The complexities of quantifiable pharmaceutical practice in
the thirteenth and fourteenth centuries are explained by Michael R.
McVaugh, *Arnaldi de Villanova Opera medica omnia II: Aphorismi de
gradibus* (Granada-Barcelona: Seminarium   historiae   medicae
Granatensis, 1975); see especially chap. 3:   "Arabic Mathematical
Pharmacy: Alkindi and Averroes," pp. 53-74.

[20] For the School of Salerno, see Paul Oskar Kristeller, *Studi
sulla Scuola medica salernitana* (Naples: Istituto Italiano per gli Studi
Filosofici, 1986), and Kristeller, "Bartholomaeus, Musandinus, and
Maurus of Salerno and Other Early Commentators of the 'Articella,'
with a Tentative List of Texts and Manuscripts," *Italia medioevale e
umanistica* 19 (1976): 57-87; also H. Bloch, *Monte Cassino in the Middle
Ages* (Cambridge: Harvard University Press, 1986), Vol. 1, pp. 98-110,
127-36.

substances.[21] Anyone searching for recipes in the translation would have had a large number from which to choose.

B. Pharmacy, Medicine, and Commerce

The late Middle Ages was a time of rapidly growing popular interest in medical learning and in the use of pharmaceuticals in general. London especially supplied a market for both medical expertise and drugs. The demand was not so much for advice about a regimen of health as for easy-to-use remedies providing a "quick fix," suitable not only for the poor, but also for anyone who lacked the leisure to regulate his or her life style in the way dietetic medicine required.

The preface to London priest John Mirfield's medical compendium, *Breviarium Bartholomei*, written in Latin before 1407, indicated how "quick fix" remedies could gain popularity over the dietetic medicine offered by learned physicians. Mirfield began his compendium thus:

> I want you to know that in many places in this piece I intend to use expedients [*experimenta*], both because they work faster, and because many sick people nowadays are exceedingly impatient: They do not want to wait around until the fourth or fifth day or longer if necessary, for the peccant matter to be digested and expelled properly, the way they used to do in the old days. Indeed, unless they feel an improvement right away the first day, they are distrustful of the physician, and reject his medicines and have contempt for them.[22]

---

[21] One of the earliest attacks on the multiplicity of medicinal substances propounded by physicians like Gilbertus comes from the next generation of natural philosophical thinkers. English Franciscan Roger Bacon wrote his *De erroribus medicorum* insisting that only a few drugs were necessary to promote health and prolong life. Their occult properties could be discovered by the study of nature's symbolism and of ancient texts. The philosopher's stone was offered as the ultimate medicine, making all others unnecessary. *De erroribus* is found in Latin in Little and Withington, *De retardatione*, pp. 150-79. An English translation is Mary Catherine Welborn, "The Errors of the Doctors according to Friar Roger Bacon of the Minor Order," *Isis* 18 (1932): 26-62. For medicine and alchemy, see *The Opus Majus of Roger Bacon*, ed. J. H. Bridges (London, 1900), vol. 2, pp. 204-13.

[22] My translation. The Latin text of the preface and another English translation are found in Percival Horton-Smith Hartley and

Mirfield called attention to three types of pharmaceutical practice. The first was embodied in dietetic medicine, based on natural philosophical principles, and requiring careful regulation in the hands of an educated physician who had an intimate knowledge of the life style of the patron. The second was that of *experimenta*, expedients that worked quickly, and did not involve a lengthy regimen, but were nonetheless approved by reason and by the ancient authorities. The third type of pharmaceutical practice, which Mirfield called another kind of experiment, was neither tested by reason nor approved by the ancient authorities, but instead was founded on empiricism alone. Mirfield rejected this altogether, as dangerous and deceptive, citing the first aphorism of Hippocrates for support.[23]

Mirfield also called attention to what had always been a difficulty with humoral or dietetic medicine. In order for it to operate successfully, the entire life style or regimen of the person had to be analyzed and carefully regulated.[24] Pharmaceuticals were employed as a part of this regulation, but ideally they were very mild ones used only in a preventative fashion. Mirfield wrote his book for St. Bartholomew's Hospital, Smithfield, London, where the sick were poor patients instead of rich patrons, whose life style did not permit the leisure of a well-regulated regimen of health.[25]

Harold Richard Aldridge, *Johannes de Mirfeld of St. Bartholomew's, Smithfield*: *His Life and Works* (Cambridge: Cambridge University Press, 1936), p. 50. For Mirfield's sources, see Faye Getz, "John Mirfield and the *Breviarium Bartholomei*: The Medical Writings of a Clerk at St. Bartholomew's Hospital in the Later Fourteenth Century," *Soc. Social Hist. Medicine Bull.* 37 (1985): 24-26.

[23] See Hartley and Aldridge, *Johannes de Mirfeld*. The first aphorism of Hippocrates warns that experience is deceptive: *Hippocratic Writings*, ed. G. E. R. Lloyd (London: Penguin Books, 1978), p. 206. The Middle English Gilbertus uses the word "experience" in still a different way, simply meaning a text or trial. See the Glossary: *experience*.

[24] According to Bacon: "Regimen sanitatis debeat esse in cibo et potu, somno et vigilia, motu et quiete, evacuatione et retentione, aeris dispositione, et passionibus animi; ut haec in debito temperamento habeantur ab infantia": Roger Bacon, *Opus majus*, ed. Bridges, p. 204. Bacon believed that the best advice on regimen of health was found in a set of letters supposedly sent by Aristotle to his student Alexander the Great, the *Secretum secretorum*. A summary of the history of the *Secretum* is found in *Secretum Secretorum*: *Nine English Versions*, ed. M. A. Manzalaoui, EETS 276 (1977), ix-1.

[25] Medieval hospitals served a broader function than their modern counterpart. Although some provided medical treatment, others also served the poor, the traveler, or the unwed mother. Several were notable educational institutions, and cared for orphans. Medieval hospitals thus must be seen as charitable institutions, and not exclusively as medical centers. A description of the workings of a medieval London

Just as the care of patients at London hospitals did not easily allow the use of dietetic medical advice, the burgeoning market economy of London demanded drugs, and information about drugs, for an instant cure, rather than advice about regulating life style, advice that required the leisure and riches of a king to be effective. And as Mirfield said, medical practitioners felt pressure to provide these expedient cures, lest the sick person lose confidence in the practitioner and his or her type of care.

The effect of market demand on medical practice was most apparent in medieval London, which in size and wealth dwarfed England's other urban centers. It was to London that the ill came, looking for treatment, drugs, or advice.[26] It was also in London that the medical profession established itself.[27] London's urban growth brought

---

hospital is Martha Carlin, "The Medieval Hospital of St. Thomas the Martyr," *Soc. Social Hist. Medicine Bull.* 37 (1985): 19-23. Also, see Carlin, "Medieval English Hospitals," in *The Hospital in History*, ed. Lindsay Granshaw and Roy Porter (London: Routledge, 1989), pp. 21-39, and Carole Rawcliffe, "The Hospitals of Later Medieval London," *Medical History* 28 (1984): 1-21. Rawcliffe points out that London hospitals were much more concerned with regimen for the well-being of the soul than for that of the body (p. 11).

[26] A London coroner's inquest in 1300 was held into the death of William Wattepas, who had come to London from Essex to be treated for an arm wound. Another in 1325 investigated the death of Thomas de Hodesdone, who was struck in the head during a fight and was brought to London for treatment: *Calendar of Coroners' Rolls of the City of London, A.D. 1300-1378*, ed. Reginald Sharpe (London, 1913), pp. 1, 116-7. John Paston III requested John II that he send "by the nexte man that comyth fro London ij pottys of tryacle of Jenne--they shall cost xvj d.; for I haue spent ought that I had wyth my yong wyff and my yong folkys and my-sylff. ... I prey yow lette it be sped. The pepyll dyeth sore in Norwyche": *Paston Letters and Papers of the Fifteenth Century*, ed. Norman Davis (Oxford: Clarendon Press, 1971), vol. 1, p. 616, dated 1439.

[27] In 1423, London physicians and surgeons petitioned the mayor and aldermen to grant ordinances to a *comminalte* of practitioners to survey practice, inspect apothecary shops, judge disputes, and treat the poor: R. Theodore Beck, *The Cutting Edge: Early History of the Surgeons of London* (London: Lund Humphries, 1974), pp. 63-67. The *comminalte* oversaw one dispute (Beck, p. 69), but by November 10, 1424, lord mayor John Mitchell repudiated the ordinances: *Calendar of Letter-books ... Letter-book K*, ed. Reginald Sharpe (London, 1911), p. 36. On a suit brought before the *comminalte*, see Michael Walton, "The Advisory Jury and Malpractice in 15th Century London: The Case of William Forest," *Jour. Hist. Medicine* 40 (1985): 78-82. A college of physicians finally was founded in London in 1518: Charles Webster, "Thomas Linacre and the Founding of a College of Physicians," in *Essays on the Life and Work of Thomas Linacre, c. 1460-1524*, ed. Francis

with it another condition that favored the medical practitioner and medical commodities: the spectacle of mortality and morbidity presented by epidemics. Sylvia Thrupp has provided a catalogue of the epidemics that rocked the capital, beginning with the plague of 1348-9, which reoccurred three times in the 1360s. At the same time there was an outbreak of a disease characterized by *pokkes*, and in 1407 a return of the plague so severe that one chronicler reported thirty thousand people died in London alone. The 1420s brought an epidemic of something like influenza, and the 1420s and 1430s saw six more outbreaks of plague, which came again twice between 1450 and 1470. Between 1471 and 1474 a dangerous disease struck called the *styche*, which might have been a kind of dysentery, and another called *le flux*, said to be new in England, broke out at the same time. In September 1485 came a new fever known as the sweating sickness, which was caused, according to contemporary medical doctor Thomas Forestier, by corruption of the air coming from the stench of rotting beasts in deep caverns, by the close proximity of London's drinking water to its privies, and by the stench of the entrails of dead animals thrown into the Thames. The century ended with two more outbreaks of the plague, beginning at Westminster in 1487.[28] Legal records reported that mountebanks and quacks preyed on the terror of the citizenry, as did the more respectable practitioners.[29]

Maddison, Margaret Pelling, and Charles Webster (Oxford: Clarendon Press, 1977), pp. 198-222.

[28] Sylvia Thrupp, *The Merchant Class of Medieval London* (Ann Arbor: University of Michigan Press, 1962), p. 201. A recent survey of the demographic consequences of epidemic disease in medieval England is John Hatcher, *Plague, Population and the English Economy, 1348-1530* (London: Macmillan, 1977). French physician Thomas Forestier's tract on the English Sweat is found in British Library, Add MS 27582, a late-fifteenth-century medical compendium, ff. 70-77.   Forestier attacked what he called *false lechys*, who advertised their cures on gates and church doors (f. 70), cures that were without effect, or worse, harmful. The tract is discussed by Michael Walton in "Stinking Air, Corrupt Water, and the English Sweat," *Jour. Hist. Medicine* 36 (1981): 67-68, and "Thomas Forestier and the *False Lechys* of London," *Jour. Hist. Medicine* 37 (1982):   71-73.   The sweat seems to have endured in England for some time. William Paston IV, about 1495, wrote to John Paston II that he was staying with Sir John Fortescue away from his studies *be-cause they swet so sor at Cambrygg* (Davis, *Paston Letters*, Vol. 1, p. 670). On the sweat, see J. A. Wylie and L. H. Collier, "The English Sweating Sickness (Sudor Anglicus):   A Reappraisal," *Jour. Hist. Medicine* 36 (1981): 425-45.

[29] "Sir" John Scarle, parson of St. Leonard, Foster Land, Aldersgate Ward, London, was indicted on Christmas Day 1421 for a number of moral crimes, including taking advantage of his flock "bycause that he presentit hym self a surgeuon & a viscioiun to disseive the peple with is false connyng, that he sheuithe unto the peopl, by the whiche craft he hathe slayn many a man": *Calendar of Select Pleas and Memoranda ...*

Many medieval English people seem also to have been preoccupied with thoughts of death and disease. "An anxious curiosity" is what Eleanor Prescott Hammond called it,[30] and this fascination with information about mortality and morbidity penetrated into both the literature and the art of the period.[31] This curiosity may be extended to interest in disease and cures among the growing numbers who were literate and able to afford books and doctors.[32]

Among other types of written sources, legal documents demonstrate that, at least from the twelfth century, medical learning existed on many levels of society. For example, according to early curia regis rolls, lay people were considered qualified to make medical

---

1413-1437, ed. A. H. Thomas (Cambridge, 1943), p. 127. The struggle of the city of London against medical opportunists is outlined in Carole Rawcliffe, "Medicine and Medical Practice in Later Medieval London," *Guildhall Studies in London History* 5 (1981): 13-25. See also Rawcliffe, "The Profits of Practice: The Wealth and Status of Medical Men in Later Medieval England," *Soc. Hist. Medicine* 1 (1988): 61-78. Rawcliffe's works reminds one that, although London was doubtless predominant in trade in late-medieval England, other urban centers such as York played an important part in the development of medicine and commerce.

[30] *English Verse between Chaucer and Surrey* (1927; rpt. ed. New York: Octagon Books, 1965), p. viii. Philippe Ariès refers to the "great flowering of the macabre" and "the great macabre voices of the fourteenth and fifteenth centuries" in *The Hour of Our Death*, trans. Helen Weaver (New York: Knopf, 1981), p. 111. Other useful sources are T. S. R. Boase, *Death in the Middle Ages: Mortality, Judgment and Remembrance* (London: Thames and Hudson, 1972), and R. C. Finucane, "Sacred Corpse, Profane Carrion: Social Ideas and Death Rituals in the Later Middle Ages," in *Mirrors of Mortality: Studies in the Social History of Death*, ed. Joachim Whaley (New York: St. Martin's Press, 1981), pp. 40-60.

[31] The topic is explored in detail by Philippa Tristram, *Figures of Life and Death in Medieval English Literature* (London: P. Elke, 1976).

[32] Robbins postulates a sixfold increase in the number of medical MSS in the fifteenth century over the fourteenth: "Medical Manuscripts," n. 2. Bennett has noted that the "growth of vernacular literature is perhaps nowhere more notable than in the multiplication of medical manuscripts in the fifteenth century. ... It is clear that English homes and English readers (professional or lay) were making use of vernacular instruction on what hitherto had been very largely written in Latin only, and were doing so to a considerable extent": "Science and Information in English Writings of the Fifteenth Century," *Modern Language Review* 39 (1944): 3. The fifteenth century was also the time during which England's medical faculties established themselves. See Getz, "The Medical Faculty at Medieval Oxford," in *The History of Oxford University*, vol. 2, ed. Jeremy Catto (Oxford: Clarendon Press, forthcoming).

judgments. Matrons certified that a posthumous heir was expected (a widow could not inherit her husband's property unless as the guardian of an heir). Lepers were presented before the barons of exchequer for inspection, and in the case of essoin of bed sickness, which excused a person from appearing in court for a year due to illness, four knights of the shire were required to view sick persons and say how long they would be ill.[33] Knights could also determine whether or not a person was mad.[34] Lay judgment on medical matters seems to have led to the establishment of fixed standards for compensation of the victims of violence. The size of a wound or the number of bones that were extracted from it determined how much an injury was worth, and if possible the victim showed a jury the wounds in open court.[35]

Coroners' rolls also give the picture of lay persons making fairly advanced medical judgments without the aid of medical experts. Many diseases mentioned in the Middle English Gilbertus appear as causes of death in coroners' inquests.[36] These included epilepsy, which took John de Bristowe in 1300 when he was praying, while the *festre* that had been bothering William Hampnie caused a vein to burst in his leg and he bled to death. In 1301 Roger le Brewere died of *tisik* (phthisis), and in the same year Richard de St. Albans died of *morbus squinacie* (quinsy). There are also accounts of death from a quartan fever; and Isabella, wife of Robert de Pampesworth, hanged herself as a consequence of *frenzy*, from which she had been suffering for two years. Finally, Alexander de Hadleye died of a long-standing *postume* (apostem).[37] Another set of coroners' rolls gives more information. *Morbus paraliticus* (paralysis) following a slight head injury was said to have killed a person in 1301, while in 1266 a man was reported to have been accidentally wounded, to have recovered, and then died of *fluxus ventris* (diarrhea). The jury returned that it was not as a consequence of the wound.[38]

Medieval English legal records demonstrate that medical knowledge similar to that found in texts such as the Middle English Gilbertus was by no means confined to medical books or practitioners, and that people who were apparently not medical practitioners offered legal judgments about medical matters. London's growth as an urban

---

[33] *Introduction to the Curia Regis Rolls, 1199-1230*, ed. C. T. Flower, Selden Society 62 (1944): 380-83.

[34] *Borough Customs*, Vol. 2, ed. Mary Bateson, Selden Society 21 (1906): 156-57.

[35] See for examples *Select Pleas of the Crown, Vol. 1: A.D. 1200-1225*, ed. F. W. Maitland, Selden Society 1 (1888): pp. 2, 3, 4, 58; also *The Mirror of Justices*, ed. W. J. Whittaker, Selden Society 7 (1895): 24-25.

[36] A formula for conducting such an inquest is given in Whittaker, *Mirror of Justices*, pp. 29-33.

[37] Sharpe, *Calendar of Coroners' Rolls*, pp. 5, 11-12, 16, 22-23, 24-25, 36-37, 209-10.

[38] *Select Cases from the Coroners' Rolls, A.D. 1265-1413*, ed. Charles Gross, Selden Society 9 (1896): 69, 4-5.

center, however, provided an impetus for the city not only to control medicine and surgery as it did other trades, but to identify groups of practitioners whose unanimity of training and ethics set them apart from the quack or opportunist, and qualified them to exercise judgment and control over the craft. The city of London, too, appointed persons of recognized expertise to prevent the diseased from entering into the city, its prisons, or its baths. These experts were usually barbers.[39] Medical experts increasingly were employed by civil authorities to judge the qualifications of a person accused of cheating, injuring, or killing a patient.[40] A practitioner might also be asked to examine medicinal substances being sold retail, or arriving at one of London's ports.[41]

Adulteration of medicinal substances was a dangerous problem, and the purity of spices and related substances was important both for the doctor and for the cook. In 1394, William Witman was charged with having delivered to one Thomas Keys, merchant, "divers false powders for good ginger, and tansy seed for good worm seed." He was condemned to the pillory, "the false powders to be burnt under it."[42] In about 1475 one John Davy was condemned to the pillory and to imprisonment for fabricating a powder called "saunders" (sandalwood).[43] The letter-books also relate that the Grocers' Company received from the mayor and aldermen the directive that no spices be sold before they had been garbled (inspected and sifted of refuse) by someone appointed

---

[39] Letter-book D recorded that in 1310 Gerard the Barber was sworn keeper of the gate of Newgate: *The Annals of the Barber-Surgeons of London*, ed. Sidney Young (London, 1890), p. 25. See also Jessie Dobson and R. Milnes Walker, *Barbers and Barber-Surgeons of London: A History of the Barbers' and Barber-Surgeons' Companies* (Oxford: Blackwell Scientific Publications, 1979), for the history of the company.

[40] In 1354 the mayor summoned London surgeons to give testimony concerning an apothecary (John le Spicer of Cornhill) in his treatment of a jaw wound, and in 1369 the mayor charged four master surgeons with the duty to present to him "the defaults of others undertaking cures ... [and that the surgeons should] attend the maimed or wounded" to give testimony to the city officials as to whether or not they were in peril of death: *Memorials of London and London Life*, ed. Henry T. Riley (London, 1868), pp. 273-74, 337.

[41] The mayor and aldermen of London called together all the physicians and surgeons of the city to examine William, rector of the church of St. Margaret Lothebury, who had claimed a cask containing four putrid wolves, imported for the purpose of curing a disease called *le lou* in 1299-1300. The doctors came and "said that they could not find in any of their medical or surgical writings any disease against which the flesh of wolves could be used": *Calendar of Early Mayor's Court Rolls*, ed. A. H. Thomas (Cambridge, 1924), p. 51.

[42] *Calendar of Letter-books of the City of London, Letter-book H*, ed. Sharpe (London, 1907), p. 42.

[43] *Calendar of letter-books ... Letter-book L*, ed. Sharpe (London, 1912), p. 130.

by the grocers, whose company then embraced the apothecaries,[44] while seventeen named apothecaries and two physicians were charged by the mayor and aldermen in 1472 to investigate the importation of barrels of treacle, a medicinal preparation then enjoying a great vogue. They found the treacle unwholesome, and it was burnt publicly in Cheapside, on Cornhill, and in Tower Street.[45]

London regulated its trade by means of a guild structure, which was responsible for educating and policing each guild's own members, and in return received from the city a monopoly on trade. By contrast, the services of medical practitioners were never successfully controlled in medieval London. Although attempts were made, no one could create a consensus about what standards should be, and who should enforce these standards. Instead, the municipality handled infractions on an *ad hoc* basis, concerning itself almost exclusively with cases in which a practitioner was accused of murder, mayhem, fraud, or failure to fulfill a contract. The standards for pharmaceutical trade, on the other hand, were well established, and apothecaries were organized and regulated.

The apothecaries of the city of London were part of another organization, the Company of Grocers, and their association with the suppliers of food reflects the close relationship medieval medicine held between pharmacy and diet. By the middle of the fourteenth century, apothecaries, spicers, grocers, and pepperers were all grouped together in what was called the Fraternity of St. Anthony,[46] and the apothecaries did not receive a separate charter until 1617. Very little is known about the individual affairs of apothecaries, but we can trace them as an association from the fourteenth century. They appointed surveyors in 1365,[47] and from their names it is apparent that many came from outside England.

The first apothecary about whom much is known is one Robert de Montpellier, spicer to Henry III, who came from a family of French apothecaries. Robert lived in Milk Street, near the Spiceria, the Cheapside spice market. He was a merchant trader, and owned warehouses and market stalls. Robert's medical duties, if any, are not known, but the king's physician, Robert de Neketon, was required to prepare the wines and claret at the king's table in the apothecary's

---

[44] *Letter-book H*, ed. Sharpe, pp. 400-401.

[45] *Letter-book L*, ed. Sharpe, p. 103. The popularity of this panacea, which often came from Genoa, is amply attested in the Paston letters. Margaret Paston requested her husband in 1451 to send "a potte wyth triacle in hast, for I have been ryght evyll atte ese" (Davis, *Paston Letters*, Vol. 1, p. 243). John Paston II sent her "iij triacle pottes off Geane, as my potecarie swerytht on to me, and mooreouyre that they weer neuer ondoo syns þat they come from Geane" (Vol 1, p. 512).

[46] Matthews, *Royal Apothecaries*, p. 5.

[47] Leslie G. Matthews, *History of Pharmacy in Britain* (London: Wellcome Institute, 1962), p. 34. For areas outside London, see T. D. Whittet, "The Apothecaries in Provincial Gilds," *Medical History* 8 (1964): 245-73.

absence.[48] There is also evidence of apothecaries being called on by the city to give expert opinion, once in the case of a shipment of treacle, as has been shown.[49]

One of the best sources about ordinary fifteenth-century English apothecaries is the inventory of John Hexham, London apothecary, given at an inquisition in London before Mayor William Crowmer on April 30, 1415.[50] Hexham had been hanged for counterfeiting coin. He possessed a still, and seems to have dealt in the main with ready-made drugs: unguentum agrippa, borage syrup, and oil of laurel (all common substances in medieval recipe collections). Each drug was weighed and valued in the inventory, and the approximately thirty substances came to a little more than £4. The total value of the inventory was £5. 3s. 7d., compared to £5.11s.6d. for a jeweler's shop in 1381 and £3. 10s. 7d. for a haberdasher in 1378.[51]

Far from existing in isolation, then, recipe collections grew in numbers along with demand for useful medical knowledge in the commercial sphere.[52] The pressure of market demand for cures, rather than for lengthy regimens of health, was already apparent in late medieval English society, and this pressure was ultimately to help change the character of medical practice altogether.[53]

II. THE PRACTICE OF MEDICINE IN THE MIDDLE ENGLISH GILBERTUS ANGLICUS

The Middle English Gilbertus is a practice of humoral medicine arranged from the head downward and divided into nineteen chapters. The medieval translator made every effort to provide a medical work that was an independent unit. He explained difficult terms and arranged the translation for easy reference. This discussion rearranges the material of the text under various subject headings recognizable to the

---

[48] Matthews, *Pharmacy*, pp. 8-9.

[49] See n. 45 above.

[50] The inventory, found in London, PRO E 153/1066/1, is printed with explanatory notes by G. E. Trease and J. H. Hodson in "The Inventory of John Hexham, a Fifteenth-Century Apothecary," *Medical History* 9 (1965): 76-81.

[51] Ibid., pp. 77-78.

[52] Robbins has suggested, "It appears very likely that collections of medical recipes were written in commercial scriptoria for speculative sale." "Medical Manuscripts," p. 413.

[53] See Harold J. Cook, *The Decline of the Old Medical Regime in Stuart London* (Ithaca: Cornell University Press, 1986), esp. chap. 1: "The Medical Marketplace of London," pp. 28-69.

modern reader, and provides translated excerpts of the Middle English text.

A. Anatomy

The organs of the body's trunk are divided into two sections. The organs above the diaphragm that are involved with respiration, such as the lungs and the heart, are called spiritual members (f. 144v). These are distinguished from those below the diaphragm, such as the liver (f. 154).

More attention is given to the anatomy of the brain than to that of any other organ. The brain is divided into three parts, each having its own functions and diseases. An affliction of the front of the brain caused frenzy; loss of reason came from a disturbance in the middle of the brain; and lethargy was caused by disease in the rear of the brain (f. 52). The brain is white (f. 58) and cold (f. 66v), and its diseases affect the emotions, senses, and thought (ff. 53, 59-59v, 61-61v). It also contains hollow spaces (f. 64v) that allow fumes to "fly around" (f. 52), and it can turn inside the skull (f. 52v).

The senses serve to carry information to the brain. The eyes see by the agency of "spirits, that are small bodies in a person's eye; and they are the instruments that the sight sees with. For such spirits receive the light of those things that a person sees" (f. 101), while the tongue is the organ of both taste and speech (f. 138v). The instruments of the voice are the lungs, chest, and throat (f. 147). The heart is notable for its "compassion" for other parts of the body, and feels pain in sympathy (ff. 184v-185). Like the eye, the heart contains spirits, and its affliction with bad humors causes fever to spread throughout the body (ff. 184-184v).

The stomach contains the appetite, to sustain itself and the rest of the body (f. 224v). "In the top of the stomach there is feeling. And when the humor melancholy drops onto the top of the stomach, the stomach feels the sharpness of this melancholy and wants and desires more food naturally" (f. 225). The guts contain feces and excrete them (f. 264v). "A person has six guts in the abdomen: three small and three large" (f. 269). One is called the colon, which "lies around the navel and in the direction of the genitals; sometimes on the right side, sometimes on the left side. Sometimes it goes sideways, over the abdomen as if it were a belt. Sometimes it lies toward the front, sometimes toward the back" (f. 264). Another, a small gut, is called "ilion" (f. 264). A third is "called 'longaon,' and that gut goes down to a person's rectum" (f. 272v).

The liver, "a noble and worthy organ" (f. 204), is located on the right side (f. 169). Its shape is characterized by "hollowness" and "gibbosity" (f. 207). The liver contains four openings or "pores." "One is in the direction of the veins that come from the guts. Another is in the top of the liver where it swells out. Another is toward the gall bladder. And the fourth is on the way to the spleen" (f. 202).

The spleen is on the left side, and "it is intended to receive melancholy that comes from the liver" (f. 210v). The by-products of the spleen's function are "purged through the bladder with the urine" (f. 215). The gall bladder is mentioned once as "the bladder that hangs onto the liver, receiving choler and gall that comes from the liver" (f. 210v). The function of the kidneys was to "soak up moisture from the veins that come from the liver" (f. 291). This moisture "passes ... to the bladder" (f. 291.), which "receives the urine" (f. 210v). The penis contains sperm (f. 301) and became erect through "fleshly desire" (f. 300).

Hemorrhoids "are five veins that connect to the anus to rid the body of useless melancholy blood that would harm other organs" (f. 305v). Their bleeding is thus regarded as a normal function: "And when the blood may not be expelled as it should be, it returns to the liver and predisposes a person to dropsy" (ff. 305v-306). Other veins are also named, and although the Latin text distinguished veins from arteries, the Middle English translation does not. Veins contain blood (f. 96v) and are observed to swell under certain conditions (f. 72). The practice of bloodletting made the location of many veins a necessary thing for the practitioner to know (ff. 99, 277v). Some veins are given special names: "the vein of the arm that is called basilica" (f. 155v), or the vein in "the left arm in the 'saluitica' of the left hand" (f. 216). Bloodletting could draw offending matter into the veins, which was to be avoided (f. 122). Natural bleeding, such as that from the nose, could be caused by "sharpness and keenness of the blood that pierces the veins," or from an excess of blood (f. 125, also f. 288). It was for the practitioner to determine whether this bleeding was nature's way of ridding the body of excess blood, or if in fact the bleeding was unnatural and needed to be stopped.

B. Physiology

The Gilbertus translation, unlike the Latin text, is exclusively concerned with disease and treatment, and not with the theoretical or natural philosophical aspects of medicine. For this reason, much of what can be gathered from the translation about the functioning of the body comes from descriptions of abnormal conditions. If the central metaphor for our understanding of modern human physiology is the heart as a pump, its medieval equivalent must be the fire as mechanism of digestion. Food was cooked in the stomach, and was distributed in increasingly refined form throughout the body. Faulty coction (i.e. cooking) or the failure of the body to rid itself of the superfluities, or by-products, of this cooking caused most disease. For instance, those with headache are cautioned against eating cumin or anise "for they will send up smokes into the head that would increase the ache" (ff. 51-51v). "Cathalempsie" comes "from a poisonous smoke that comes from a remote place into the head" where it is cooled by the naturally cold brain, which is in turn adversely affected by the smoke's heat (f. 66v). The smoke from this coction, if not allowed to escape, could cause a variety of illnesses. "Ringing in a person's ears, or other noises like blowing horns occurs in different ways. Sometimes, it comes from thick windy matter that is in the ear, and moves up and down and all around inside and cannot find its way out" (f. 116), while "windiness of the spleen" is caused when humors "prevent the wind that is in the spleen from getting out" (f. 213v).

The most common type of superfluity, however, is a liquid one, which travels throughout the body either simply through falling, or as the result of the actions of heat, cold, moistness, or dryness. A head cold, for instance, is caused when "rheum falls down into the nose." This could set off a kind of chain reaction: "Sometimes it falls into the cheeks, and makes them swell and ache. Sometimes, it falls down into the roots of the teeth, and then it makes them ache and rot. Sometimes, it falls down into the chest, and makes the chest tight. Sometimes, it falls down into the lungs, or into the stomach, or into the kidneys, or into a person's guts. And unless the organ is strong enough to expel it, it will make an apostem there. Sometimes it falls down among the veins and guts in different places of the body. And sometimes it rots and heats the veins and makes a person have a fever" (ff. 120v-121).

A comparable chain of events is set off in the urinary tract by the action of heat and dryness in diabetes, which is marked by excessive urination and weight loss: "Diabetes is an immoderate passing of urine that comes of excessive dryness in the kidneys, for when the kidneys are very dry, they soak up much moisture from the veins that come from the liver, and the liver in turn much from the guts, and the guts much from the stomach" (f. 291). This process is caused by too much heating of the body, either from excessive labor, "too much meddling with women," exposure to hot temperatures, or applying of hot ointments over the kidneys (f. 291.). Any of these factors could have the effect of upsetting the delicate balance necessary for the body's function. It was the maintenance of this balance that was the basis of health. A defect in diet or regimen, a predisposition, or a wound could lead to disease.

Diseases are most often differentiated by the humors (blood, choler, phlegm, melancholy) or qualities (hot, cold, moist, dry) that are their cause. Each of these humors or qualities revealed itself in a different way. When the tongue has an apostem, "if it is caused by too much blood, the tongue is swollen, and red, and hot, and soft, and aching. And if it is from choler, the tongue is very hot, and citrine, that is to say, a dark red. The ache is more acute than that from blood, and the swelling and softness are less than from blood. But if it is from phlegm, the tongue is cold, and swollen, and soft, and of a white color. From melancholy comes coldness, and a dark yellow color (f. 139, also ff. 58-59).

The qualities of each humor are explicitly described: Blood is hot and moist (ff. 78-78v), choler is hot and dry (f. 48v), phlegm, cold and moist (f. 48v), melancholy, cold and dry (f. 49v). When the humoral cause of a disease has been determined by the "signs of the humors," treatment, usually by opposites, is advised. For example, if heat has enfeebled the stomach, the patient should be cooled by opposites: "let him have rest, and sleep, and cold air. And anoint his stomach with oil of roses and of violet. And give him cold syrups to drink, for example syrup of violet and roses" (f. 226).

The desire for balance pervades the preparation of drugs, as well as the conduct of everyday living. For example, to make oxymel squillitike, the outer skins of the onionlike squill bulb are discarded, "because they are too hot. And throw away as many of the innermost skins, for they are too cold" (f. 50). Certain kinds of headache could be corrected by doing the opposite thing to what caused the trouble: "If the headache comes from staying awake too much, make him sleep. And if it comes of sorrow or of anger, or of much fasting, make him leave such things and draw him to do the contrary things" (f. 50v).

The concept of the apostem is closely associated with medieval ideas of how the body functioned. This text offers little straightforward explanation, but it can be generalized from a number of passages that an apostem occurs when an organ or part is too weak from cold, an injury, or from some other debilitating cause to digest a particular humor it needs for its nourishment. This humor then lies in a part (f. 165), rots (f. 247v), and varying degrees of swelling, changes in color, and pain occur, as can be seen from the example given above for apostem of the tongue. When the apostem matures, it ruptures, emitting pus. The maturing and rupture of an apostem were an important part of its cure (f. 208). The formation of an apostem could account for a number of medical phenomena: abscesses, tumors, ulcers, rashes, and many similar afflictions.

C. Diagnosis

Since the primary cause of illness is an imbalance of humors, the obvious method of diagnosis is to recognize which humor is at fault and then work to purge that humor. This method accounts for the two most popular forms of medical treatment in humoral medicine: bloodletting and what is variously called pharmacy, physic, or laxing, by which is meant the giving of laxative drugs to purge the offending humors.

The discovery of the true cause of a disease was the first step to treatment. But this was not always a straightforward process. A remote affliction could cause a symptom in another part of the body. For instance, "if the headache comes of the sickness of the stomach or of any other member, heal that sickness and then the ache will go away" (f. 50v). Each disease had its own special signs or symptoms. For example, a man dying of lethargy can be known because "a water leech will not stick to such a man to suck out his blood" (ff. 61v-62). There were also general aids to diagnosis. The pulse was the monitor of the state of the spiritual or respiratory organs and of the body's heat. The cardiacle (heart attack) is distinguished, for instance, by a fast pulse (f. 185), while the urine was especially useful in diagnosing the state of the spleen and liver. The feces indicated the state of the guts (ff. 254v-255v).

Diagnosis of an illness could be aided by certain prognostic signs. Bleeding from the ears could come "every third or fourth day" (f. 113v), and some kinds of nosebleeds have "a certain time that they flow, such as every second or third day" (f. 125v). When phlegm affects the lungs, "the illness is more severe at night than in daytime, and in winter more than in summer" (f. 163), since both coldness and nighttime would accentuate the phlegm, which is also cold and wet. When the lungs are affected by choler, however, "they are worse in the daytime than at night, and in summer more than in winter" (f. 163v).

The practitioner or patient could aid in diagnosis by being aware of any predisposing conditions that may have led to the disease. Gonorrhea resulting from sperm that is too watery and leaks out will reveal itself according to a man's diet and constitution (f. 301), while "diampnes" (urinary incontinence) commonly affects those going barefoot or who catch a chill in cold weather (f. 294). A person would know he had caused a prolapsed rectum if he "had sat on a marble stone or on some other cold stones when it was cold" (f. 274v).

Physical examination of the patient was of course one of the simplest and best ways to tell what was wrong, but the Gilbertus translation also suggests several interesting "experiences" or tests as aids to diagnosis. A number of tests "to find out whether there is an apostem in the lungs" are given on f. 166. In another test, which humor has contaminated hemorrhoidal blood is known thus: "Put some of the blood on a linen cloth and wash away the blood, and the cloth will take on the color of the humor affecting the blood" (ff. 306-306v).

The most important thing for a practitioner to know is whether or not a patient would survive. The Gilbertus translation gave the practitioner many prognostic signs as to the outcome of a disease. For example, numerous "signs of death" in phthisis are offered (f. 176v). Then, an "experience" is given to determine if the person would recover: "Let them spit in a basin and the next morning add hot water and stir it; and if there is thick matter at the bottom, he is incurable" (f. 176v).

Pain and numbness could characterize an illness (ff. 294, 276), as could disruptions in sleep (f. 106v). Those suffering from melancholic mania had an array of emotional and visual disturbances They had "much sorrow; and they fear what they ought not to fear, and think about things they ought not to think about. And it seems to them that they see dreadful things when nothing is there. And it seems to them that they see black devils or monks that would slay them. And some think that the sky will fall down on them, and some think that the earth will fall under them. And they hanker after doctors and medicines. But when they have them, they put little faith in their words. And they want to be in dark places and by themselves" (ff. 58v-59).

D. Therapeutics

The Gilbertus translation was designed primarily for treatment of easily identifiable conditions, and by far the largest part of the text is occupied with instructions for treatment of these conditions. These treatments were broken down into diet, regimen (life style), surgery, and pharmacy.

Diet, like pharmacy, is used to correct an imbalance of the humors, although the dietary advice could sometimes be as simple as eating foods easy to digest (f. 78). A headache from phlegm or melancholy is treated by avoiding "melancholy foods" of which numerous examples are given (ff. 49, 67v). Mania from melancholy is treated in the same manner, with the addition of moist foods to counteract the dryness of that humor (f. 59v). If a person has lethargy and has no fever, the diet should help maintain innate heat and moistness, and not upset the balance of bodily qualities. The diet should thus be "temperate, that is, hot and moist" (f. 64), while if there is a fever the diet should be cooling: "and let his diet be cold, that is to say, not too cold" (f. 63). Some foods could thicken the blood, such as "rice and hard boiled eggs" (f. 127), while some make "little blood, like herbs and fruits" (f. 127). The close relationship between diet and pharmacy is of course reflected in these treatments.

Many medical and natural historical texts give complex reasons for why certain foods possess certain qualities. The Gilbertus translation seems to operate on a simpler system, classifying foods according to the way they look, feel, or taste. White, wet, and cold fish were bad for people with phlegmy illnesses (f. 132), while "good wine warmed" was hot and moist (f. 160). Often advice for diet and regimen appeared together. The man suffering from spitting of blood should "beware of anger, and being with women, and vigils, and fasting, and sour foods, and salty ones, and sharp ones, and of getting too hot, and of bathing, and of hard work, and of much thinking, and activity, because all these things heat the spirits" (ff. 172-172v).

Regimen, like diet, was used to counteract an excess of heat or cold, with rest and sleep being considered as cooling, and thought and activity as heating. The frenzied person is warned to "keep silence and do not speak" (f. 57), while the sufferer from headache caused by heat should "abstain from many vigils, and much thought, and from the company of women, and much bathing" (f. 48). The cold sufferer is to be given no medicines (f. 121v). "And let him beware of excessive eating and drinking, and of late suppers, and especially of late drinking, and much sleep. ... And also beware of much light, and much smoke" (f. 122). Regimen could also include simple exercise. A patient could disburse hardened matter filling the spleen if he would "stir well his left arm like ringing a bell or blowing bellows. And let him work from dawn until it is fully light. And let him make a habit of walking in hilly places in the morning until he sweats" (f. 215v).

Fainting required what might be called a form of physical therapy: "If there are too many spirits enclosed around the heart and they come from outside into the heart ... let someone bind his fingers with thongs and his toes as well, so that the spirits and the blood may be drawn away from the heart. And hold his nose, and open his mouth so that the fume can come out of his mouth. And wring him hard by the nose, and pull him by the hairs of his beard and also of his head. And let some friend of his kiss him who tenderly loves him. And rub his hands vigorously, and this shall make him rise up from his attack" (f. 191v).

Surgery encompasses shaving, bleeding, leeching, cupping, scarifying, and treatment by surgical operation and manipulation. The translator left out most such procedures, his interests lying largely with the medical aspects of treatment. However, there are several notable exceptions to this. The victim of frenzy, which was usually a hot disease, comes in for a variety of surgical treatments, staged in increasing severity according to the disease. After giving the patient an enema, it is recommended that the doctor "shave his head and lay on it a warm plaster of cooling herbs to drive away the smoke that comes to the brain." From this, the remedies become more severe (f. 56v).

Like frenzy, pain in the eyes could be "cooled off" by phlebotomy. The process described in this instance is cupping, that is, drawing blood to a place by suction, in this case, with an animal's horn. "Let him be cupped in the back of the head or between his shoulder blades. Or let him bleed from the vein of the elbow. And set a horn around the elbow and cup him there. But remember that all these bloodlettings shall rather be done when the ache comes from heat than from cold" (ff. 84-84v). Another type of bloodletting is scarification, in which small cuts were made in the skin's surface and blood was sucked out of them with a horn or a cup. Such a treatment was recommended for epilepsy (ff. 68-68v).

Surgery is very pointedly recommended only as a last resort, and surgical procedures are never described in detail. For mania, if a number of medicines fail to work, "the last remedy is to slit the skin and open the skull" (f. 61). A similar finality is expressed in treatment for the toothache: "If the ache does not stop using all these medicines, then use stupefactives, such as henbane and opium. And if they do not stop the ache, draw out the tooth" (f. 138). The utility of surgery to deal with wounds is clearly expressed in the admonition that, if spitting of blood "comes from a blow, let that be treated by surgery" (f. 172). Cautery is recommended only once, for the nosebleed. First very mild remedies are suggested, then strong chemicals, and finally, the practitioner is told, "lay a hot iron on it" (f. 128). The only surgical appliance mentioned is the truss, which is suggested for a hernia. A mixture of powders is prepared, "and lay on it a piece of leather and put it on the sore place, and on it lay a piece of lead and bind it up. And let it lie there forty days, for by that time it will be soothed" (f. 297v).

E. Preparation of Medicines

The system of apothecary Troy weights is used to measure drugs. This consists of pounds, ounces, drachms, scruples, and grains (1 pound = 12 ounces; 1 ounce = 8 drachms; 1 drachm = 3 scruples; 1 scruple = 20 grains; 5,760 grains = 1 pound). Although this system is used in most recipes, less specific amounts are also employed. The major ingredient of a recipe, water, for instance, is often given in the amount of "what is needed." (f. 150v). The amount is sometimes not specified (f. 307), or is given as "a good quantity" or "a little" (f. 62v). "Ana" or "alike much" denotes that the same amount of each ingredient ought to be used (ff. 274-274v). A spoonful, a handful, an exage, which is about three ounces, proportions such as two parts to one or three to one, and such comparisons as "the size of a walnut" (f. 174), "the size of three peas" (f. 245v), and "an eggshellful" (f. 161v) are common. The quantities these recipes would yield are for the most part very large. Most yield in excess of two pounds (ff. 76-77), although the measures are too imprecise in most cases to say exactly, just as it would be impossible to give the precise weight of the ingredients given in a cookbook of the same period. Furthermore, the recipes assume a high level of expertise on the part of the preparer, many being entirely innocent of any instructions for preparation.

As is true in cookbooks, substitutions and adjustments are occasionally offered. A fumigation of three hot seeds and wheat bran is suggested for a cold, "and if you do not have all of them, use what you can find" (f. 123). In a similar manner, a *quid pro quo* is given for the preparation of medicine for dysentery (f. 258v). Just as the nobility of the heart and liver demanded noble medicines, the rich required expensive drugs. For a man suffering from liver trouble, if he were rich, he should use expensive electuaries; if he were poor, less expensive alternatives would do (ff. 198v-199).

Sometimes a dosage, time, or method for administering a drug is specified. A salt recommended for a number of purposes should be given "in the morning 3 drachms with wine or mead" (f. 55), while a man with sore eyes should be given a stew "five or seven times" (f. 84). Saffron is added to a drug "if it is winter" (f. 105), and an interval of fourteen days should elapse between the administering of two types of medicine (f. 159v).

The long lists of general classifications of foods and drugs according to their actions which appear especially at the beginning of the Gilbertus translation point to the notion that the practitioner was meant to create his own compounds. General rules for the preparation of ingredients are given throughout the text. The juice of herbs ought to be clarified with the whites and shells of eggs (f. 69) much in the same way as campers clarify coffee today. How to make powders very fine is explained (ff. 94v-95), as is how to dissolve gums in water (f. 156v). A remarkable set of directions for the preparation of corrosives and how to increase their power is given along with a long list of such drugs (ff. 88v-90).

General directions for how to fit the treatment to the patient appear in a number of places. Enemas "should be given to people with strong constitutions, but a person may take suppositories even though very sick and feeble" (f. 64). General directions for the giving of enemas are also offered (ff. 259-259v). A useful piece of advice for the doctor treating diseases of the lungs: "In all your medicines, you must take into account how hot the sick person is, and also the acuteness of his fever. And afterwards, you must order your medicines according to their hotness and coldness" (f. 170).

A practitioner treating his patient with the aid of the Gilbertus translation had a wide variety of methods of administering drugs available. Many are described. Ointments contain wax or oil or both and are applied externally (ff. 157v-159). Pills usually have a gummy substance to hold them together and are described in sizes such as a bean or a pea (ff. 123-123v). They can be held under the tongue (ff. 149v-150), swallowed with a liquid (ff. 60-60v), or put into the nostrils with wine (f. 77). Electuaries are pastelike substances that contain sugar or honey, are prepared over a fire (f. 180), and are eaten, or held in the mouth until they dissolve (f. 153v). An amount often given for an electuary is a gobbet the size of a walnut (f. 174).

Enemas and suppositories are prescribed for a variety of ailments (f. 259v), as are plasters (ff. 168-168v). To make a syrup, the herbs must "simmer ... in water until their virtue is in the water. Then strain it and add sugar or honey, that is to say, a fifth of your liquid must be sugar or honey. And then set it over a fire until it has simmered a little while softly. And take the whites of three or four eggs and beat them well, and add them. And keep skimming it until it is clear. Then take it off, and strain it clear so that no dregs remain in it. And then put it in a closed vessel" (ff. 167-167v). A gargarism is a gargle (f. 145), but this text departs from others written in English, because it is clear that sometimes a medicinal preparation held in the mouth "to gnaw on" (f. 136v), or "to chew in his mouth" (f. 139v), is also meant.

A fumigation is treatment by smoke arising from substances burnt over hot coals (ff. 160v, 308-308v). A stew or stuff is treatment by steam from a boiling pot containing medicine (ff. 108-108v, 122v), while baths could also be used for a number of ailments (f. 257). For nosebleed, the smell "of stinking things is good, such as swine manure, and the hairs of a hare burnt, or other hairs, or of horns burnt" (f. 127v). What is called in Latin *fomentatio*, a cloth soaked in a hot medicinal preparation, helps, for instance, toothache (f. 137).

Most of these medicines are intended in some way or other to purge the humors, and can be labeled according to what humor they eliminate. For a man with sore eyes from choler, "give him a cologoge, that is to say, a medicine that can cleanse him and purge him of choler" (f. 77v), while a cough caused by cold humors can be treated if the patient is purged "with a fleumagoge or with a malagoge" (ff. 159-159v), since phlegm and melancholy cause coldness. Phlebotomy was the most obvious way to purge the body of excess blood, but the Gilbertus translation adds, perhaps to allow the practitioner to avoid bloodletting if possible, "that thing that purges choler purges blood" (f. 54).

Apart from the humors they purge, medicines are classified as general or specific. For example, at the beginning of the text are given medicines good for general purposes, including "a profitable salt and a thing that purges all humors in a person's head, and it is good for aching of the joints, and for the gout, and for dropsy" followed by another, "that purges the head, and takes away dimness of the sight, and gets rid of earache, and is good for palsy" (ff. 54v-55). Sugar of borage "is good in every illness caused by melancholy" (f. 55), while sugar of roses "is good for every flux of the belly and for all troubles that come of choler" (f. 48v). Sugar of violets "is good for all manner of unnatural heats, and for sickness of the chest, and of the sides, and of the lungs, and of the liver, and for the heart attack, and for the tertian fever" (f. 48v). In addition to these panaceas are specifics against particular diseases, and these are suggested throughout the treatise (f. 183).

Medicines are also classified by whether they are simple or compound: "Simple medicines are those made of one herb alone, or of one water that is made of one herb, or of honey, or of olive oil, or of one gum, or of one spice by itself. Compound medicines are made of two things, or three, or of many things mixed together" (f. 79v). As with many other general statements about medicines, the translator of the Gilbertus text presents this information very early on in the text.

How various medicines accomplish their purpose is explained by a lengthy series of names descriptive of drugs' actions. General terms such as "cold," "sharp," and "biting" are used, but more numerous are technical terms. Again, the four qualities hot, cold, moist, and dry underlie the actions of drugs, and the imagery used is of freezing and melting. For example, a list of drugs is prefaced by the fact that they are "dissolutives, that is to say, hot medicines that can dissolve the matter of the sickness just as the sun dissolves ice or snow into water" (f. 78v). Repercussives are explained as drugs that "repel from the eye the humor that is the cause of the ache" (f. 78v). "Strong repercussives are called stupefactives because they stupefy a part through their cold and so they make it lose its ache and its feeling. And because of their great violence, you shall not take them in the ache of the eyes nor in any other ache unless the ache is very violent and dangerous" (f. 80v). "Feeble repercussives are called mitigatives because they assuage the ache and comfort the part" (f. 80v).

Confortatives "comfort the part that aches" and should be used to mitigate the action of harsh drugs, "for unless a part is strong enough to function on its own, the strength of the medicine will do little good. The medicine is only a helper, and the principal actor is the part that is sick" (f. 79).

Strictories are used in nosebleed "to staunch the blood" (f. 126v), and "to staunch the flowing of the humor that comes from the head" in a toothache (f. 135). After a person is purged of the humor causing a flux, "then you shall staunch his flux by medicines that are strictories" (f.

256v). Laxatives have the opposite effect (f. 86), and mollificatives are used "to make that soft that is hardened," while lenitives "make that smooth that was rough, and sharp, and hard through dryness" (f. 149v). Healing is accomplished by "consolidatives, that is to say, such things that have the power to soothe a thing that is cut or broken" (ff. 96v-97), while mundificatives are used "to cleanse" (f. 112). An apostem is made "to wax ripe" with maturatives (f. 110v), and "diuretic herbs are those that have the property of opening pores in a person's body that are stopped" (ff. 197-197v). Subtilatives are drugs that make "the matter subtle, so that it may the more easily come out and the wound the more easily be dried" (f. 178v).

Throughout the Gilbertus translation, the proper order of administering drugs is emphasized. Confortatives at the beginning of a sickness should be followed with consolidatives and dissolutives (f. 79). In the case of hardness of the spleen, "you shall give him no laxative medicine by mouth, nor diuretic medicine, nor a medicine that is very dissolutive, neither internally nor externally, until you have given him mollificatives to make the spleen soft; otherwise, the matter that is subtle would vanish away and the spleen become harder than it was before" (f. 215).

The theory of drug action is further explained with regard to the treatment of pain in the kidney. Opium, a stupefactive, or very cold drug, is used in the medicines to treat pain in the kidneys because by its extreme coldness it will not be dissolved on its way to the kidneys and can carry another drug to them (f. 278v).

III. THE MIDDLE ENGLISH GILBERTUS ANGLICUS AND ITS RELATIONSHIP TO MIDDLE ENGLISH RECIPE COLLECTIONS

The Gilbertus translation demonstrates an important aspect of Middle English recipe collections. A comparison of its recipes with those found in other collections shows that the Latin Gilbertus was the source not only for its Middle English translation, but also for many recipes found outside that translation in other recipe collections. As with the various witnesses to the Middle English Gilbertus, it is impossible to prove a set of direct links for this deployment of material. But, a commonalty of shared material can be demonstrated.

The demonstration begins with the late Roman writer Marcellus of Bordeaux. Marcellus was a learned compiler of recipes whose work was adopted by Gilbertus himself in his *Compendium* and was also translated into Old English. Marcellus' recipe for the earache is as follows:

Fraxini tenerrima folia tundes et exprimes
sucum eorum atque auribus dolentibus
tepidum infundes. Fraxini recentem surculum,

id est umore proprio adhuc madentem, ex una
parte in foco pones. Cum per aliam partem
sucus ebulliet, suscipies eum diligenter et oleo
addito tepefactum auribus instillabis. Cardui
siluatici semen ex oleo coques ita leniter, ne
uratur. Quod postea colabis per linteolum et
tepidum infundes dolenti auriculae ac deinde
lana purpurea obturabis.[54]

In the Latin Gilbertus, it appears thus:

Item bacculi fraxinei virides ponantur in ignem,
et liquor distillans a capite capiatur ad
plenitudinem teste ovi cui addantur olei
communis vel butyri duo coclearia; et de succo
barbarum porrorum, coclear .i.; et de succo
sempervive .ii.; de melle claro .i.; et de lacte
mulieris masculum nutrientis ad masculum
femine ad feminam .i. coclear. Commisceantur
et colentur, et auri infundatur una gutta vel due
et obturetur auris. Item sagimen anguille et
succus sempervive ana commisceantur et
infundatur. (F. 148v)

The Middle English translation found in W is:

Or take þe bowes of green asshes and leye on
þe fyer, and take of þe watir þat comeþ at þe
endes of hem þe quantite of a sponeful and
halfe, and put þerto ii° sponful of oile or of
bottir and oon sponful of þe iuse of synegrene,
and ii° sponful of hony, and a sponful of
womanes mylke þat norissheþ a man childe.
And medle alle togedre. þen put a drope or ii°
in þe ere and stoppe it. Or take þe ius of
syngrene and þe fatnesse of an eel yliche
moche, and put þerof in þe eere. (Ff. 119-119v)

The same recipe also appears in many Middle English and Welsh recipe
collections.[55]

---

[54] *Marcelli de medicamentis liber*, ed. Max Niedermann and
Eduard Liechtenhan, 2d. ed. (Berlin: Corpus medicorum Latinorum 5,
1968), p. 170. The Old English translation is found in Thomas Oswald
Cockayne, ed., *Leechdoms, Wortcunning and Starcraft of Early England*,
Vol. 2, rev. ed. (London: Holland Press, 1961), p. 42.

[55] They include the six fifteenth-century collections in Fritz
Heinrich, *Ein mittelenglisches Medizinbuch* (Halle, 1896), pp. 66-67;
Wellcome MS 542, f. 1; Wellcome MS 409, f. 17; Wellcome MS 408, f.
47; Herbert Schöffler's edition of John of Burgundy's practice of physic:
Mittelenglischen Medizinliteratur (Halle, 1919), pp. 195-96; George

Other recipes found in the Middle English Gilbertus can be traced in a similar manner. The "red snail" recipe on f. 94 of W appears in G. Müller (p. 55), Schöffler (p. 194), and Henslow (p. 80). This affiliation has led the editors of most Middle English recipe books to demonstrate at great length considerable similarity among Middle English recipe collections, and Margaret Ogden's comment in the *Liber de diversis medicinis* that "the material contained in these late vernacular collections is more stereotyped than has usually been recognized" can be extended to include the Gilbertus translation also.[56] To present an edition of a single witness of a medical text containing recipes, giving due attention to the role both that witness and others like it played in the transmission of medical learning, would seem to be the only method of edition that has any chance of producing a text that will be of lasting value.[57]

Henslow, *Medical Works of the Fourteenth Century*, rpt. ed. (New York: Burt Franklin, 1972), p. 109; Robert M. Garrett ed., "A Middle English Rimed Medical Treatise," *Anglia* 34 (1911): 163-93, this recipe, p. 186. In Gottfried Müller's *Aus mittelenglischen Medizintexten* (Leipzig, 1929), the recipe appears twice in similar form, suggesting that the collection was taken from at least two sources: pp. 91 and 110. In *A Leechbook or Collection of Medical Recipes of the Fifteenth Century*, ed. Warren R. Dawson (London: Macmillan, 1934), it is found three times: pp. 22, 98, and 100. Margaret S. Ogden's edition of the *Liber de diversis medicinis*, rev. EETS 207 (1969), reproduces the recipe twice: pp. 6-7 and 13. In *The Physicians of Myddfai*, edited by John Williams (London, 1861), it appears twice, once for deafness and once to improve hearing (pp. 314-15 in English, pp. 105-6 in Welsh). A more scholarly edition of this text with modern French translation is *Le plus ancien texte des Meddygon Myddveu*, edited by P. Diverres (Paris, 1913). See also Ida B. Jones, "Halfod 16: A Mediaeval Welsh Medical Treatise," *Etudes celtiques* 7, fasc. 2 (1955): 270-399, where the recipe appears on p. 274, English translation on the facing page. It would seem that medieval Welsh recipe books were similar to Middle English ones, and may be translations of them. I am grateful to Dr. Dorothy Watkins Porter and Dr. Neil Morgan for assistance in translating Welsh.

[56] Ogden, *Liber,* p. xxvii.

[57] A recent discussion of the difficulties involved in editing Middle English recipe collections is Henry Hargreaves, "Some Problems in Indexing Middle English Recipes," in *Middle English Prose: Essays on Bibliographical Problems*, ed. A. S. G. Edwards and Derek Pearsall (New York: Garland, 1981), pp. 91-113.

IV. THE MIDDLE ENGLISH GILBERTUS ANGLICUS AS A TRANSLATION

A. The Mechanics of Translation: A Comparison of the Middle English and Latin Texts

The translation of Latin texts into Middle English was the principal means of conveying medical information in the vernacular in the fifteenth century.[58] Although translators and copyists felt free to adapt their material in various ways and by that adaptation achieve a result that was in some ways "original,"[59] Latin was still the preferred language of discourse for learned practitioners and Middle English was dependent on it.[60]

The simplest method of demonstrating some of the ways in which the Gilbertus translator handled his material is the placement of a Latin passage alongside its Middle English counterpart. In the following passage, the translator has turned the Latin into idiomatic English, leaving out very little and employing few Latin loan words. Only the

---

[58] Some unpublished Middle English medical texts that are translations of Latin exemplars are Bernard Gordon, *De prognosticis*, Sl 5, ff. 61-63; Bernard Gordon, *Phlebotomia*, London, British Library, Sloane MS 6, ff. 33-40; Constantine the African (?), *De natura humana*, London, Wellcome MS 290, ff. 1-41; Copho, *De anatomia porci*, ibid., ff. 41-48v; Galen, *De ingenio sanitatis* (extracts), Sloane MS 6, ff. 183-203v; Haly Abbas, *Liber regius*, ibid., ff. 43-50v; Johannitius, *Isagoge*, ibid., ff. 1-9; Petrus Hispanus, *Thesaurus pauperum*, Cambridge, University Library MS Dd. x. 44, ff. 116v-118; Roger of Parma, *Chirurgia*, Sloane MS 240, ff. 1-47v; Trotula of Salerno (extracts), Douce 37 (Bod. SC 21611); William of Parma (Saliceto), *Chirurgia*, Sloane MS 6, ff. 53-140v.

[59] For a discussion of this process as it took place within the Latin tradition and especially as regards writers such as Gilbertus, see Luke Demaitre, "Scholasticism in Compendia of Practical Medicine, 1250-1450" *Manuscripta* 20 (1976): 81-95.

[60] English was only one of a long series of languages to receive what was originally Greek medical learning in the medieval period. Translation of Greek, Syriac, and Arabic medical texts is discussed in the following entries in the *Dictionary of Scientific Biography*, 16 vols, ed. Charles Coulston Gillispie (New York: Scribner, 1970-80): Michael McVaugh, "Constantine the African," Vol. 3, pp. 393-95; Richard Lemay, "Gerard of Cremona," Vol. 15, pp. 173-92; G. C. Anawati and Albert Z. Iskandar, "Hunayn ibn Ishaq," Vol. 15, pp. 230-49. Also, see Marie-Thérèse d'Alverny, "Translations and Translators," in *Renaissance and Renewal in the Twelfth Century*, ed. Robert L. Benson and Giles Constable, with Carol D. Lanham (Cambridge: Harvard University Press, 1982), pp. 421-62.

finer and more complex points of uroscopy are glossed over. In the Latin:

> Calide discrasie sine humoris vitio: signa sunt arsura et punctura sub dextro ypocondrio, lingue et palati siccitas, sitis continua, urina intensa rubea vel subrubea vel ultra quandoque obumbrata cum spuma crocea, citrinitas faciei, et color viridis aut emulus, habutudinis extenuatio et maxime cause prolongate; frigida prosunt, calida obsunt; frequens ventris constipatio, et egestionis paucitas, et fastidium, et sompnus brevis. Semperque in somnis os habent apertum. Adest nausea, fastidium, et in augmento oculorum, et faciei infectio, et ycteritia, et tunc sequitur universalis pruritus et scabies, cum sanguis exuritur vel incenditur, et tunc valde tabescunt. Si autem sit cum humoris vitio, aggravatio sentitur sub dextro ypocondrio. (F. 235)

In W:

> Distempering of þe lyuer þat comeþ of hete haþ þes tokenes: brenyng and pricking vndir þe riȝt side, dreines of þe tunge and of þe roof of þe mouþe, continuel þrist, þe vryn is of an hie colour, þe face is citryn and oþirwhiles grene. Colde þingis comforten him and hote þingis noien him. He is ofte costif, and whan he shetiþe, it is but litil. He volateþ his mete, and slepiþ but litil. And whan he slepiþ, he holdeþ his mouþ open. And oþirwhiles his visage and his yȝen ben infecte with a ȝelewe colour. And þen he haþ a grete ycching ouer al þe bodi and a scabbe. And if þis distempering be of sum corrupt humour, þei felen heuynes vndir þe riȝt side. (F. 194v)

In the second example below, considerable modification has taken place, as the translator introduced an explanation for the anglicized Latin term "spiritual member" into advice on respiratory diseases:

> Et nota quod isti pleuretici et peripleumonici et laborantes vitio spiritualium debent esse iuxta ignem carbonum a longe ut aer tepefiat inspiratus. Omnia enim actu frigida apostematibus sunt inimica. (F. 178v)

> And vndirstonde þat þo þat han greuaunce in
> her þrote, eiþir in her breest, eiþir in her
> spirituel membris, þat is to sey, in þo membris
> þat ben above þe mydrif, as þe herte and þe
> li3te, shullen be ny3e an hoote fier, þat þe eyr
> þat þey resceyven in drawing breeþ be hoot, for
> al colde þingis ben noiful for postems. (F.
> 144v)

The same sort of expansion has taken place with the Latin word *ptisana*, which is glossed in Middle English as "ptisane is watir þat barliche is soden yn" (f. 149). Latin *consolidativa* is also explained: "consolidatiues, þat is to seie, suche þingis þat haþ vertu to souden a þing þat is y-kitte or broken" (f. 97); and a medicinal ingredient is described as "þe wilde gorde þat is clepid in Latin collaquindida" (f. 68). The word *gourdes* is explained again further on: "watir of gourdes, not of þe sedis þat is in þe grete gourdes, but of þe herbe þat Y clepe gourdis in al þis tretis" (f. 150).

At times the translator employed a kind of shorthand, using pairs of synonyms to translate a Latin word. This can be seen in the Middle English Gilbertus when, for instance, Latin *corrosiva* is rendered *corisiuf and freting*, leaving the reader in little doubt as to what the word meant.

Explanations were not always given, however, as when an almost total adoption of Latin names of medicinal substances into Middle English took place. In the Latin:

> Debiliter dissolutiva sunt vitellum ovi, succus
> mente, basiliconis, sansuci, verbene, endiue,
> foliorum rubi, mica panis tritici tepida aspero
> vino vel aqua rosarum, succus feniculi,
> eufrasie, hedere terrestris, licium, succus
> prunellorum, sarcocolla, acatia, muscus, aqua
> vitis, mel, sanguis columbe vel pulli gallinacei,
> limatura auri. (F. 132)

In W:

> Feeble dissolutiues ben, þe yolke of an egge, þe
> iuse of myntes, of basilicon, of sansuke,
> verueyn, endiue, þe leues of madir, hote
> crummes of whete brede y-springed wiþ wyne
> or wiþ watir, also þe iuse of fenel, of eufrace,
> of hayhoue, of licium, þe iuse of sloon,
> sarcacolle, acacia, muske, þe watir of a vine,
> hony, þe blood of a coluer or of an hen or
> cheken, and lymail of golde. (Ff. 80-80v)

Passages such as these, which are very common in the Middle English Gilbertus, are much less translations than importations, and they assume some sort of familiarity on the reader's part with the names of medicinal substances, a familiarity far more developed than that with other types of medical vocabulary. In the first example given above, the translator removed the more subtle and complex material, and it is this sort of simplification that is one of the cardinal characteristics of this translation.

An example of how the translator understood his text and then apparently decided to edit it down can be seen in the description of mania. The Middle English version conflated "mania" and "melancholy" at the expense of the original, the reason being, it would seem, not that the Latin was too difficult, but that the two medical conditions seemed much the same. The English gives no more information than simply naming the disease "melancholy" (f. 58), but the Latin reads: "mania est infectio anterioris cellule capitis cum diminutione ymaginationis ... Melancolia est infectio medie cellule cum diminutione racionis. Isti morbi non differunt nisi in positione materie" (f. 102v).

Another characteristic of this translation is the consistent omission of the name of every authority found in L. For instance, where the Latin explains the three kinds of dysentery thus: "quedam fit in superioribus intestinis, quedam in infimis, quedam in mediis, qui ut dicit Galienus in Tegni," the Middle English says, "oon is in þe ouermost guttis, anoþer is in þe middle guttis, and þe þridde is in þe neþermost gutis. And in oon maner ..." (f. 254v).

The translation is also marked by the literal and concrete imagery added to the text that does not appear in Latin. For example, vertigo "makeþ a man semen þat al þinge þat he seeþ as it semeþ to dronken men: þat þe house goeþ aboute hem and þat þe weie reseþ up a3enst hem" (f. 52v), while the Latin only remarks that "videntur enim ei quod omnia vertantur in girum." Discharge from the eyes is described in Middle English but not in Latin as being *viscous as bridlym* (f. 75v), and the list of such examples need not end here.

Additionally, the translation omits large chunks of material that do not follow the strict head-downward order (fevers, for example, or the section on the senses). It would also appear that on occasion text has been brought forward or moved backward from other sections of the Latin.[61] At other times, the copyist seems to have regarded the text as a kind of recipe collection, adding here and there material from elsewhere.[62]

Also added to the translation are short introductory summaries of nearly all the nineteen chapters. These are the greatest departure from the Latin text and are the most powerful simplification of its technical material. These introductions most closely resemble the prose in the medical sections of Trevisa's translation of Bartholomaeus Anglicus. In addition, the translator seems either unwilling or unable to confront the complexities of Gilbertus' technical Latin. For example, Gilbertus' subtle explanation of the mechanics of epilepsy, describing the anatomy of the brain and of the nerves, the finer points of humoral

---

[61] For example, the recipe for rose sugar on ff. 48-48v.

[62] For example, on f. 51v.

distinctions, proximate and distant causes, the role of the moon, and other matters, is condensed by the translator into a few short sentences, making the text shorter, easier to understand, and less faithful to the original.[63]

Finally, the reader is given a summary guide by the brief bits of explanatory material placed at the beginning of the text concerning the nature of the humors, the actions of drugs, and the preparation of generally useful medicines. For example, the recipe for *pillules of diacastor* (ff. 76-76v), which would appear to be good for nearly everything, has been placed into the Middle English text from a section of Latin not otherwise translated.

B. Neologism in the Middle English Gilbertus Anglicus

Medicine was one of the first bodies of technical material to enter into the vernacular, and as is hardly surprising, a text the length of the Middle English Gilbertus displays a number of first usages, especially of plant names, technical terminology, and the names of medicinal substances. The glossary to this edition indicates exactly what these are, and at times, how they confirm or contradict entries in the *Middle English Dictionary*. These new words come exclusively from Latin, and in many cases are defined in the translated text. An example is the first known usage of the word "gonorrhea":

> Gomorra, þat is flowing of a manis sede agenis
> his will, and þis is of plente of blood, eiþir of
> palesie of þe stones, eiþir of grete feblenes of a
> man þat mai not wiþholden his sede, eiþir it
> comeþ for þe sede is þinne and flowiþ oute
> lightli. (Ff. 300-300v)

Among words that seem not to survive the translation or were supplanted by other words, the plant name *camapiteos* (*Ajuga chamaepitys*, or ground pine) finds its only known English usage in the Middle English Gilbertus, as do such words as *carpobalsamum*, the fruit of the balm tree, and *alipiados*, the spurge laurel. Because many names were adopted from Latin into Middle English more or less intact, not only Middle English herbals but also Latin ones must be used for modern identification.[64]

---

[63] L: ff. 109v-110v; W: ff. 64v-66v.

[64] To the Middle English herbals found in the bibliography to this edition can be added the following ones in Latin: J. L. G. Mowat edited two Latin plant glossaries that are also useful for the identification of disease names: *Sinonoma Bartholomei* (Oxford: Anecdota Oxoniensia, Mediaeval and Modern Series, 1882), and *Alphita* (Oxford: ibid., 1887). Also useful is *The Herbal of Rufinus*, ed. Lynn Thorndike

C. The Lexicon of the Middle English Gilbertus Anglicus

The guiding principle of the glossary for this edition has been that the Middle English Gilbertus is a translation of a Latin text, and every entry was defined keeping that in mind. Difficult words were compared with their counterparts in the Latin text, and this comparison has allowed certain generalizations to be made about how the translator rendered his subject matter into Middle English and about the number of translators whose work appears in the text of this edition.

First, the names of diseases are most often anglicized versions of Latin terms. Words such as Middle English *frenesy* (L *frenesis*), *lithargie* (L *litargia*), and *analempsy* (L *analempsia*) were all adapted from Latin in the same way as Trevisa had done in his translation (see Seymour, pp. 348, 350, and 354). There are also several instances when the translator does succeed in using an English translation for a Latin word. Middle English *pose* (L *coriza*), *stiches* (L *dolor laterum*), *turnyng of þe brayn* (L *vertigo*), *stering of þe hert* (L *sincope*), and *festre* (L *fistula*) are notable examples and are by no means unique to this text.

The medicinal substances named in the Middle English Gilbertus have, however, provided the most information about the nature of this translation. Where two Middle English words appear to have been used to translate the same Latin one, the question of multiple translators must arise. For instance, L *crocus* is translated variously as *saffren* and *citre* (see the Commentary, 311/23). L *malva* appears as *hocke, malue,* and *mallewis,* while L *bismalue* is rendered *holy-hock* and *bismalue*. However, no particular pattern emerges from these "inconsistent" translations. Just as a medieval herbal glossary could give a number of names for the same plant--"camedreos, quercula minor, germandria idem"[65]--so translators seem to have varied their translations of a single Latin word without attaching any particular significance to this.

With other sets of "inconsistent" translations, however, the use of different names for the same plant gives evidence about the nature of the text itself. In the case of Middle English *bawme/melisse* and *gromel/milium solis/palma Christi*, the first word in each group is a translation from L, while the word or words following in all likelihood indicate the same plant but appear in recipes that were added to the Middle English Gilbertus by its copyist after the translation was made and are from sources other than L. The modern identification of Middle English plant names can thus provide evidence about the structure of a text containing a large number of them.

(Chicago: University of Chicago Press, 1946), which was written in Italy but summarizes many of the herbals popular in England. The first two glossaries, although largely in Latin, also give a number of English and French equivalents for Latin plant names.

[65] Mowat, *Sinonoma Bartholomei*, p. 14.

For the purposes of this edition, English plants are assumed to have been used in preference to foreign ones, and the possibility of fraud or adulteration (as in the case of *mummie*, for example) has been ignored. In the case of difficult plant identifications, much weight has been given to the fact that the Middle English Gilbertus is a translation of a Latin text. Medicinal plants have been given by far the most attention. They are listed by botanical family, genus, and species where possible in the Glossary, and are listed by botanical genus and species in alphabetical order after the Glossary. Their modern botanical names have been standardized by use of A. R. Clapham, T. G. Tutin, and E. F. Warburg, *Flora of the British Isles* 2d ed. (Cambridge: Cambridge University Press, 1962); and L. H. Bailey, *Manual of Cultivated Plants*, rev. ed. (New York: Macmillan, 1977).[66]

The listing by genus and species allows the plant lexicon of the Middle English Gilbertus to be compared with a Middle English text in which the identification of plants rests on much firmer ground: Gösta Brodin's edition of *Agnus Castus: A Middle English Herbal* (Cambridge: Harvard University Press, 1950). Brodin's text gives descriptions and alternate names for plants, and he lists them by genus and species on pp. 307-13. I have compared his list with mine in a section that appears after the Glossary, indicating with an asterisk on my list every plant that is found both in the Middle English Gilbertus and in *Agnus Castus* (some plants in Brodin's text are not entered in his list and were sought in his glossary). The correspondence is remarkably close, and if all plants that come from tropical climates are eliminated from the list in the Middle English Gilbertus, the correspondence is almost total.

This correspondence points toward the existence of a fairly standardized English herbal pharmacopeia encompassing a remarkable variety of substances. In the Middle English Gilbertus, approximately three hundred plants are mentioned, classified into nearly eighty modern botanical families. If the medicinal substances derived from nonvegetable sources are added to consideration, the medieval pharmacopeia as represented by the Middle English Gilbertus rises to comprehend nearly four hundred substances, making it one of the most important sources for medical vocabulary in Middle English.

---

[66] Also useful are *Index plantarum medicinalium totius mundi eorum synonymorum*, ed. Giuseppe Penso (Milan: O. E. M. F., 1983), and Maud Grieve, *A Modern Herbal*, 2 vols. (New York: Penguin, 1978).

*D. Modification of the Middle English Gilbertus Anglicus by the Copyist of
Wellcome MS 537: The Removal of References to Diseases of
Women and Children*

So far, we have examined the modification of the Latin
Gilbertus by means of translation into Middle English.[67] It has in
addition been shown how the translator added or subtracted material
and how the Wellcome copyist added recipes from elsewhere to the text.
It is also possible to demonstrate how the Wellcome copyist
systematically edited out most references to the diseases of women and
children. Collation of W with Add 30338 and Sl 5, which represent two
branches of the "family" of Middle English Gilbertus manuscripts, shows
exactly what these omissions were, and the material that was left out is
supplied in the Commentary to this edition. Two scribal cancellations
make it possible to show that this omission took place in W and not any
earlier.

The first is found in W, f. 56, where the word *postem* is followed
by "of þat skynne þat a childe þat a childe is conceyvid yn" canceled in
red. The corresponding reading in Add 30338 follows W to the word
breest and then has "oþer in a womman of þe posteme of þat skyn þat a
chyld ys y-conceyfed yn" (f. 15), after which agreement with W resumes.
A similar false start corrected by cancellation occurs on f. 64 of W, where
the scribe began to copy the first ingredients of a recipe he wanted to
omit of a suppository for men or women. He canceled these ingredients,
realizing his mistake, and returned again to the intended recipe. These
deliberate omissions are sustained throughout the Middle English
Gilbertus in W and can be as short as that of the phrase "and of þe

---

[67] For a more general treatment of translation, the development
of English prose, its triumph over French as the vernacular of choice,
and the influence of various writers on it, see H. S. Bennett, *Chaucer and
the Fifteenth Century*, rev. ed. (Oxford: Clarendon Press, 1970); Peter
Murray Jones, "Four Middle English Translations of John of Arderne,"
in *Latin and Vernacular: Studies in Late Medieval Manuscripts*, ed.
Alastair Minnis (Woodbridge: D. S. Brewer, 1989), pp. 61-89; S. K.
Workman, *Fifteenth-Century Translation as an Influence on English Prose*
(Princeton: Princeton University Press, 1940); William Matthews'
introduction to his edition of *Later Middle English Prose* (London: Peter
Owen, 1962), pp. 1-27; John H. Fisher, "Chancery and the Emergence of
Standard Written English in the Fifteenth Century," *Speculum* 52 (1977):
870-99, and his "Chancery Standard and Modern Written English," *Jour.
Soc. of Archivists* 6 (1978-79): 136-44; Malcolm Richardson, "Henry V,
the English Chancery, and Chancery English," *Speculum* 55 (1980): 720-
50.

moder after emeroids,"[68] or as long as the description of the special nature of a woman's epileptic seizure.[69]

Anyone who is familiar with medical compendia will be aware of the careful attention medical writers paid to the diseases of women.[70] In the discussion of medical compendia containing the Middle English Gilbertus that appears below, it is shown how often Rowland's text on gynecology appeared with the Middle English Gilbertus. These deliberate omissions from W are, alongside this, very unusual indeed.

The exact purpose for which W was intended as well as its ownership in the medieval period is unknown and this can be said for most MSS of its kind. We may guess, however, from the style of binding and the amount of illumination that W may have been intended for monastic use. What is certain is that the Wellcome copyist felt free to change the text by insertion or deletion of material and that these changes were not accidental or the result of carelessness. They were instead the result of a deliberate attempt on the part of the copyist to adapt the material before him better to suit his own needs or the needs of the patron.

---

[68] Add 30338, f. 137; W, f. 295.

[69] Add 30338, ff. 22-22v; W, f. 72v, omitted after the word *up*.

[70] Although women must have performed much if not most medical care in the Middle Ages, their contribution is not easy to document. Eileen Power, "Some Women Practitioners of Medicine in the Middle Ages," *Proc. Roy. Soc. Medicine* 15 (1921-22): 20-23, discusses a certain Joan, petitioning Henry IV for protection in her practice of physic. She is probably the same as Johanna, who appears in the Westminster Infirmarer Rolls, 1407-09, as Johanne Leche, *mulier* (Talbot and Hammond, p. 100). A family of men and women practicing medicine together is documented in Edward J. Kealey, "England's Earliest Women Doctors," *Jour. Hist. Medicine* 40 (1985): 473-77. For a fifteenth-century illustration of a woman practicing phlebotomy, see Jones, *Medieval Medical Miniatures* (London: British Library, 1984), fig. 56 (Sloane MS 6, f. 177). See also *Medieval Woman's Guide to Health*, ed. Beryl Rowland (Kent, Ohio: Kent State University Press, 1981), which reproduces a number of interesting illustrations from "women's" medical texts. An excellent general bibliography is Monica Green, "Women's Medical Practice and Health Care in Medieval Europe," *Signs* 14 (1989): 434-73. On pp. 464-67, Green compares Rowland's edition with that of a similar text edited by M. R. Hallaert, "The '*Sekenesse of Wymmen*': A Middle English Treatise on Diseases of Women," *Scripta* 8 (1982).

V. GILBERTUS ANGLICUS AND THE LATIN TEXT

A. The Writings of Gilbertus Anglicus

Compendium medicinae of Gilbertus Anglicus is one of the longest medical works ever written in Latin.[71] It was written about 1240.[72] The text is divided into seven books. The ordering of material is roughly head to toe, with the exception of the chapter on fevers, which concern the entire body. However, Gilbertus also had in mind an arrangement by various systems. Since fever was a general topic, it went first. The second book is about the brain, the wits (senses), and diseases near to the brain. The Middle English translation begins in the second book, with the chapter heading *De dolore capitis et eius speciebus.* The third book is about the organs of sense and diseases affecting parts near to them. The fourth is about the "spiritual" members, that is, those parts of the body having to do with respiration, which in medieval physiology included the heart. The fifth is about the organs of digestion. The sixth deals with organs handling the "watery substances" of the blood and adjusting the humors in the body. The seventh deals with the reproductive system and anything else that was left out of previous chapters, including diseases of women, advice for travelers, how to light fires, and antidotes to poisons.

The principal MSS of the *Compendium* are as follows: TK 3: Bruges, Belgium, Bibliothèque Publique MS 469 (dated 1271), 244 ff.; Cambridge, Pembroke College MS 169 (13th/14th c.), ff. 1-233v; Cambridge, Peterhouse MS 52 (13/14th c.), ff. 1-92v; London, British

---

[71] See Henry E. Handerson, *Gilbertus Anglicus: Medicine of the Thirteenth Century* (Cleveland, Ohio, 1918). Ernest Wickersheimer lists Gilbertus in his *Dictionnaire biographique des médecins en France au moyen âge* (1936; rpt. Geneva: Librairie Droz, 1979), pp. 191-92. He is also listed in Talbot and Hammond, pp. 58-60. A study of Gilbertus is found in Charles Talbot, *Medicine in Medieval England* (London: Oldbourne, 1967), pp. 72-87. Talbot compares Gilbertus' plan in the *Compendium medicinae* to Aquinas' in the *Summa theologica*, discussing his "syllogistic reasoning, based on Aristotelian logic ... typical of university education for the medical student of the time" (p. 74). For a modern English translation of part of the Latin text, see Michael McVaugh, "Gilbert the Englishman: The Symptoms of Leprosy," in *A Source Book in Medieval Science*, ed. Edward Grant (Cambridge: Harvard University Press, 1974), pp. 752-54.

[72] The dating of the *Compendium* rests largely on the use Gilbertus made of new Latin translations, especially of Averroes. Gilbertus' sources are discussed by Talbot and Hammond, p. 59, and with greater precision by Marie-Thérèse d'Alverny's review of Talbot and Hammond in *Cahiers de civilisation médiévale* 13 (1970), p. 393.

Library, Sloane MS 272 (14/15th c., in which the *Compendium* is called *Laurea anglicana*), 262 ff.; TK 380: Oxford, Bodley MS 720 (SC 2634) (early 14th c.), ff. 1-156v; Florence, Biblioteca Riccardiana MS 731 (14th c.), ff. 1-231v; TK 881: Cambrai, Bibliothèque Publique MS 906 (14th c.), 247 ff.; Vienna, National-Bibliothek MS 2279 (14th c.), ff. 1-239v; TK 1115: Rouen, Bibliothèque de la Ville MS 984 (14th c.), 225 ff.; beginning like the 1510 printed edition with the incipit *Incipit liber morborum* is Oxford, Merton Coll. MS N. 3. 9 (Coxe MS 226) (14th c.), ff. 207, which once belonged to Simon Bredon, Oxford MD. There are also two MSS in Spain about which detailed information was not available: Madrid, Biblioteca Nacional MS 1199; Madrid, Biblioteca Universitaria MS 120. These references were found in Guy Beaujouan, "Manuscrits médicaux du moyen âge conservés en Espagne," *Mélanges de la casa de Velazquez* 8 (1972): 185.

    Extracts from the *Compendium* and other works attributed to Gilbertus are as follows: commentary on the uroscopy of Gilles de Corbeil, TK 79, 442, 821, 1483, 1588, 1616; *Antidotarium Gilberti*, TK 54; *De febribus*, TK 553; *Practica*, TK 715; *Quedam de lepra*, TK 1086; *Emplastrum magistri Gilberti Anglici* (not in TK), found in London, British Library, Royal MS 12 D xii (15th c.), f. 64.

    The *Compendium* was printed at least once, in Lyons, by Jacobus Saccon for V. de Portonariis, 1510. Another printing, Geneva 1608, is recorded by early bibliographers (Fabricius, vol. 3, 160, for example), and this has been picked up by later writers. I could find no copy of it and it is not recorded by Shaaber.[73]

    Sections of the *Compendium* were translated into languages other than Middle English during the medieval period. I have found extracts from it incorporated into the writings of Ortolf of Bavaria in New High German (London, Wellcome MS 120, ff. 18-48 and elsewhere).[74] It appears also in fourteenth-century Hebrew,[75] and in Catalan.[76]

B. *Gilbertus Anglicus and His Reputation*

    The background and career of Gilbertus Anglicus are obscure. A manuscript dated 1271 (Bruges, Bib. Pub. MS 469), about twenty years

---

[73] M. A. Shaaber, *Check-list of Works of British Authors Printed Abroad, in Languages Other than English, to 1641* (New York: Bibliographical Society, 1975); 1510 ed.: no. 311, p. 83.

[74] I am grateful to Prof. Dr. Gundolf Keil for his advice on this translation; Prof. Dr. Keil is preparing a critical edition of Ortolf's works.

[75] Moritz Steinschneider, *Die hebraeischen Uebersetzungen des Mittelalters,* rpt. ed. (Graz: Akademische Druk-und-Verlagsanstalt, 1956), pp. 798-99.

[76] Beaujouan, "Manuscrits médicaux," p. 185.

after he was dead, refers to him as Gilbertus de Aquila, Anglicus, and from this may be drawn, first, that he had a reputation beyond England and, second, that he could have come from one of the prominent English families of that time named Aquila. From other documents it may be gathered that he was a cleric in major orders and physician to the king by 1207.[77] It may be further inferred that he was educated abroad, because English universities were unable at that time fully to educate a medical doctor. Some have offered that he must have studied at Salerno, but Paris, Bologna, or Montpellier are also possible.[78]

Theodoric of Lucca gave an early citation of Gilbertus in his surgery (ca. 1267) when he spoke of *oleum benedictum* made by him,[79] and it was again his remedies that prompted French surgeon Guy de Chauliac to remark in his surgery (1363), "I have taken litel of emperykes and of charmes, of the whiche þinges plente is founden in Gilbertyn."[80] From Guy's remark and from the way in which he is cited, it would seem that by the fourteenth century Gilbertus was at best known as the "surgeon's physician" and at worst as a collector of recipes and not a medical theorist. It was probably this reputation that led to his being chosen for translation into Middle English, and to his recipes being so often included in Middle English recipe collections.

The best-known testimony to his learning outside the medical tradition is Chaucer's description of the physician in the General Prologue to the *Canterbury Tales*:

> Wel knew he the old Esculapius,
> And deyscorides, and eek Rufus,
> Olde Ypocras, Haly, and Galeyn,
> Serapion, Rhazis, and Avycen,
> Averros, Damascien, and Constantyn,
> Bernard, and Gatesden, and Gilbertyn.[81]

---

[77] Talbot and Hammond, pp. 58-60.

[78] Evidence for where Gilbertus may have studied is weighed in Wickersheimer, *Dictionnaire biographique*, pp. 191-92. From a reading of Gilbert and his sources, Talbot finds it likely that Gilbert "was a product of Salerno and Montpellier": *Medicine in Medieval England*, p. 73.

[79] Theodoric is in many ways the surgical equivalent of Gilbertus in Latin. He relied heavily on recipes, combined medical and surgical treatment, and gave detailed directions for preparation of medicaments. His surgery has been translated into English as *The Surgery of Theodoric*, 2 vols., ed. Eldridge Campbell and James Colton (New York: Appleton-Century-Crofts, 1955 and 1960). The reference to Gilbertus is in Vol. 2, p. 221.

[80] Middle English translation in *The Cyrurgie of Guy de Chauliac*, ed. Margaret S. Ogden, EETS 265 (1971), pp. 533-34.

[81] Geoffrey Chaucer, *Works*, ed. F. N. Robinson, 2d ed. (Boston: Houghton Mifflin, 1957), ll. 429-34.

Of the last three, so often mentioned as a group, Bernard Gordon wrote his *Lilium medicinae* about 1305, and John Gaddesden wrote his *Rosa medicinae anglicae* about 1314.[82]

Gilbertus' reputation in English medical literature did not fade with the end of the manuscript tradition. He is named in a recipe collection entitled *The treasurie of hidden secrets: commonly called, the goodhuswiues closet of prouision, for the health of her houshold, gathered out of sundry experiments, lately practised by men of great knowledge,* attributed elsewhere to John Partridge.[83] Yet another citation to Gilbertus appeared in 1671. Mr. Henry Stubbe engaged in printed correspondence with George Thomson, MD, on the subject of bloodletting. Stubbe cited the efficacy of phlebotomy in the treatment of smallpox, according to "the old English practise, directed by Johannes Anglicus de Gadesden in his Rosa medicinae, and Gilbertus Anglicus, almost three hundred years ago; and their directions are as positive and ample, as those I cite out of Avicenna."[84]

To label Gilbertus' writings, whether in Latin or in their English translation, as part of a popular tradition might seem to some more a condemnation than an evaluation. It is perhaps better to say that his writings had a popular appeal. His encyclopedic approach and his attention to practical matters not only attracted the notice of the translator, but kept him a part of English medical literature for over four hundred years.

VI. DESCRIPTION OF THE MANUSCRIPT

A. Binding

Contemporary with the MS. Alum-tawed sheepskin (or deerskin) turned in, over oak boards, original sewing, projecting bands. Three leather thongs stitched with thread pass horizontally under the spine. Thongs pegged into three parallel grooves enter boards around outside of inner edge. Clasp on front missing, hole on back for boss, boss missing. Squares do not project. Book was probably closed with a leather thong. Stitching at top and bottom of the spine.[85]

---

[82] Luke Demaitre, *Doctor Bernard de Gordon* (Toronto: Pontifical Institute, 1980), p. 51; Talbot and Hammond, p. 148.

[83] London, 1627 (first ed. 1573), f. 16.

[84] George Thomson, *A Letter Sent to Mr Henry Stubbe* (London, 1672), p. 12. I am grateful to Prof. Harold Cook for calling these two references to my attention.

[85] Material for this description is arranged according to the suggestions offered in Graham Pollard, "Describing Medieval

B. Physical Description

Ff. v + 327 + iv. Paper, save for 1^4, 40^{12}, 41^{14}, which are parchment. Page size 135 x 100 mm, save for f. 322: 145 x 100 mm, and ff. 324-335: 125 x 90 mm. Difference in page sizes accounted for by booklet structure of codex. Writing space ca. 90 x 70 mm, ca. 20 long lines per page. Ruled with hard point on four sides, save for tables and ff. 324-336, which are pricked along the three outer edges. Collation: 1^4, 2^{10}, $3-6^8$, 7^7 wants one, $8-39^8$, 40^{12}, 41^{14} plus one leaf of parchment that was a pastedown that has been ripped up. The codex is composed of six booklets that were bound together in the medieval period. Employing the numbers of the gatherings used above for collation, the booklets are as follows: I(1) + II(2) + III(3-6) + IV(7-39) + V(40) + VI(41). Modern pencil foliation is incorrect: moves from 37 to 39. Narrow strips of parchment strengthen each central opening. F. 5 has the upper right corner missing and f. 70 the lower right corner missing. The upper third of f. 337 has been cut away.

Ff. 6-10v in one hand. F. 10v l. 13-f. 14v in one hand. Ff. 15-44v l. 1 in larger, less formal hand of a similar script, with initials in red and paragraph heads with red ornament. F. 44v l. 2 - f. 46v l. 4 in same or similar hand to ff. 48-310v l. 16. F. 46v ll. 5-11 in same hand as f. 310v l. 17-f. 311. This hand is also that of one of the marginal glossators. Ff. 47-47v blank. Ff. 48-310v: running chapter heads with initials decorated in red; titles framed in red. Marginal notes with initials in the same hand as the text and framed in red. Chapter headings have initials in gold leaf (rare for this type of MS): ff. 74v, 103v, 105v, 120, 129, 133, 138v, 146v, 162, 184, 194, 210, 221, 253v, 275v, 300, 305v; decorated in black, green, blue, red, and white over the blue, with white touched with gray over the red. Foliage often filled in with gold leaf. Titles after each chapter in blue with red decoration. Colored capitals cued in margin. Paragraph marks in red. Ff. 311v-315 blank; ff. 315v-318v col. 1, tables in red and black; ruled in black ink ff. 315v-317 and ruled in red and black ink on ff. 317v-318v. Text of f. 318v col. 2-f. 319v in similar hand to ff. 48-310v. F. 318v col. 2, 3-line initial in red, capitals touched with red. F. 320, tables in red and black, ruled in black. F. 321v, tables in red and black, ruled in red. Text on f. 321v col. 2, 3-line initial and first two lines in red. Text of ff. 321v-322v in same hand as ff. 318v-319v. Ff. 323-325v blank. F. 326 in new hand with initials in red. Ff. 326v-333, tables in red and black, ruled in black. Ff. 333v-336v blank. F. 337 in new hand. F. 337v shows traces of red and green wax, used as paste.

Medieval foliation: ff. 6-14v, marked i-iiii; catchword at bottom of f. 13v is not at the end of the gathering. Ff. 15-47v, foliation ai-diiii, mostly cut off; catchwords. Ff. 48-310v, foliation aii-ggiiii, catchwords. Foliation in gathering qi-qiiii (ff. 151-158v) corrected from li-liiii by

Bookbindings," in *Medieval Learning and Literature*: *Essays Presented to Richard William Hunt*, ed. J. J. G. Alexander and M. T. Gibson (Oxford: Clarendon Press, 1976), pp. 50-65.

scribe. Gathering pi-piiii (ff. 159-166v) corrected from mi-miiii as above. Si-siiii (ff. 183-190v) corrected from pi-piiii. First two leaves of ti-tiiii (ff. 191-198v) corrected from qi and qii. The scribe has written *ca^m x* below folio marking piiii (f. 162). F. 152v, chapter head *The Coughe*, is out of order. The scribe has written in the margin, "*Al þis is voide hederto.*" The page is completely independent of the preceding and following pages and is not a duplicate. F. 158 is marked by the scribe *vacat*. Ff. 167-174v are out of order in the gathering owing to reversal of leaves qiii and qiiii. This error was not caught by the scribe or binder. Rubrication is missing on ff. 192v and 197, and ff. 193v and 196. Each pair is conjoined in the gathering. Ff. 202v-203v are copied out of order; the scribe indicated their proper ordering writing "verte ad aliam partem folii subsequentis" at the bottom of f. 202v and marking the pages with the letters *a*, *b*, *c*, and *d*. On f. 221, at the beginning of the chapter on the stomach, is written by the scribe: "Aftir trev stonding, þis chaptir shulde stonde nexte aftir þe title of sincopis; and nexte þis: þe chaptir of þe guttis, and aftir þat, þe chapitir of þe liuer; and aftir þat, þe chaptir of þe spleen; and þen þe chapitir of þe reines; and soforþ as it is written." The MS is described briefly in S. A. J. Moorat, *Catalogue of Western Manuscripts on Medicine and Science in the Wellcome Historical Medical Library*, Vol. 1: *MSS written before 1650 A.D.* (London: Wellcome Institute, 1962), 394-95.

C. Contents of the Manuscript

Booklets are indicated by roman numerals. Incipits are in bold. Each text is given an arabic number, and line numbers are indicated only when several short texts appear on a single page. The division of one text from another is to some extent an editorial judgment.

I. Ff. l-5v booklet blank.

II. Ff. 6-14v booklet contains two groups of texts, 1-7 and 8-17, each in a different hand.

1. Ff. 6-9 *Canon pro medicinis dandis et recipiendis.* **Ad sciendum quo tempore debet dari medicina laxatiua ...** [f. 9] *preter martem. quere veritatem.* [excerpts from commentary by unknown author on astrological-medical works, citing *Thelit* (Thabit ibn Qurra), *Haly* (Ali ibn Ridwan), and *Ptolemy*.[86] Similar to a tract found with a Latin Gilbertus in Cambridge, Peterhouse MS 52, ff. 115v-118v. See also *The Kalendarium of Nicholas of Lynn*, ed. Sigmund Eisner (Athens: University of Georgia Press, 1980), pp. 209-23, for a longer but similar Latin text. TK 61. See also Manzalaoui, *Secretum Secretorum*, pp. 63-64].

---

[86] Dr. Charles Burnett of the Warburg Institute was kind enough to give me his advice on the names found in this text.

2. F. 9v **Nota quod luna est planetarum infima** ... *13 horis, 18 minutis, 38 2^{is}*. [on the properties of the moon. See Seymour, pp. 489-95].

3. Ff. 9v-10 **Nota quod sunt dignitates accidentales** ... [f. 10] *dicunt astronomi fortissimum esse.* [aspects of various planets. See Seymour, pp. 460-65].

4. F. 10 *Nota bene de ponderibus.* **Scopolus** [i.e., *obulus*] **ponderat xx grana** ... *per pondera iacentia.* [on weights and the difference between Troy weights and other systems; similar to the text found in *Medical Works of the Fourteenth Century*, ed. Henslow, p. 131, and many others].

5. F. 10v ll. 1-3 **Corpus solis continet tre cencies** ... *corpus terre 7^{es}.* [relative volumes of the planets].

6. F. 10v ll. 4-6 **Nota ab origine mundi** ... *xli minuta.* [age of the universe *secundum Alfonsum.* See "Extracts from the Alfonsine Tables and Rules for their Use," in Grant, *Source Book,* pp. 451-487].

7. F. 10v ll. 7-12 **Menses per circulum anni** ... *Maius 13 gemeni.* [which month is associated with which sign of the zodiac].

8. Ff. 10v-11 **This is þe forme and maner** ... **Take a potel of þe beste aquevite** ... [f. 11] *wel and close, et cetera.* [how to make Quinta Essencia, in this recipe, a kind of medicinal liqueur. See *Aus mittelenglischen Medizintexten*, ed. Müller, p. 27 and following].

9. Ff. 11-12 **These ben þe uertues** ... **If a man haue þe pallesy** ... [f. 12] *feyr vertues. deo gracias.* [properties of Quinta Essencia. See also *The Book of Quinte Essence,* ed. F. J. Furnivall (1866; rpt. EETS 16, 1965)].

10. F. 12 ll. 6-10 *For þe stomake* ... **Take rede myntes** ... *þou shalt be hole.* [recipe].

11. F. 12 ll. 11-20 *For þe stomake* ... **Take þe rote of radiche** ... *and sanaberis.* [recipe].

12. Ff. 12 l. 21-f. 12v l. 3 *For sekenes in þe splene* ... **Take verveyn** ... [f. 12v] *and sanaberis.* [recipe].

13. F. 12v ll. 4-13 *For a feuer* ... **Take grene mader** ... *at euen, et cetera.* [recipe].

14. F. 12v ll. 14-16 *For an axes vppon digestion* ... **Recipe borage** ... *and use it.* [recipe].

15. Ff. 12v-13v *Menses per circulum anni cum signis eius pertinentibus.* **Januarius. Sol in aquario xi videlicet die erit. si tonitrus hoc mense** ... *ventos validos* ... [f. 13v] *sol erit in capricorno.* ["book of thunders" telling what to expect if thunder is heard in a particular month; TK 652, attributed to Bede: **Presagium tonitruorum in quolibet mense**; in TK 1466, the same text is anon.].

16. Ff. 13v-14 **Yemps calida estas procellosa** ... [f. 14] *fenum multum erit.* [prognostication by the quality of winter and summer weather, with seven possibilities given, marked A-G. See

Stuart Jenks, "Astrometeorology in the Middle Ages," *Isis*
74 (1983): 185-210 for similar texts].

17. F. 14v *Notandum est quod* **si aliquis vulneratus in capite** ... *pedes
facti sunt.* [safe days for bleeding; same as text found in
John of Arderne: *Treatises of Fistula in Ano* (1910), ed.
D'Arcy Power, EETS 139 (1968), p. 16; similar to TK
1441, **Si aliquis efficitur**].

III. Ff. 15-46v booklet contains mainly urine and fever texts, two
topics found in L that the Middle English translator
appears to have removed; this booklet repairs that
omission.

18. Ff. 15-40v *Here begynneþ þe practise of þe sighte of vrynes.* **Hit is to
vndurstonde þat whoso wille loke an vryn** ... [f. 21] *Here
endeþ þe significacion of þe colours of vryns. Nowe we
wille* [f. 21v] *declare and telle of þe cercles of vryns and
begynne at þe hede of man.* **A cercle þat is grete** ... [f. 23]
Here endiþ þe cercles [f. 23v] *of vryns with her
significacions. And now foloweþ þe contents of hem and þe
passing excesse of hem and þe open declaryng of hem which
ben gode and holsom and commendable.* **Eche vryn is
clensing of blode** ... [f. 35v] *Here endeþ þe treatise of þe
cercles of vryns with her significacions and also þe propirtes*
[f. 36] *of vryns and ouerpassing excesse of hem. And nowe
foloweþ remedy and medysyn for meny of hem þat ben
rehersid.* **Medisyn for colour as camellis flesshe. Take þe
croppe of sauge** ... [f. 40v] *And þus þis practis of fisike
endeþ.* [compilation of four uroscopies (incipits in bold)
with some repetition of material and with links added
between the texts; the copyist/translator summarized his
material freely from the Latin; see Gundolf Keil, *Die
urognostische Praxis in vor- und frühsalernitanischer Zeit*
(Freiburg: Institut für Geschichte der Medizin, 1970), for
Latin analogs].

19. Ff. 40v-41v **Of every sekenes thre tymes þer be** ... [f. 41v] *by þe grace
of god.* [on critical days of febrile sickness; similar to TK
997, **Omnis egritudo habet**].

20. F. 42 *For him þat is traueled* ... **Take camylmelle** ... *þe selfe wise* [fever
recipe].

21. F. 42v ll. 1-10 *Forto swage and abate þe malice of þe hote axes* ... **Take
mandrake** ... *in a short time.* [fever recipe].

22. F. 42v ll. 11-17 *For him þat pisseþ blode* ... **Take wilde sage** ... *use þe
drinke.* [recipe].

23. Ff. 42v-43 *For dymnes of yen* ... **Take centuary** [f. 43] *to þy bedde.*
[recipe].

24. F. 43 *For þe coughe* ... **Take elemini** ... *firste and laste.* [recipe].

25. Ff. 43-43v *Electuary for þe coughe* ... **Take cynamum** ... *and use hit.*
[recipe].

26. F. 43v *Gargarismus for purgyng of þe hede* ... **Take mustard** ... *til þou
be esid.* [recipe].

27. Ff. 43v-44v *For a collerike man* ... **Take borage** ... [f. 44v] *and sanaberis.* [recipe].

28. F. 44v *Gargarismus for þe hede* ... **Recipe nigelle** ... *super umbilicum.* [recipe in Latin].

29. Ff. 45-46 **Ther ben iiii Ages** ... [f. 46] *soupe is þeir quarter.* [relationship of the four ages of man to the four seasons, winds, and humors; see Little and Withington's edition of Roger Bacon's *De retardatione,* p. 199, where this information is presented in the form of a wheel; and Seymour, pp. 291-93].

30. F. 46 *Nowe foloweþ þe reigning of þe complexiouns* ... **Fro þe iii of þe clocke** ... *is most greuid.* [the relationship of the four complexions to the hours of the day].

31. Ff. 46-46v *For þe morfu.* **Wasshe al þy body** ... [f. 46v] *be wel usid.* [recipe].

32. F. 46v *For þe iaundice.* **Take greynes** ... *at ones.* [recipe, same hand as nos. 34 and 35].

     IV. Ff. 48-310v contain the Middle English Gilbertus and a recipe added in a later hand (no. 34), which is related in content to the recipe added at the beginning of V (no. 35).

33. Ff. 48-310v ... *superfluites and moche slepe* ... [f. 310v] *and stonis. deo gracias.* [practice of medicine arranged from the head downward; translated from Gilbertus Anglicus; cf. Seymour, pp. 343-411].

34. F. 310v *A medisyn for þe stoon* ... **Take karewaye** ... *of a conseruatif.* [recipe in the same hand as nos. 32 and 35].

     V. Ff. 311-322v [recipe in later hand plus tables for practice of astrological medicine].

35. F. 311 *Anoþer maner making is þis.* **Take alle þese** ... *þes dissesis.* [recipe in same hand as nos. 32 and 34].

36. Ff. 315v-317 [Golden Numbers for calculating the dates of the new and full moon in metonic (nineteen-year) cycles; useful for prognostication and for explaining the past onset of illness; most commonly used to calculate the date of Easter].

37. Ff. 317v-318v [Dominical Letters for calculating the date in any year upon which the first Sunday would fall; useful in the practice of astrological medicine in as much as certain zodiacal signs govern certain days of the week; ecclesiastical use].

38. Ff. 318v-319v **Quicumque cursum lune** ... [f. 319v] *eorum tractavimus.* [signs of the zodiac; useful in practice of astrological medicine].

39. Ff. 320-321v [lunar tables telling which signs of the zodiac the moon will be in; especially useful for bloodletting and administering medicines; same as Power, *John of Arderne,* pp. 18-19].

40. Ff. 321v-322v *Regula pro precedentibus.* **Si scire vis sub quo signo luna est** ... [f. 322v] *in antedictis membris.* [how to use the above lunar tables; same as Power, *John of Arderne*, p. 16].

VI. This booklet certainly was constructed to exist independently; ff. 323 and 336 form its covers, are blank, and are larger in size than the material in between.

41. F. 326 **In this qwair be conteyned alle the chaunges of the moone** ... *ccc.lxv et sex hore.* [instructions for the following tables; dated 1462 and useful until 1519].

42. Ff. 326v-333 [lunar tables used to determine when the moon will be full; more exact than no. 36].

D. *Watermarks*

The paper in every booklet except III bears a watermark consisting of a bull, on foot, head turned forward, with a tail in three strands, no. 2785 in Allan Stevenson's edition of C. M. Briquet's *Les filigranes: Dictionnaire historique des marques du papier* (Amsterdam: Paper Publications Society, 1968). It is listed: Bordeaux 1460. The paper in III is marked by an arrow pointing downward with two circles, one on each side of the arrow, which are connected by a horizontal bar. This mark is not in Briquet.

E. *Dating and Script*

The codex is copied throughout in an English cursive bookhand characteristic of the second half of the third quarter of the fifteenth century.[87] The Wellcome Middle English Gilbertus is throughout the work of one scribe. If the watermark dating is correct, the greater part of the codex could not have been copied before about 1460. Section 41 contains an introductory sentence stating that the table "was made and drawen in þe 3eer of our lorde a thousande cccclxii" (f. 326). The mixture of paper and parchment writing surfaces, the differing watermarks, the booklet structure of the codex, and the fact that the dated section could have been copied at a time later than the original make a precise dating impossible.

---

[87] Dr. M. B. Parkes, Fellow of Keble College, Oxford, and Prof. A. G. Watson, Reader in Manuscript Studies, University College, London, assisted me with their opinions on the nature and dating of this script.

F. Provenance

The MS was deliberately defaced with a cutting tool after the eighteenth century, removing any evidence of previous ownership. In addition to the missing first page of the Middle English Gilbertus, several other pages have been damaged, but not necessarily at the same time. The location of this damage has been described above. A date and possibly a signature in an eighteenth-century hand have been cut out of f. 5, and f. 337 shows the mutilated signature "Galfrydus Halle" in a medieval hand not found elsewhere in the codex. It is followed by a series of *probationes pennae* in the same hand. An armorial bookplate has been ripped off the inside front cover so that only the crest remains. The Royal College of Arms in London was unable to identify the owner of the crest and it does not match the bookplates of any of the people known to have seen the book or to have owned it.[88]

The MS's history in the nineteenth century is more clear. It belonged to Joseph Payne (1808-76), best known as England's first professor of education, who sent it to the antiquarian Francis Douce for his opinion as to the date of copying. An inscription in black ink on the inside front cover states, "Mr. Douce says this MS was written about A.D. 1400--before 1450."

The MS is accompanied by a letter dated May 13, 1858, and written to "J. Payne" by Thomas Wright, author of several pieces on medieval science. Wright dated the MS to "the reign of Hen. VI and Ed. IV."

The MS passed to Joseph Frank Payne, Joseph's son (1840-1910), a physician who was the author of "English Medicine in the Anglo-Norman Period" in the *British Medical Jour.* 2 (1904): 1281-84. Dr. Payne's collection of rare books and MSS went on sale at Sotheby's in 1911 (July 13, this MS, item no. 406). The MS was described in the catalogue as having been damaged. The Wellcome Library bought the book and it remains in their collection. No record survives of the purchase price.

G. Scribal Correction and Glossing

The Middle English Gilbertus found in Wellcome MS 537 was corrected by the scribe after the text was copied. His cancellations are highlighted by the rubricator, whose hand, in the few examples there are of it, is very similar to that of the scribe, and the two may be one and the same. Interlineations and marginal insertions, also many times

---

[88] I am grateful to the Royal College of Arms and to the British Museum Department of Prints and Drawings for their assistance in my attempts to identify the bookplates.

highlighted by the rubricator, are made in the ink of the text and are most usually indicated by carets or three dots arranged in a triangle. If the scribe discovered that he had copied large sections, for example entire pages, out of order, then he used letters of the alphabet to indicate the correct sequence. The scribe's method of handling a major reordering of material, entire chapters, for example, is discussed above.

At least two fifteenth-century hands appear as glossators of the codex as a whole. The most prominent is the same hand that added the recipes numbered 32, 34, and 35 above. This neat, formal hand provided marginal glosses that are almost always repetitions in Latin of material in the text. In the chapters of the translation on lethargy and epilepsy, however, this writer appears to have drawn corrections from the Latin Gilbertus, inserting for example *citri* after *þe rynde of* on f. 64v, where W here agrees completely with other witnesses. Another far less formal hand inserts an occasional marginal note, and often draws a hand-like form in the margin beside recipes or signs for diagnosis. This hand is more common in the uroscopy text earlier on (no. 18).

H. Dialect and Orthographical Peculiarities

The Middle English Gilbertus in Wellcome MS 537 is written throughout in the late transitional English of the southeast Midlands that can best be described as standard English. In this respect the language of the text is unremarkable. It presents such southern characteristics as OE *a>o* in words such as *also, colde,* and *holsum*; weak plural nouns ending in *-en*: *children, lambren, y3en*; past participles prefixed with *y-* or *i-*: *y-passid, y-grounden,* and *i-medlid*; *ben* used exclusively for the present indicative plural of *to be*; and *w* for *v*: *clowes,* and *wp*. Typical eastern Midland characteristics include *-ch* for *-k*, as *ache*; and *þei, hem, her,* for modern English *they, them, their*.

If it is assumed that the scribe's zeal for maintaining fidelity to his exemplar is greatest at the commencement of his work, W supplies a few clues to the linguistic characteristics of that exemplar. For instance, there are anomalies such as *wexit* (f. 48) for the more usual *waxiþ*, and numerous instances of *k* for *c* or *qu*: *kembe his hede with an yuery kombe* (f. 48), *kaste þerto* (f. 50), and *hony wol keke al maner medisyns* (f. 51).

Some of the scribe's concerns about orthography are betrayed by his corrections. The insertion of the letter *i* is frequently encountered, and the textual notes to this edition call attention to the number of times correction occurs. The letter is added to such words as: *aisshe, armoniac, fleisshe, neisshe,* and *waisshe*.

The letter *w* seems to have given this scribe a great deal of difficulty. False starts *solow-* for *swolle,* as well as simultaneous use of two words for modern English *sweat--soot* and *swete* on the same folio indicate how this scribe reflected the as yet unsettled state of his language.

VII. EDITING THE MANUSCRIPT

A. Editorial Procedures

The Middle English Gilbertus exists in about a dozen MSS, all within about fifty years of each other, and presents challenging problems for the editor. In this edition, a methodology has been employed to convey, apart from the content of W itself, three things. The first is that the text is a translation from a Latin exemplar. The second is that the translator and copyists of the Middle English text felt free to modify the text in a number of ways in order to adapt it to their particular needs. For instance, they added recipes or left them out, divided the material in new ways, systematically left out subject matter, may have incorporated recipes from the Middle English Gilbertus into other collections, and, most important, they included the text in compendia, many of which share other texts in common. The third is that the Middle English Gilbertus is part of a larger tradition, that of vernacular medical translations and recipe collections.

The freedom with which the translator and copyists modified their respective exemplars has made the establishment of common and uncommon texts by critical edition impractical. What is more, new MSS of the Middle English Gilbertus are sure to be identified as the nature and scope of Middle English medical literature are increasingly realized.[89] The presentation of a single witness seems under these circumstances to be the best procedure and the one chosen for this edition.

Evidence from witnesses other than W has been used in the following way. All known versions of the Middle English Gilbertus have been divided into three groups. The first group contains W as well as other complete versions that have now or once have had the incipit *A mon þat woll help men in her sykenesses*. The second group of witnesses contains two MSS that begin with the chapter on *scotomy* and thus with respect to the first group are incomplete. They have the incipit *Scotomye is such a sekenes*. The third group contains fragments of the text that are parts of medical compendia.[90]

---

[89] A catalogue of incipits of Old and Middle English medical and scientific texts is being prepared by Prof. Linda Voigts and Dr. Patricia Kurtz. An edition of the section of the Gilbertus translation on epilepsy is being prepared by Prof. George Keiser using H. It will appear in *Practical and Popular Science of Medieval England*, edited by Lister Matheson.

[90] Fragments of the Gilbertus translation that are not incorporated into recipe collections are as follows:

1. Har 2375, mid-fifteenth century contains the chapter on the liver, the spleen, the kidneys, and the bladder (ff. 4-19). A fragment

One witness roughly contemporary with W from each of the first two groups-- for the first, London, British Library, Additional MS 30338, and for the second group, London, British Library, Sloane MS 5--have been collated with W. W has also been collated with the Latin Gilbertus Anglicus printed in Lyons in 1510. These collations have established several things: first, it is possible to isolate short sections that the Wellcome copyist has added to his text that do not appear in the Latin or in the other Middle English versions; second, it is possible to determine how the Wellcome copyist edited out certain material; third, it is possible to verify the remaining text as being common to two or three witnesses.

Other MSS apart from Add 30338 and Sl 5 containing the Middle English Gilbertus have been examined with the following aims. First of all, certain passages have been checked to determine if any clear hierarchy of all witnesses exists. A clear hierarchy was not apparent. Second, the passages the Wellcome copyist has added to the text were sought in other witnesses. The result of this search was to verify that these passages are unique to W (although as yet unidentified MSS may show otherwise). Third, other MSS containing the Middle English Gilbertus were examined in order to determine whether these MSS had in common any other texts apart from the Middle English Gilbertus. The result of this examination is that the first and second groups of MSS discussed above share a number of texts within their respective groups.

The textual information gained by the examination of the Middle English and Latin Gilbertus texts has been presented in the following way. The text of the edition of W contains not only the folio numbers from the Wellcome MS, but also a rough guide to the folio numbers of the Latin 1510 edition. The folio numbers of the Latin text are enclosed in square brackets. This Latin text is available for detailed comparison with the Middle English version in a number of libraries and

---

of the Middle English gynecology edited by Rowland is also present, and it is followed by a Middle English uroscopy.

2. Sl 442 is compiled from many booklets from the late fifteenth century. It has the first pages of the Middle English Gilbertus to the recipe for compound oxymel. It then has scraps from the chapter on apostem of the kidneys. The Middle English Gilbertus material extends from ff. 38 to f. 40v.

3. Har 3407 has a single gathering of the Middle English Gilbertus concerning the spleen and kidneys on ff. 68-79v. It is badly damaged. The gathering is bound with other medical fragments from the fourteenth and fifteenth centuries in English and Latin.

4. Sl 3553, from the mid-fifteenth century, begins the Middle English Gilbertus defectively with material just before the chapter on ophthalmia and ends defectively with the chapter on diarrhea. The text covers ff. 21-95v. It is bound with other Middle English texts on astrology.

is on microfilm available from the Wellcome Library.[91]   The printed
Latin text has been compared with a fifteenth-century MS that is nearly
contemporary with the date the Gilbertus was translated (London,
British Library, Sloane MS 272) and no significant differences were
apparent. The Commentary to this edition notes with question marks
sections that apparently have been added to the Wellcome MS by its
copyist. The Commentary also contains sections that are missing from
the Wellcome MS that are found in Additional MS 30338 within the
following boundaries. All missing material removed from W by damage
has been supplied either in the Commentary or in the printed text in
brackets. All material relating to the diseases of women and children
that the Wellcome copyist left out has been noted in the Commentary.
All material of a theoretical nature missing from W has been supplied in
the Commentary. The rest of the missing material consists of short
recipes, and unless these are of more than three lines in the text or are in
some way significant, they have been ignored.

B. Transcription Procedures

The letter *i* is represented as written, either *i* or rarely *ij*. The
letter *3* most often represents the yogh and is shown as such.
Occasionally it is the long-tailed *z*, and in such cases appears as *z*. *Ff* and
ff are shown as *F*; *u* and *v* are represented as written.
Minim letters are ambiguous in form, although the *i* is almost
always stroked. Context has dictated the distinction between *f* and long
s; *c* and *t* often cannot be told apart and likewise the ligatures *cc* and *tt*.
Some instances of final *e* in the text are the result of editorial
expansion. A horizontal stroke through a final ascender or ascenders
(*all*) has been expanded to *e* or *is* according to context, although this is
done with the understanding that such a stroke may be without meaning
in certain words. Also dictated by context is the expansion to *e, er, ir,* or
re of the curl after letters such as *r* and *þ*. Neighboring scribal practice
has been allowed to resolve the ambiguity of such ambiguous expansions,
but it should be remembered that words such as *plastre/plastir/plaster*
can vary in spelling even within a page, while words such as *watir*,
although frequently used, are almost never spelled out in full; indeed, it
may be that the scribe rarely if ever visualized words such as *watir* in any
form but the abbreviated one.
Other abbreviations are *p* = *per* or *par*; stroke over a vowel for
m, n, or sometimes *u*; backward *c* for *con* or *com*; superscript *a* for *ur*.
Superscript letters indicate that the one before has been left out (*þ*ᵗ for
þat) and have been silently expanded. The stroke over words ending in

---

[91] The 1510 edition of the *Compendium* is the one used by the
Dictionary of Medieval Latin from British Sources, edited by R. E.
Latham (London: Oxford University Press, 1975-86).

-ion is probably otiose and has been ignored except where scribal practice has expanded it elsewhere to *-ioun*. These cases are rare.
In the system of apothecaries' weights used in the text, $\mathfrak{Z}$ = ounce, $\mathfrak{Z}$ = drachm, and $\mathfrak{D}$ = scruple. *Quart* is expanded to *quartron*, *li* to *libra*, *m* to *manipulus*, *aq* to *aqua*. A long *s* with a backstroke through the center representing the Latin *semis* has been written as 1/2. *&* has been expanded to *and* except in certain cases within recipes. *q* followed by a long *s* with a backstroke through the center has been expanded to *quantum sufficit*.
Medieval capitalization and punctuation have been altered to suit modern usage. The medieval paragraph sign has been retained. Chapter division follows the scribe's intentions except where indicated in the textual notes. Running heads found in the manuscript have been reproduced in the edition as closely as possible. Division of words in the MS has occasionally not been respected (MS *man is* = *manis*). Short and obvious dittographies without textual significance have been silently removed. These dittographies occur most frequently at the end of one line and at the beginning of the next.
The very good condition of W has made emendation rarely necessary. All material imported into the text is both enclosed in brackets and indicated in the textual notes. Obvious eyeskips, *malage* for *malagoge*, for instance, occur from time to time, and where the word has been imported from Latin and has not survived into modern English, positive evidence for emendation has been derived from the spelling closest to the Latin original. The very few cases where damage to the MS has made the use of other MSS necessary to restore a reading are shown in the notes. Fortunately, these restorations can be offered with some confidence, with the exception of the missing first page of W, which has been supplied from Add 30338 and appears in the Commentary.

VIII. THE MIDDLE ENGLISH GILBERTUS ANGLICUS AS PART OF A COMPENDIUM

A compendium is a compilation of a number of texts from various sources into a single MS.[92] The Middle English Gilbertus is usually contained in compendia, and a large number of these have in common texts other than the Middle English Gilbertus. This commonalty of texts may point to an original compendium, now lost, containing the shared material. These compendia also contain unique

---

[92] The expense of collecting books appears to have led to the compiling of compendia. In Latin, these often appear under the heading of guides for the poor. The most popular and enduring example is John XXI's *Thesaurus pauperum*, often translated into vernacular languages. See also Demaitre, "Scholasticism," where the Latin tradition is outlined.

texts not shared by the other MSS. Comparison of several MSS containing the Middle English Gilbertus allowed these common and uncommon texts to be established.[93]

A. MSS Containing the Middle English Gilbertus with the Incipit A mon þat woll help men in her sykenesses.

W belongs to a group of MSS that now have or once had the incipit for the Middle English Gilbertus *A mon þat woll help men in her sykenesses*. Other MSS belonging to this group are as follows.

Add 30338 is from the mid-fifteenth century. It is described in *Catalogue of Additions to the Manuscripts in the British Museum in the Years 1876-1881*, rpt. ed. (London, 1968), pp. 70-71. The Middle English Gilbertus is found on ff. 11v-149, beginning *A man that wolle helpe*. It ends with a recipe for iron rust.

Sl 3486 dates from the mid-fifteenth century. The Middle English Gilbertus is found on ff. 91-139. It begins defectively with what is in this edition chapter I, part 2: *In a mannes hede*. There is a gap in the text after the section on mania labeled chapter 17. The text resumes with f. 25, which concerns epilepsy, and which was bound in error with a Middle English surgical text running ff. 18v-57v. Chapters 20-24, on the eyes, are confused in their ordering. From chapter 25 on watery eyes, until chapter 77 on the liver, the text is complete. There is material missing from the section on the liver, after which the numbering of chapters becomes confused. The text ends as does W with a chapter numbered 93. The MS is in the main concerned with surgery, and is badly defective. Ff. 148-49v contain a table of contents to the entire MS in the same or similar hand as copied the MS's texts. On f. 148 is an explicit, much damaged and crossed out, naming Thomas Betrisden as putting together the material preceding *ex arte phisicali*. The surname was crossed out and replaced in the right-hand margin by a later hand.

Hu U.7.1 is described by John Young in *A Catalogue of the Manuscripts in the Library of the Hunterian Museum in the University of Glasgow* (Glasgow, 1908), pp. 245-6. The script and initials indicate a

---

[93] See especially Malcolm B. Parkes, "The Influence of the Concepts of *Ordinatio* and *Compilatio* on the Development of the Book," in *Medieval Learning and Literature: Essays Presented to Richard William Hunt*, ed. J. J. G. Alexander and M. T. Gibson (Oxford: Clarendon Press, 1976), pp. 115-41. Parkes observes that *compilatio* "operates at two levels: at one level it involves the adoption of a general scheme or structure in which the compiler can incorporate most conveniently the particular materials he has selected; and at another level it involves the choice of a critical procedure by which the diverse *auctoritates* can be divided up and redeployed according to the nature of the subject matter" (p. 128).

date of copying between 1400 and 1450. The binding, which was described by Young, was removed in 1971. The text is copied in one hand. Ff. 13-145v contain the Middle English Gilbertus, beginning *A man þat wole helpe men in her syknesse,* and ending as does W. There is damage to ff. 13v, 14, 14v, 15v, 16, 18. Most of the other texts concern pharmacy and bloodletting.

SoA is contemporary with Hu U.7.1 and is written in a single hand. It is described by N. R. Ker in *Medieval Manuscripts in British Libraries,* Vol. 1 (Oxford: Clarendon Press, 1969), p. 312. The Middle English Gilbertus is found on ff. 7v-76v, and begins *A man þat wolle helpe men;* it ends in the same way as does W.

H is from the first half of the fifteenth century. It is described by Ralph Hanna, *A Handlist of Manuscripts containing Middle English Prose in the Henry E. Huntington Library. Index of Middle English Prose, Handlist I* (Cambridge: D. S. Brewer, 1984), pp. 40-41. I follow Hanna's description. Hanna neglected to note that the text was the Middle English Gilbertus, and this omission is carried forward in the Huntington's catalogue to its entire collection. The Middle English Gilbertus runs ff. 16-237v and begins *A mon þat wol helpe men;* it ends with a recipe for iron rust. The other texts concern pharmacy.

Other witnesses containing the Middle English Gilbertus in a complete or nearly complete form are as follows. Hu V.8.12 is from the mid-fifteenth century. It is described by Young, pp. 416-17. The Middle English Gilbertus runs ff. 15-167v and begins *A man þat wole helpe men;* it ends as does W. Add 25589 is from the mid-fifteenth century and contains the Middle English Gilbertus on ff. 1-73 beginning *A man that woll helpe.* It ends with the chapter on the spleen.

B. MSS Containing the Middle English Gilbertus Anglicus with the Incipit
       Scotomy is such.

Two other MSS containing the Middle English Gilbertus were copied for the most part in the same hand. Sl 5 was copied and compiled in the middle of the fifteenth century. It belonged to *Richard Dod. de London, Barbor Sorion* (f. 157), who apparently was attached to the hospital of St. Giles without Cripplegate, as the name of that hospital appears at the top of f. 157 above his name. The Middle English Gilbertus runs ff. 63v-151v, *Scotomy is such ...* [f. 151v] *of an eye. Explicit.* The Middle English Gilbertus is missing about five leaves between *gutta rosacea* and *squinancy.* The other texts the MS contains are mainly on pharmacy, surgery, astrology, and uroscopy.

TCC is contemporary with Sl 5 and has been described by M. R. James in *The Western Manuscripts in the Library of Trinity College, Cambridge,* Vol. 2 (Cambridge, 1902), 3, p. 494. The Middle English Gilbertus runs ff. 36-122, *Scotomye is such a sekenes ...* [f. 122] *white of an egge. Explicit.* The Middle English Gilbertus begins with a new hand;

the old hand resumes f. 40. The other texts in the MSS are recipes and a Middle English translation of Bernard Gordon, *De prognosticis*.

The following is a summary of the principal texts that MSS discussed in sections A and B above have in common. Incipits are in bold.

a. Anon. **It is to vnderstonde þat a man is made** [on humors, elements, qualities, urines]. Sl 3486, ff. 86-90; Hu U.7.1, ff. 1-13; SoA, ff. 1-7v; Hu V.8.12, ff. 1-15.

b. Gilbertus Anglicus, Middle English *Compendium medicinae*. All MSS.

c. Anon. On buboes. **Þer falleþ oftentymes an enpostume.** Sl 3486, ff. 139-40; Hu U.7.1, ff. 145v-148v.

d. Anon. Middle English gynecology. **Also we shal vnderstonde þat wymen.** Printed under the title *Medieval Woman's Guide to Health*, ed. Rowland. Sl 3486, ff. 140-47; Hu U.7.1, ff. 149v-165v; SoA, ff. 76v-85v; Sl 5, ff. 158-172v; TCC ff. 126-128 (imperfect).

e. Guy de Chauliac, On bloodletting. **A phisiciane bihoueþ to knowe þre maner inspeccions.** See *The Cyrurgie of Guy de Chauliac*, ed. Margaret S. Ogden, EETS 265 (1971), pp. 543-45. Sl 3486, f. 147v; Hu U.7.1, 165v-166.

f. Guy de Chauliac, On scarifying and cupping. **For garsynge and ventasynge.** See Ogden, *Guy de Chauliac*, pp. 545-50. Sl 3486, f. 147v; Hu U.7.1, ff. 166-166v.

g. Bernard Gordon, *De prognosticis*. **Age is moder.** Sl 5, ff. 61-63; TCC, ff. 31v-32v.

Witnesses to the Middle English Gilbertus that end with the recipe on iron rust and therefore could not be descended from those without that recipe unless cross-contamination took place are H, Add 30338, and Sl 2394. Neither Sl 5 nor TCC could be the ancestor of any MSS in the group containing W because they both lack the chapter on headache the others contain (barring cross-contamination).

The Wellcome Middle English Gilbertus must belong to the group that does not contain Sl 5 and TCC. Even though it wants the first page of the Gilbertus text, it still contains material missing from the other group containing Sl 5 and TCC. Furthermore, W would seem to belong to a class of MSS that contain either the Middle English Gilbertus by itself, or the text in a separate booklet. MSS fitting this description are H, Add 30338, Sl 2394, and Add 25589.[94]

Other parts of the compendia discussed above are found as separate texts. The Middle English gynecology (d) above, edited by

---

[94] Since this edition was completed, three other witnesses to the Gilbertus translation have been identified. I have not seen them, and my information is incomplete. They are: Oxford, Bod. Bodley 178, ff. 51-140v; London, Sloane 1388, ff. 1-55v (incomplete; 15/16 c.); Sloane 3449, ff. 1v-5 (introduction only). I am grateful to Prof. Linda Voigts for supplying these references.

Rowland, is very common; she discusses other MSS pp. 46-48. The encyclopedic text (a) above is also found without the Middle English Gilbertus in two Sloane MSS: 965 and 3449, both from the middle of the fifteenth century.

IX. CONCLUSION

A study of the Middle English Gilbertus demonstrates the complexity of the medieval recipe tradition. The very existence of the Gilbertus translation demonstrates that the matter of learned medicine was not confined to the sphere of Latin university texts. Nor can vernacular recipe collections be said to represent an exclusively folk or low culture tradition. A survey of the historical background to these recipe collections in England shows that medical knowledge was not the property of "experts," and that interest in, and knowledge about, the medical practice, pharmaceuticals, and vocabulary the Middle English Gilbertus represents could be found on many levels of medieval English society. Furthermore, the rapid increase in numbers of vernacular medical MSS from about 1400 is contemporary with urbanization and the growth of a market economy. Recipes, and the simple advice that went with them, became a commodity like pharmaceuticals, developing in response to social demands for expedient cures rather than impractical regimens of health.

Theoretical complexity is apparent when the recipes and ingredients found in collections like the Middle English Gilbertus are examined in the light of learned justifications for their use. These justifications could be symbolic, or part of humoral medicine; however, they have little in common with modern notions of pharmacology. Whatever the justification, historical records demonstrate that medieval people used the ingredients and recipes found in texts like the Middle English Gilbertus, and that this use stemmed from medieval understanding of the physical world.

Complexity operates on the textual level in medieval recipe collections as well. A study of the Middle English Gilbertus in various MSS shows that it could appear integrated into medical compendia reflecting the particular interests of the compiler. The text itself could be modified, with material added or subtracted at will, in the case of W, to remove references to women. Finally, the recipes found in both the Middle English and Latin Gilbertus texts share material with many if not most Middle English recipe collections, and also with collections in Welsh.

Gilbertus' *Compendium* and texts similar to it provide a matrix for adaptation: by translation, addition, deletion, and inclusion in other recipe collections and compendia. These texts are also mirrors of medical practice, supporting a range of theories and beliefs. By the fifteenth century, these texts and the material they contain had also become commodities, translated and copied for the expanding audience of medical expertise.

THE MIDDLE ENGLISH
GILBERTUS ANGLICUS
from
WELLCOME MS 537

Chapter I, The Head
Part 1, Headache

f. 48 / superfluites, and moche slepe, and moche dulnes of witte.

[89v] And of clene moystnes comeþ no grete ache.

And if it comeþ of dryenes, þe skyn wexit drye, and þer ben fewe superfluytees, and litil slepe, and moyist

5 þingis doon him gode.

Remedy
a3enst
hete

If þe hed-ache be of hete, lete him vse coolde þingis, as watir of endyue or of roses, and specialy sugur roset and sugur of violet. And let him kembe his hede with an yuery kombe oftetymes, for þat is gode in euery ache of þe

10 hede. And let him wasshen his fete with warme salte watir. And let him abstyne him from moche waking, and moche þou3t, and from þe company of women, and moche baþing.

[224v]

How
sugir
roset
is made

Sugyr roset is þus made: Take a pounde of sugir and

15 halfe a pounde of tendir roses lyues, and stampe hem wel togedir til þey be smale grounden and wel medlid with þe sugir. And þen do þat in an erþen vessel and set it in þe sunne þritty dayes aftir mydsommer. And euery day,

f. 48v styre it / twies, ones in þe morwetide and ones in þe

20 euentide. But whan xv daies ben y-passid, take halfe a pounde of sugir not ful smale-y-grounded and medle it with þe toþir with þin handes. And when þo þritty daies ben y-passid, put it in a boxe and kepe to-close. This sugir roset is gode for euery fluxe of þe wombe and for

---

1 *First page of this section missing. See Commentary.* **2 comeþ]** *prec. by* þer *underd.* **20 halfe]** *ins. above.* **21 grounded]** *corr. from* grounden. **it]** *ins. above.* **24 sugir roset]** *corr. from* oyle.

1

yuelis þat comen of coler, þat is to sey, of hete and
drienes.

     In þe same wise is sugir of violettis y-made. And
þat is gode for al maner of vnkynde hetis, and for sekenes
5 of þe breest, and of þe sydis, and of þe ly3te, and of
þe lyver, and for þe cardiacle, and for þe feuer tercian.

     But if þe hede-ache be of flevme, þat is to sei,
of cooldenes and of moystnes, let him wasshe his fete
with warme salt watir euery ny3te. And let him often
10 kembe his hede with / an yvery combe. And of þe asshis
of heyne-houe and of elern bowes in grete quantite, and
of þe asshis of egrimoyn and of betayn, make lye and
wasshe þerwith his hede, for þis is gode boþe for falling
awey of heris and to do awey þe ache. Anoynte also his
15 hede with oyle of ellern eiþir of syneuey. Also take
galbanum and do it in a pece of leþer, and ley it to

þat place þat akiþ. And make a plastir of whete mele,
and of marche, wormode, heyhoue, rwe, fenel, and louage.
And let him leve malencolious metis, as oxe flesshe and
20 veneson; and fleumatike metis, as white metis, bottir,
ches, mylke, porke; and salt fysshe, and fresshe fysshe þat
is ful fleumatik, and also elys and congir. And lete him
ete noo raw peeris ne applis, ne onyons, ne suche oþer
rawe þingis. Nottes he may ete, but not meny. And let

---

3 wise] *ins. above.* **7 ache be]** *corr. from* ake. **to sei]** *ins. above.*
11 elern] *corr. from* eldern. **14 his]** *corr. from* þe. **16 leþer]** *prec. by*
of *canc. in red.* **23-24 oþer rawe þingis]** *copied* rawe þingis oþer *and*
marked for reversal.

him vse þe sau[ce] / of garlike and of pepir, gynger, clowes, myntes, peletre, and vynegre. And gode clere white wyne is gode for him. And let him absteyne him from long fasting and also from ydelnes, from wraþþe,

5 from waking, and from colde. Baþeng is gode, but not ofte-tymes.

If þe ache be of malencoly, þat is to sey, of drines and of colde, let him vse al-þinge as þoughe it were of flevme. But let him vse oxymel to purgen him of malencoly:

10 eiþir simple oximel eiþir oxymel compovned.

Symple oxymel is made of hony and of vynegre, two

partis of vynegre and þe þirde parte of hony, y-medlid togederis and soden.

Oxymel componed is made on two maners: Summe is

15 made of oximel simple and of oþer þingis y-put þerto, as oximel squilli[ti]ke and oximel of radiche. Þe toþir

oximel componed is made of oximel / simple and of many oþir maner þingis.

Oximel squilli[ti]ke is þus made: Take an oynon of þe

20 see þat is clepid in Latin squillia and do awey þe vttir shellis of þe oynon, for þei be to hote. And as meny as þou doist awey of þe vttermest, so meny do awey of þe innemest, for þei ben to colde. Take þen hem þat ben in þe myddil, and seþe hem in vynegre, and aftirward clense hem. And kast

---

1 him] *ins. above.* **sauce]** sau. **16 squillitike]** squillike. **19 squillitike]** squillike. **oynon]** *corr. from* onyon. **21 oynon]** *corr. from* onyon. **22 doist]** *corr. from* do.

þerto þe iii part of hony and make it vp.

Oximel of radiche is þus made: Take þe rote of radiche and kit it into smale þynne rollis, and seþe hem in vynegre.   And aftir clense hem and streyne hem. And do þerto þin hony as it is seyde now.

5

Oximel componed is made of meny þingis, and it defieþ and loseþ malencoly, and departiþ it, and makeþ it þynne, and openeþ þe weies þat ben stoppid of þe lyver and also of þe spleen.   Take þe rote of marche, fenel, parcil, calamynte, tyme, rosmaryn, / syngrene, and oþer herbis þat purgen malencoly.   And if þou wilt haue it stronge, do seen þerto.   And streyne it and aftir þat caste þerto þin hony.   If þou wilt 3eue a man oximel componed, 3yue him first oximel simple.   But if þe hede-ache comeþ of þe sikenes of þe stomake or of eny oþir sikenes or of eny oþer membre, hele þat sekenes and þan þe ache wole awey. And if it comeþ of moche waking, make him to slepe.   And if it comeþ of angir, or of sorowe, or of moche fasting, make him to leue suche þingis and drawe him to do þe contrary þingis.

10

15

20

And if he haue a demegreyn, þat is, þe ache of oon side of þe hede, let him vse pillules Arabie, for þei ben gode for euery sikenes of þe hede, and for euery ache of þe hede, and purgen al noiful humours of þe

---

1 **þe**] *ins. above.*   7 **departiþ**] *corr. from* departid.   16 **þe**] *ins. above.*   24 **purgen**] *corr. from* purgeþ.

Pillules
of Arabie
ben
gode
for þe
hede

brayn, and maken / a man glad. Þei doen awey heuynes,
and sharpen a mannes wittes and a mannes sy3te, and saven
his mynde. And þei suffren not a man to be hoor tofore his
tyme. And also þei helpen a man þat haþ þe turnyng of his

5   brayn and þe demegrayn. And þei ben good for men and
women also.

     And þei ben made on þis wise: Take of alloes epatike,
dr. iiii; of brome, of mastike, of baies of lorer, of
scamonye, and of clowes, of eche of þes, oz. i. And

10   medle þes with þe iuse of caule eiþir of fenel. And
do þerto a litil hony forto kepen it, for hony wol keke

Anees
and
comyn [99]
ben yvel
for þe
hede-ache
f. 51v

al maner medisyns þat it is put to from appeiring. A
man þat haþ þe hede-ache of ony humour in his hede shulde
not eten comyn, ne anees, ne noon oþir aromatike þyngis, /

15   for þey wolen heve vp smokis to þe hede þat shulde
encrese þe ache. And if þer be ony emplastir leide to
þe hede, it must be warme, þoughe it be made of hote
herbis, to habate þe coolde of þe heed, for if it be
leide al coolde to þe heed, it wole do harme to þe brayn.

[?]

Cure
of þe
megrayn

20   For þe demegreyn: Take sangdragon and tempere it
with þe white of an eye wel-swonge, and make a plastir
as brood as þe soor is. And þus do twies or thries til
þou be hool. And in leyeng to of þe plastir and when
it is plastrid, sey þis Colet in worship of Seynt Joon

1 **maken**] *corr. from* makeþ. **þei doen**] *corr. from* it doeþ. **2 sharpen**] sharpeþ. **saven**] *corr. from* saueþ. **3 þei suffren**] *corr. from* it
suffreþ. **4 þei helpen**] *corr. from* it helpeþ. **17 of hote**] *corr. from* of
holde.

6

Baptist: Perpetuis nos domine Sancti Iohannis Baptiste;
tueri, presidere, etc. Anoþir medisyn for þe same: Take
auence, myllefoyle, and ruddes, ana, dr. iii; and þre
croppis of bawme. Stampe hem smale and drinke hem with

5   ale. And reste þe vppon þe soore side. /

Chapter I, Part 2
Other Sicknesses of the Head

f. 52

[?]

    In a mannes hede þer ben many oþer sikenessis as
wel as aches. And somme sekenessis comen of fume and
smokis þat fleen about a mannes brayn, as turnyng vp
of þe brayn and scotomy. Oþer sekenesses ben of humours

10   þat ben y-turned to postemes in sum parti of þe brayn,
as frenesy þat is a postem of coler in þe foreparty of
þe brayn; and woodnes and leesing of mannes wit and
of reson þat is a postem in þe myddel of þe brayn; and
litarg[i]e þat is leuyng of mannes mynde þat makeþ

15   him for3eful and is a postem in þe hyndir party of
a mannes hede; and epilencie þat comeþ of an humour
þat filleþ þe partis of a mannes brayn þat shulde
be voyde of suche humours, and makeþ a man for þe
tyme to leesen his wit and his meving.   And he

f. 52v   20   lieþ stil as þoughe he were / deed.   Anoþir yvel
is callid appoplixie, þat comeþ of humours þat

[?]   stoppeþ þe poores of þe brayn, and makeþ a man to
leve his wit for þe tyme and al maner meving, saaf
oonly breþing. Þat is þe difference bitwixte it and

---

5 **And**] *prec. by* and drinke it *canc. in red.* **vppon**] *prec. by* on þe
canc. in red. 6 *2-line initial in blue.* 12 **brayn**] *prec. by* hede *canc. in*
red. 14 **litargie**] litarge. **þat (2)**] *prec. by* and *canc. in red.* 22 **a man**]
in l. h. margin.

epilencie.

Scotomye is suche a sekenes of þe brayn, þat it makeþ a man to seme þat he seeþ flies or blacke þingis in þe eyer. Turnyng of þe brayn makeþ a man semen þat al-þinge þat he seeþ as it semeþ to dronken men: þat þe house goeþ aboute hem and þat þe weie riseþ vp a3enst hem. And þis sekenes comeþ of þe stomakes greuaunce, eiþir of smokes, eiþir of humours þat ben aboute þe brayn. And if it be of þe stomake, þes ben þe tokenes: Þe herte lepiþ and haþ grete greuaunce. And aftir mete, þe greuaunce takiþ a man. And when þey bowen hem doun, her brayn tur/neþ, þat is to seie, hem semeþ þat þo þingis þat lien stille rennen aboute. But if þis sikenes come of blode, þese ben þe tokenes: His temples mouen faste; hevynes of his browes; and moche þou3t of rede þingis, as of brenyng of laumpes; and bleding of þe nose; þycke vryn and rede, and derke above as blode.

Of coler, þes ben þe tokenes: bitternes of mooþ, gnawing at þe herte, þyn vryn and ful rede and ful derke above.

Of malencolie, þes ben þe tokenes: sournes of mouþe, and 3elewenes of þe vryn and þinship, and wiþholding of fluxes.

Of flevme, þes ben þe tokenes: greuaunce aftir

8

The
tokenes
of
flevme

f. 53v

[99v]

Cure of
þe
greuaunce
of þe
stomake

[99]
When
is
profitable
to lete
blode

f. 54

[99v]

Pillules
þat purgen
þe hede

mete, and ache of þe sidis, and meeting of watres, and
of reynes, and of white þingis, and vnstablenes of þou3t.
And if þe greuaunce come of þe sto/make, it lasteþ þe
whiles þe smoke comeþ from þe stomak to þe hede, and
5 aftirwarde it cesiþ.   And þer is ache, and greuaunce,
and abhominacion in þe mouþe.   And a man may feele hou
þe smoke goeþ vp into þe heed.   And þe helpe þerof is
to caste or to spue.   And grete boistous metis þat wole
not be defied li3tly, þou shalt not ete.   And leve late
10 soopers.   And grete metis, and cavl-wortis, and strong
ale, and benes, and peesen, ete þou not.   But vse þou
suche metis þat wolen eesely be defied.

If þe greuaunce comeþ of blode, leting of blode is
profitable on þe heed veyne, and so it is in euery sikenes
15 of þe hede þat comeþ of blood.   If it is so þat he þat
is sike be replet of blood or of ony oþer humour, let him
dieten him as it seide of þe hede-ache. / And let him
vse þes pillules þat purgen þe heed of yuel humours,
and also þei ben good for þe si3te and for þe hering.
20 Thus þei ben made: Take of alloes þat is wel wasshen,
oz. ii; of mirabolani, ana kebulis, indorum; reubarbe,
mastike, wormod, roses, violet, sene, agarike, cuscute,
of eueriche ylyche moche, dr. i.   Tempere al þis with
þe iuys of fenel.   And if þou wilt make it sharpe, caste

þerto dr. vi & 1/2 of scamonie y-poudrid. And make þerof
gobettis of þe gretnesse of a fygge and ȝyue of hem xi or
xiii at oo tyme, for þei ben ful laxatif. And if þou
wilt purge him of coler, double or treble mirabolani. And

5   if it be for flevme, double kebulis and agarike. And
if it be for malencoly, double ynde and sene. Þat þing
þat purgeþ coler, purgeþ blode. / A profitable salt and
a þing þat purgeþ alle humours of a mannes hede, and
it is gode for akyng of ioyntis, and for þe potagre, and

10   for þe dropesy, and is þus made: Take of salt armoniac,
of cost, xii oz.; of blacke pepir, oz. v; of comyn, of
gynger, of white pepir, of fenel, of canel, of eueriche
yliche moche, dr. iii; of clowes, of zedwale, of galengal,
of quibibis, of cardamomum, yliche moche, dr. iii; of

15   ysope, of tyme, of origanum, of carewey, of anees, of
marche, of parsil, of louage, ana (of eueriche), oz.
1 & 1/2. Make of al þes a poudir and vse it instede of
salt with þi metis. And if þou wilt make it a laxatif,
caste þerto dr. ii of scamonie and drinke it with meþe.

20   Anoþir good salt þat purgeþ þe hede, and bynemeþ þe
derkenes of þe yȝen, and it doeþ awey þe ache of þe ȝeeris,
and / is good for þe palesy: Take of salt armoniake,
oz. vi; of diagredii and euforbie, oz. i; of pepir, gynger,
comyn, fenel, anees, marche, ameos, lovage, cardamomum,

[?]
f. 54v
[100]

A
profitable
salt for
þe hede

Anoþir
maner
salt for
þe siȝt
f. 55

6 be] *ins. above.* **8 alle]** *prec. by* coler *canc. in red.* **9 is]** it. **10
armoniac]** *corr. from* armonac. **14 cardamomum]** *corr. from* car-
donoum. **15 ysope]** *prec. by* clowes *canc. in red.* **19 with]** *in r. h.
margin.* **22 is]** it.

Scotomye

parseli, of eueriche, oz. i. And make poudir of hem
and 3eue þe seke þerof on morwetide dr. iii with wyne
or with meþe.

A
purgacion
for
delicat
men

And if þou wilt make delicat purgacions for hem
5 þat ben norisshid in delitis, make hem in forme of watir
and 3eve hem to drinke. Take an herbe þat is callid
elleborus niger, and squinantum, and esula, and seene,
and seþe hem in wiyn, and distille þat wyn into watir,
and vse þat to purge þe of malencoly.

Sugir
of
borage

10 Also sugir of borage is good in euery greuaunce
of malencoly, and it is made of borage floures like-wiys
as sugir roset is made of rooses. And oken apples soden

f. 55v

in wiyn / maken þe wiyn medicinable forto destroie corrupte
humours and smokes þat ben in a mannes hede.

Chapter I, Part 3
Frenzy

þe
frenesy

15 Frenesy is a brenyng postem in þe foreparty of a
mannes brayn or in þe skynnes of þe brayn. And sum postem
is of corrupte blode, and sum of corrupt colere, and sum

[100v]

of boþe togedir. Comen signes þat folowen þis sikenes
is: moche waking, and lacking of good witt, wreeþ and
20 wodenes, and sodeyn risinggis vp, and sodeyn fallinggis
dovne.

þe
tokenes
of coler

But if it is of colere, þese ben þe tokenes: grete
wille to fi3te and to smyte, drines of þe mouþe, blacknes
of þe tonge, myche sharpe and bitter ache, and moche

2 and 3eue . . . morwetide] *in r. h. margin.* dr. iii] *prec. by and
take þerof at oo tyme canc. in red.* 11 is] *ins. above.* 15 *2-line initial
in blue.* 20 sodeyn (1 and 2)] *corr. from* soden.

stering of þe hert.   And his pisse is swarte rede and his yȝen ben swollen.

f. 56
    But þe tokenes of blood / is a clene colour of þe visage.   Þei lacken hir wit and þreten men and mysseien

5 hem.   And þei ben aboute to pullen oute strees and stickis of þe wowes.   But if it be not a very frenesy but is

Tokenes of
frenesi
and þe
cause
þerof
comen of sum oþer postem, as of þe stomake or of þe breest, þen þese ben þe tokenes: a grete pouse, and a swifte, and a þick; and þe vrin is white and þinne.   Þe cause

10 þerof is, for þe hote colerik mater þat shulde make þe vryn reed and shulde com donward with þe vryn, and it passeþ vpward into þe heed and þat makeþ a man frentike. And þis sikenes oþirwhiles is a sikenes bi himselfen, oþirwhiles it foloweþ annoþir sikenes.   If it is a sikenes

f. 56v

[102]
15 bi himsilf, it may / be þus y-holpen.   First lett him rubbe softly þe soles of his fete with vynegre and wiyn

Cures
and
remedi
for þe
frenesi
and salte.   And if he mowen not wel take a purgacion for his heed, make a clistre in þis wise: Take þe hocke and þe holy-hock, waxe, cene, fenel, salt, and mercury,

20 and seeþ al þes in watir.   And aftir þey ben soden, streyne hem and put to hem hony and oyle.   And let þe seke resceyve it by his fundement.   Aftirward shaue his heed and leie þerto a warme plastir of coolde herbis to dryue awey þe smoke þat comeþ to þe brayn.   Aftir þis is doon, if

6 wowes] *followed by* and þei lacken her wit and þreten men and missein hem *in r. h. margin.* **7 postem**] *followed by* of þat skynne þat a childe þat a childe is conceyvid yn *canc. in red.* **11 and it**] *ins. above.* **22 shaue**] *in l. h. margin.* **his** (2)] *prec. by* let wasshe *canc. in red.*

f. 57

A plastir
for þe
frenesy

Cures for
þe frenesi

f. 57v

[102v]

it nedeþ, take a ʒonge whelpe and slit him a-two. And
caste awei þe guttis and ley it al hoot to þe fore-hede.
And when he is coolde, ley to anoþir, for þe moo þat
þou ley to, þe bettir it is. But / if þou hast but oon,
5 when he is coolde, put hote watir in him and ley him to
eftsones. Aftirward take oz. i of popilion, and dr. i of
opium, and dr. ii of henbane, and dr. iii of blacke popi.
And poudir hem and medle hem with popilion, and with
þe mylke of a woman þat fedeþ a meide childe, and with
10 þe iuse of syngreen. And make þerof a plastir and ley
it warme on þe heed nyʒe his foreheed. And if his sleep
a-swagid his foly, it is a good token. And ellis, it
is yuel. And wasshe his heed with þe iuse of marche
and with vynegre, or with oyle of roses, or with þe iuse
15 of solatre, or with iuse of marche and oile of rooses.
And let him kepe cilence and speke not. And lete him
be let blode in þe v[e]yne þat is in þe myddil of þe
foreheed. And let him streyne his neck / þe while with
a towal. And if he blede not ynowe, take a watir leche
20 and kit of his taile, and do him in þe myddil of his
foreheed above þe nose or on þe templis bisidis þe yʒen.
And let him soke oute þe blood til he haue sokid as moche
as a blode-letting is. And if he is not holpe bi al þis
doyng, take þe iuse of letuse and of portulake, and medle

---

1 ʒonge whelpe] *marked for reversal.* **2 fore-hede]** ſoore-hede. **9
a (1)]** *ins. above.* **10 syngreen]** *corr. from* synegreen. **13 þe]** *ins.
above.* **17 veyne]** vyne. **18 þe]** *prec. by* if þou hast but oon *canc. in
red.*

hem with oyle of rooses or of violet, and a dramme and
an half of opium. And anoynte þerwiþ his templis and his
forheed. And if litarg[i]e comeþ to a frentike man, it is
a token of deeþ. But if þe frenesi come to him þat haþ þe

5 litarg[i]e, it is a good token. And it is profitable to
strawe his house wiþ colde herbis and to make col/de
watir to renne ny3he his chambre. And in euery sikenes
if it be ful grevous in þe begynnyng, worche with stronge
medicyns. And if þe sikenes be easi, bigynne with esy

10 medicynes.

f. 58

Chapter I, Part 4
Mania

Mania is an-oþer sikenes of þe myddil party of þe
brayn and comeþ of a postem in þat parti. But oþirwhiles
it is a sikenes himsilf, and oþirwhiles it foloweþ anoþir
sikenes. And summe comeþ of blood, and sum of coler, and

15 sum of malencoly. But of clene flevme it comeþ neuermore,
for flevme is white as þe brayn is and þerfor it may not
appeiren it. And if it comeþ of blood, þe greuauce is with
lawghing. And if it be of coler, it is with a fers wode/-
nes. And if it be of malencoly, it is with moche drede.

20 And if it is of coler and malencoly medlid togedir, he
lawgheþ and fi3teþ togedir. And so if it is of oþer
humours, it haþ þe propirtees of þo humours. But comonly
þo þat han þis sikenes of malencoly, þei han moche sorowe,
and dreden myche of þing þat is not to drede, and þenken

f. 58v
Condiciones
malencoli

on þing þat is not to þenke on.   And hem semen þat þei seen dredeful þingis when þei seen no-þyng.   And hem semen þat þei seen blacke develis eiþir monkis þat shulden slee hem.   And sum wenen þat hevene wole falle dovne on hem

5 and sum þat þe erþe wole falle vndir hem.   And þei han myche desire aftir le/chis and aftir medicynes.   And when þei han hem, þei 3eue litil feieþ to hir wordes.   And þei desiren to be in derke placis and bi hemsilfen.   But þo þat han þis sikenes of blood loven to walke aboute

10 ryvers, and in þe feldis, and in fair gardens, and in li3t placis.   And þei loven compeny and myrþe.   And if hem lackiþ suche þing, hem semen þat þei ben ny3e deed.   But þo þat han it of coler loven wrastlyngis, and fi3tingis, and lepingis, and oþer dedes of hardynes, and crieng, and

15 myche noise, and suche oþir þingis.

   And if þis sekenes be of coler or of blood, it is y-holpen as þe frenesy eiþir þe heed-ache þat comeþ of heet. But if it is of malencoly, he muste leve / malencolious metis and vsen metis þat ben moiste, as fisshe, and ripe

20 fruytis, and borage, and suche oþer, and herbis þat ben inscisif, as calament, and herbis þat ben dissolutif, as fenel and parsily.   But he shal not euermore vse moiste metis, lest his blode be corrupte and his complexion appeirid be þerbi.   And þes erbis ben profitable for hem:

f. 59

Condiciones
sanguinei

[?]

Condiciones
colerici

f. 59v

[104v]

Be-ware of
continuel
vsyng of
moiste
metis in
þis sekenes

---

8 **desiren**] *corr. from* desire. **11 myrþe**] *prec. by* li3t *canc. in red.*
12 ben] *ins. above.* **17 þe** (2)] *in r. h. margin.* **24 be**] *ins. above.*

arage, letuse, spinage, betis, purslane, oynons, carses, carloke, anet, fenel, mynte, calament. And þes metis þat ben moiste ben profitable, as lambren, and kiddis of oon 3eer, and sooking beestis, and hennes, and chekenes,

5 and partriche, and suche oþer; also fisshes of ryvers smale and grete, and þe fyss[h]es þat ben not fat, ne fisshes of stony placis. And let him vse his metis y-di3t / wiþ gynger, and cardamomum, and saffron, and clowes, and coliandre, and carewei, and comyn. And let him blede

10 in þe necke-pitte. And comforte him with myrþe to do awei his heuynes. And if þei fomen at hir mouþ as a wode dogge þat were y-bete, it is a token of deeþ withyn vii dayes. And if he castiþ moche and volatiþ boþe mete and drinke, and þat litil þat he resceyueþ stondeþ him

15 but in litil profite, ne he may not suffre hete of þe sunne ne of þe fyer, ne he may not slepe but litil and lieþ doun-ri3t, þes ben þe tokenes of deeþ. And if he haue not þes signes, 3yue him pillules made of wiyn drastis and of whete flour whan he is fasting. Also take of anyse,

20 oz. i; of parsely, oz. iiii; of pepir, oz. iiii; of epityme / þat is þe flour of tyme, oz. iii; mel, quasi semis; and 3yue it him wiþ watir. And euery-þing þat is good for þe feuer quarteyn is good for þis sekenes. And in euery sekenes and lesing of a mannes witte, aftir his

f. 60

[105v]

The tokenes of deeþ

f. 60v

[106]

---

1 oynons] *corr. from* onyons. **6 fysshes]** fysses. **10 do]** *ins. above.*

What is to
be doon to
him þat
haþ lost
his wit
in þe
beginning
of his
passion

purgacion, let him be cuppid in þe two neþir sidis of þe

hede a litil aboue þe necke, eiþir bitwene þe two shuldir-

bladis.   And in euery lesyng of a mannes witte, make him a

clistre in þe begynnyng of mynte, and rwe, and suche

5   oþir þingis.   And it profiteþ to suche men to baþen hem

oþirwhiles, but to dwelle þerin a litil while.   And a

special medi/cyn for þis sikenes is lapis armenicus y-

3oven in pillulis eiþir in decoccions, y-wasshe eiþir

vnwasshe, but vnwasshe it wole make a man to caste.   And

10   if alle þese medicyns helpiþ him not, þe laste remedy is

to slitte þe skyn and open þe skulle.

Chapter I, Part 5
Lethargy

Litargye is a sekenes þat makeþ a man so for3eteful,

þat when he haþ do a þinge, he ne haþ no mynde þat he did

it.   And þis sekenes comeþ oþirwhiles of to moche corrupte

15   fleume in a mannes hede, oþirwhiles of a posteme þat is in

þe hyndir parte of a mannes hede þer-as his mynde is.

And if it be a postem, þes ben þe tokenes: a continuel

fever, myche sleep, for/3etefulnes.   When þei ben clepid,

vnneþe þei wolen answere.   And when her mouþ is opened,

20   vnneþe þei moun close it.   And þis sekenes is called

a coolde frenesy.   But if it comeþ of flevme, þes ben þe

tokens: His vryn is troble, is mere pisse.   His pouse is

soofte and greet; his sleep is deep and heuy; his breþing

is slowe and greuous.   If it comeþ of flevme and of coler

5 it] *corr. from* if it. **8 pillules**] *corr. from* pulleules. **12** *2-line initial in blue.* **13 ne haþ**] *in r. h. margin.* **16 þer-as**] *prec. by*
Eiþirwhiles *canc. in red.* **20 þei**] *ins. above.* **22 is (3)**] *corr. from* and.

Of
flevme
and of
coler

y-medlid togedir, þen þe tokens of hem ben y-medlid,
for his vryn is more rede and his pouse is swifter.
Tokenes of deeþ in þis sekenes ben 3elewenes of þe face,
and qwaking and tremblyng of a mannes body and of a mannes

5 face, and sweting of þe hede when þe body swetiþ not
byneþen. Also a watir le/che wole not cleuen on suche
a man to souken oute his blood.

f. 62
Tokenes
of deeþ

A
purgacion
for þe
litarg[i]e

A purgacion to purgen suche mannes heed: Take of
alloes, oz. i & dr. ii; of agarike, of sticados, of
10 eueriche, dr. iii; of mastike, spike, cassie, canel,
clowes, squinantum, gynger, of eueriche, dr. i & 1/2.
And make þerof pillulis of þe quantite of an ey and 3yue
him þerof at oones dr. iii with warme watir. And make
him to snese with castory, piretre, pipir, staphie, nygil,
15 and suche oþir. And let him chewe þe same þingis in
his mouþe. And make a plastir on þe mouþe of þe stomake

A plastir
for þe
litarg[i]e

of sum hote oyle, as oyle of rwe or suche oþir, and shepis
wolle þat was y-shore vnwasshed. And anoynte his heed
with oyle of rwe and with þis oynement: Take of euforbie,

f. 62v 20 piretre, sineuei, / affodille, castorie, long pipir,
of eueriche, oz. i. Seeþ hem in þe iuse of rwe and in

An
oynement
for þe
litarg[i]e
of þe heed

a good quantite of oyle til þe iuse be consumed. And
putte þerto a litil wexe and ley it on his hede warme.
Also oyle of castorie, and oyle of piretre, and oyle

3 **Tokenes**] *corr. from* Tokens. 6 **a**] *ins. above.* 9 **& dr. ii**] *in r. h.
margin.* 14 **nygil**] *corr. from* nigel. 18 **was**] *in r. h. margin.* 20
castorie] *corr. from* castore.

Anoþir
for þe
same

[108]

Anoþir
for þe
same

f. 63

of ellern ben good for þis sikenes. Anoþir for þe same:
Take of affodille, piretre, sineuei, of eueriche, oz.
i & dr. vii; of castorie, of euforbe, of eyþir, dr. vii.
Tempere hem with þe iuse of wormod and of sansuke. And
5 anoynte þerwiþ þin hede in þe hyndre parti. Anoþir for
þe same: Take clay þat is bake in an ouene and medle
it with þe iuse of rwe and of suche oþer hote erbis.
And ley it on þin hede. But if þe litarg[i]e be with a
feuer, it makeþ him boþe heuy of sleep and for/ȝeteful.
10 And þat feuer comeþ of a postem in þe hyndre parte of a
mannes hede. And þen þou shalt leye him in a liȝt place
þer-as he may beholde waking. And let him haue moche
talking and moche noyse aboute him to let him fro sleep.
And lette his dieting be with coolde, þat is to sey, not

The dieting
of hem þat
han
þe
litarg[i]e

15 to coolde. And let him vse colde sirupes, as of violet
or of roses, and sugir roset or sugir of violet. And
let him rubbe wel his feet and his handis with vynegre and
salte. And let him smelle oþirwhiles sum stinking þingis,

[108v]

as þe smoke of a qwenchid candel, or of a mannes heer y-
20 brent, or of hertis horne y-brent. And in noon litarg[i]e

Be war þat
þou f. 63v
lei no-þing
þat is
cold to þe
hed þat is
greued with
litarg[i]e

ley coold þingis on þe heed, but let / shaue þe heed
and anoynte it with þingis þat been temperat, as castorie
y-temperid with þe iuse of marche or of fenel.

A clistir to make þe mater nesshe and þe more able

8 **litargie**] litarge. **11 þen**] *in r. h. margin.* **15 coolde**] *ins. above.*
20 litargie] litarge. **21 let**] *followed by* þe *canc. in red.*

[108] to be y-clensid: Take betis, and hockis, and mercury,
and violettis,   and mallewis, ana; and seeþ hem wel in
watir.   And aftirward streyne it, and put þerto an handful
of whete branne, and lete it boile.   Þen strene it and put

5 þerto oyle of violet or oyle de olijf and a litil bottir.
And medle hem togedir and let þe seek resceyue of þis
licour at oo clistring þe wei3te of a poond. And if þou
wilt, seeþ þeryn hocke rootis, and femygreke, and lynseed.

A clistir mundificatif: Take wormod, and souþerenwode,
10 and calamynte, and origanum, and mynte, and mercury, and
seeþ hem in salte watir.   Þen streyne it and put þerto

whete branne.   And streyne it eeftsones and / put þerto dr.
iii of hony, and dr. ii of mete oyle, and dr. i of salt
gemme, and medle hem togedir.

15 A suppository for þe litarg[i]e: Take iiii sponeful
of hony and oon sponful of salte.   And when it waxiþ
harde, þen it is yno3w. Þen put it a-while in colde
watir and take it oute.   And make þe tentis and shape
hem aftir þe gretnes of þi litil fyngir, and put it in

20 his fundement.   Forto make suppositories esily to entre

yn: Anoynte hem with oyle or with bottir and þat shal
make hem slyder.

And vndirstonde þat clisters and supositories shullen
be 3oven to men þat ben costif and to hem þat han feble

2 **mallewis ana**] *ins. above.* **3-4 and put . . . strene it**] *in l. h.
margin.* **6 And medle . . . and let**] *in l. h. margin.* **14 and medle hem
togedir**] *in r. h. margin.* **15 litargie**] litarge. **Take**] *followed by* hony
and seeþ it til it be þicke *canc. in red.* **15-18 iiii . . . tentis**] *in r. h.
margin.* **22 make him slyder**] *copied as* hem slyder make *and marked
for reversal.*

delyverance byneþe. But clisters shulen be y-ȝouen to strong men of complexion, suppositories a man may take þouȝghe he be riȝt seke and feble. And men þat han þe litarg[i]e withoute feuer shullen be dietid with þingis

5 þat ben temperat, þat is, hot and moyste.

An electuarie þat restoriþ a man-is mynde and

f. 64v comforteþ his brayn and / al his body: Take of canel, roses, violet, gynger, cardamomum, of eueriche, oz. ii; of dragagantum, antos, bawme þat is an herbe, maioran,

10 þe rynde of myrtille, ciperi, liquoris, siler, of eueriche, oz. ii; of squinantum, spike, clowes, quibibis, folii, galange, auence, borage, sene, bean, spodie, coral, mastike, macropipir, storax, brent silke, of eueriche, oz.

[109] 1/2 & sc. i; of sirep of roses, quantum sufficit.

Chapter I, Part 6
Epilepsy

15 Epilencie is þe falling yvel, and it comeþ of a

Epilencie moyste humour þat fulfilliþ þilke placis of þe hede þat shullen be voyde, and stoppiþ þe hyndre parte of þe hede þer-as is þe begynnyng of þe sekenes, and febliþ þe senewis. And þerfor when þe accesse of þis sikenes comeþ to man,

f. 65 20 it makiþ him for a tyme to leese his felyng / and his mevyng. Oþirwhiles þis sikenes comeþ of humours þat ben

[109v] in þe hede, and þan it is clepid epilencie; and oþirwhiles

Analempsie of fumes þat comen into þe heed oute of his seeke and feble stomake, and þanne it is callid analempsie. And

---

1 **shulen be**] *corr. from* shulben. 4 **litargie**] litarge. 9 **antos**] *corr. from* anteos. 15 *2-line initial in blue.* 16 **fulfilliþ**] *prec. by* falliþ *canc. in red.* **þilke**] þicke. 18 **þe** (1)] *ins. above.* **febliþ**] *prec. by* it *canc. in red.* 20 **it**] *corr. from* and. **him**] *ins. above.*

Cathalempsie

[110]

f. 65v

[110v]

f. 66

oþirwhiles it comeþ of greuaunce of oþir membris, and
þanne is it callid cathalempsie.   But of epilencie þer
ben ii kyndes, þe more and þe lasse.   In þe more epilencie,
þe principal places of þe brayn ben al-togedir y-stoppid.

5   Wherefore in her accesse, þei felen no-þing, and þei
fomen at her mouþe, and al her bodi qwakiþ, and it is ful
harde to helen hem.   In þe lasse epilencie, þe principal
placis ben y-stoppid, but not al-/togedir, and þerfore
in her accesse þei felen sum-what, and al þe bodi ne

10   qwakiþ not, but þe hyndre parti of þe heed.   And in
epilencie, tremblyng of þe bodi is an yuel signe, but
in þe palesie it is a good signe.   Fomyng here is a good
signe, but in appoplexie it is an yvel signe.   And þe
ofter þat þei fallen dovn and risen vp soon aȝen, þe

15   bettir signe it is and þe raþir þei movn be y-heelid.
And if þe sekenes be of þe humours þat ben in þe heed,
þese ben þe tokenes: hevynes of þe heed and confusion
of her wittes, slouþe, dymnes of þe yȝen, bitinge of her
tunge, and her pisse, and her kynde, and her dritte passen

20   awey fro hem aȝenes her wille, and so þei fallen doun /
and mown feel no-þing, and namely in þe grettir epilencie.
And if þis sekenes be of flevme, þou maist knowe it by
þe tokenes of fleume, as by softenes, and whitnes, and
slouþe, and myche slepe.   And if it be of malencoly,

---

6 and (2)] *ins. above.* **17 of**] *corr. from* in. **19 her** (2)] *in l. h.*
margin.

þou maist knowe it by blackenes, and lennes, and oþer tokenes of malencoly.   If it be of hem boþe togedir, þe tokenes ben y-medlid togedir.

5 Analempsy comeþ of a fume or of a smoke of þe stomake [þat is] malencolike. The tokenes herof ben abhominacion to mete and to drinke, tremblyng of þe herte, pricking of þe stomake, and flevmatike metis and malencolious

metis doeþ hem harme. And oþirwhiles / þey fallen not, but ben ful feble aboute þe tyme of her acces. And þeir

10 sekenes may be of flevme, of coler, and of malencolye. Of whiche of hem it is, þou maist knowe by þe signes of þe humours.

Cathalmepsie comeþ of a venemous smoke þat comeþ from fer into þe heed and þer he is coolde. And þis

15 smoke comeþ of a blood þat is bri3te and brenyng in summe partie of a mannes body. And þerfore it makiþ a man ful hoot withouteforþe and to haue a swifte breþing. And it afraieþ ful moche his y3en and oftentymes makiþ him to sowne. And he haþ oþirwhiles a feuere þerwiþ. And

20 if he be callid in þe tyme of his acces, he 3eueþ noon

answere. And if he speke, it greueþ him soor. / And his y3en watren and ben ri3t soor and he haþ an hote swete in þe delyuerance of his axes. And his breþe stynkiþ oþirwhiles. And if eny of þes þre maneris fomen moche

---

2 of hem] *ins. above.* **5 þat is]** *or of.* Add 30338: of a fume oþer of smoke of þe stomak þat is fleumatyk oþer malencolyk. *L:* ex fumo flegmatico vel melancolico abundante in stomacho. **6 tremblyng]** *corr. from* teremblyng. **9 þeir]** *prec. by 1 canc. in red.* **18 his]** *corr. from* her. **him]** *corr. from* hem. **20 he (1)]** *prec. by* þey *canc. in red.* **22 swete]** soot *in r. h. margin with dots indicating it should replace* swete, *which is not canc.*

Nota bene
diversitate
infirmorum

white fome when þei ben y-fallen a-dovne, and streynen her
teeþ togedir, þen it is of flevme.   And if he closiþ
his y3en as þoughe he slepte and fomeþ no-þing, but ariseþ
vp soone, þen it is of coler.   But if he wexiþ blacke,

5   and turneþ asidis his mouþ, and streyneþ his handis togedir,
and lieþ stille as þoughe he were deed, and fomeþ but
litil, þen it is of malencoly.

[111]

Men þat han epilencie or analempsie shullen be dietid
with metis þat ben temperat coolde.   And þes metis ben

Hou he þat
is in
þis   f. 67v
sekenes
shuld
be
dietid

10   good for hem: hennes, feisantis, and partriches, and
suche / oþer, and shalid fisshe, and also borage, and
parsely, and fenel, and good clere wiyn of Gasqwyn, but if
it be for hem þat han cathalempsie.   And let hem absteyne
hem fro malencoolies metis, as beef and al maner of caul-

15   wortis, fro benes and peses, and mylke and oþir white
metis, and fro betis, and marche, and oþir salt metis,
and also fro rostid or fried, and from watir foules,
and fysshes of myry watris, and from hertis fleisshe,
and shepes fleisshe, and swynes fleisshe, and from notis

20   and applis, and barliche brede and rye bred, and from
baþing, and cumpanye of wymen, and from wreeþ and crieng.

And 3yue him þat haþ þis sekenes oximel squillitike,
or oximel of radiche, or þis oximel þat now foloweþ to
defie þe mater of his sekenes: Take þe seedis of pyonye,

17 fro] *ins. above.* **22 þis]** *in l. h. margin.*

24

The Epilencie

and sauge, wormod, nete/les, horehone, lauendre, auence, carses, and seen. Make of þes oximel likewise as þou makist þes oþir oximellis. And put to þis oximel þe seedis þat breken þe stoon. But to hem þat han cathalempsie,

5 put borage, and ypericon, and cuscute, and epithyme.

An-oþer oximel for þis sikenes

An-oþer oximel: Take þe poudir of euforbe, and staphie, and peretre, and puliol, and suche oþir, and seeþ hem in vynegre and wiyn. And aftir make vp þin oximel.

10 Aftir al þis, ȝyue him a purgacion: Take alloes, þe wilde gorde þat is clepid in Latin collaquindida, bdellie, opoponac, eleborus niger, gumme arabike, of eueriche, oz. ii; of euforbe, oz. 1/2. Make of þes pillulis with þe iuse of horehovne. Also lapis armenicus

15 is good for him þat haþ þis sekenes. And aftir foure daies, let him blede at þe hede veyne. And if he haue

f. 68v

moche blode, let / him be garsid and y-cuppid in þe necke.

A good pocion: Take a porcion of sauge, of pyony in

A pocion

20 lasse quantite þen of sauge, of castorye lesse þen of piony, of antimonye lesse þen of castorie.

Anoþir: Take opoponac, castore, sandragun, antimonie, of eueriche yliche moche, and ȝyue þe seke in what maner þou wilt.

19 good pocion] *marked for reversal.*

The Epilence

Special þingis for þis sikenes ben, crowes eiren
y-eten, antimonie, piony, and ysope y-ete or y-dronke.
For children: Piony and ysope ben beste herbis, to hange
pyony aboute þeir neckis, and to ȝeue hem ysope to ete or
5 to drinke.

For þe falling yuel

[112]   Whan a man is fallen doune by þe falling yvel, sle
a dogge and ȝeue him þe galle to drinke. And he shal
[111v]   not falle nomore of þis sekenes. And let him bere rwe
alwey in his honde and oftentymes smelle þerto. Anoþer:
f. 69   10   ȝy/ue him in drinke antimonye, castorie, olibanum,
[112v]   houndistonge, fenel root, of eueriche yliche moche.
[113]   Anoþir, when he falliþ dovne, ȝeve him to drinke of
valerian, of sanicle and of rwe, and he shal neuer haue it
more.

A sirip for þis sikenes

15   A sirup for þis sekenes: Take þe seed of pyony, and
[112v]   sage, wormod, nettelis, and horehoune, and seeþ hem in

Hou þe iuse of herbis shal be clariefied

wiyn. Or ellis clarifie þe iuse and wiyn y-medlid togedir
with þe white and þe shellis of eggis ouer an esy fier.
And aftir it is clensid, ȝyue him to drinke. Thus þou
20   shalt clarifie al maner iuse of herbis, with þe white and
shellis of eggis. And if þe seke be costif, ȝyue him of
watir of a clisterie þat centorie, and anet, and camemyl,
and mellilot ben y-soden yn, or make him a biting
f. 69v   suppository. / An oynement for þis sekenes, and if a man

11 houndistonge] houndistoinge. **22 watir]** *prec. by* þe *underd.*

haue þe epilencie, þou shalt anoynte his rigge-boon; and
if it be analempsie, þou shalt anoynte his wombe before þe
stomake; and if it be catalempsie, þou shalt anoynte þe
membre fro whom þe sekenes comeþ: Take of castore, oz. ii;
5 of piretre, of oyle de bay, of staphyne, of euforbe, of
eueriche of þes, oz. i & 1/2; of syneuey, nytre, pepir, of
eueriche, oz. i; of oyle and waxe, quantum sufficit.

[112]

Anoþer onement: Take hondistonge, planteyn, betes,
souffri watir þat brymston is medled wiþ, as watir of
10 hoot baþes or oþir watir þat begynneþ to seþe, and put in
þis watir fenel, louage, sisymbre, violet, centrum-galli,
sage, and oold sowes grees, and lete it seþe a good while.
Aftir it is wel y-soden, gader al þat þat hoveþ aboue /
þe watir and anoynte him þerwiþ. And vndirstond þat

15 bitter medicynes been good for þe heed and for þe stomake,
and speciali þo þat han myche of alloes. Also let hem
þat han þe epilencie ete bytymes, for fasting is yuel for
[113]
hem, and loking in glas, and yuel smellis and stinkes, but
if it be of rwe, or castore, or amoni, or of antymony.
20 And loking on gith y-poudrid wole make hem falle doun
anoon. But to loke on gite hool doeþ hem good, and it
wole make hem to rise vp soon. But to hem þat [han]
analempsie, it is good to faste, if [her he]dis be not
feble. It is good f[or hem þat] han epilencie to be let

5 piretre] *corr. from* peretre. **22** *Corner torn from f. 70. Bracketed
readings supplied from Add 30338 in the usual spelling of W.* **23 to**]
ins. above.

blood [on þe] veyne þat is bitwene þe þomb[e and þe fin]gir þat is nexte him.

f. 70v

An [oyle þat dis]solueþ coolde humour[s and wastiþ] / hem is þus made: Take a povnd of lorel leves, of Englisshe

5   rwebarbe, and lauriole, ana, libra i, and stampe hem and þen seþe hem in a povnd of wiyn and in a povnd of oyle.

[113v]   And seeþ hem so long, til þat þe wiyn be wastid.   In epilence, anoynte her hedes with þis oyle; in analempsie her stomake; in cathalempsie, þe place þat þe sekenes

10   comeþ fro.   And þis oyle is also good for aking of þe heed þat comeþ of coold, and for [þ]e palesye, and for þe crampe þat comeþ [of] plente of humours aboute þe senewis, and for cold govtis.

Chapter I, Part 7
Apoplexy

[114]   [A]poplexie is a sekenes þat com[eþ o]f stopping of

15   þe principal pla[cis þat b]en in a mannes brayn þrow [sum co]rrupte humour.   And þis [sikenes b]ynemeþ a mannes

f. 71   wit / and his felyng for þe tyme and al maner meving wiþouteforþe, saaf only breþing.   Ther ben þre kyndes of

Ther ben þre maners of appoplexis

þis sikenes, a more, and a lasse, and a mene bitwene hem

20   two.   The more sleeþ a man þe first day, for it is incurable.   The meen sleeþ a man withyn þre daies, or ellis turneþ into a palesie; þe lasse withyn vii daies, or turneþ

[114v]   into palasie.   And þis sikenes comeþ of moche flevme or of moche corrup blode þat filliþ þe principal places of a

9 þe (1)] *prec. by* he *canc. in red.*

mannes brayn. And if it be in so grete plente þat it
filliþ al þe brayn, þen it makeþ a man to leese his wittis,
as his sy3te, his hering, his tasting, his smelling, and
his meving also. Þis is þe more apoplexie. But if þe

f. 71v   5   humour stoppe not but þe hyn/dre place of þe brayn þer-as
þe senewes han her begynnyng, þan it bynemeþ not a mannes
wittis, but his meving. And þis is þe lasse apoplexie. Þe
meen is þe more violent þen is þis, but not so violent
as þe grete. And þis sikenes falliþ to fleumatike men,

  10   or to men þat han to moche blode, and lyven in moche ease,
and eten moche, and drinken moche, and waisshen moche, and
kemben moche her heed. And þis sikenes is y-knowe by
certeyn signes as oþir sikenessis ben, as by heuynes of þe
heed, and stronge breþing, and aking of þe heed withouten

  15   eny encheson or cause, a feuer, slouþe, turnyng of þe
brayn, deerkenes of si3t. And if it is of blood, þe face
is rody, and pale if it is of fleume. Þe face is 3elow or

f. 72   blacke if it is of malencoly. / And mysturnyng of þe face,
also falling dovne to grounde, is a grete token. But þat

  20   comeþ in epilencie and in sekenes of þe herte þat is

[115]   callid syncopis. But þoughe falling a-doun be a token of
al þes sekenessis, it is not in oon maner in hem alle.
For in apoplexie, a man wexiþ reed when he is y-falle.
And his veynes swellen aboute his templis and his y3en,

---

    13 sikenessis] *corr. from* sikessis. **19 grounde**] *prec. by* þe *canc. in*
red. **21 of**] *corr. from* in.

and þoughe his y3en ben open, he seeþ no-þing. And he
fomeþ at his mouþe, but þat is a token of deeþ. And his
axes dureþ longe, as a day or two. In epilencie, summe
partis of þe man han þe crampe and is y-turned aside.

5 And his body trembliþ and qwakeþ, and oþirwhiles he
fomeþ, and þat is a good token, and þat his axes is ny3e
doon. Falling of syncopis is wiþ discoleryng of þe face.
And he lyeþ as þoughe he were deed, withouten crampe and

f. 72v with/outen tremblyng and fomyng also. And soon he riseþ
10 vp. Apoplexie þat comeþ in þe waxyng of [þe] moone is
incurable, and namely if it be þe more apoplexi. But if it
comeþ in þe wanyng of þe moone, it is not so greuous. And
if he desireþ diuerse metis, and as soon as he seeþ hem, he
haþ abhominacion of hem, it betokeneþ deeþ. And if he
15 haþe not suche tokenes, he may be y-holpen by medicynes.
And if it be of blode, let hem blede in þe heed veyne
of þe arme, if he be of stronge complexion. And þat
is a souereigne remedy in eche apoplexie, of what humour
þat it be. If þe body be ful of humoures and if it be
20 of eny oþir humour þan of blode, let his body be purgid

Pillulis
for þis
sikenes
f. 73
wiþ stronge medicynes, as with iera [a]logodion, or
iera pigra, or theodo/ricon, or stomaticon, or with
þes pillules if it be of fleume or malencoly: Take
of alloes and of euforbe yliche moche, and medle hem

---

5 **trembliþ**] *corr. from* tremblid. **6 þat** (2)] *ins. above.* **8 he** (1)]
ins. above. **were**] *prec. by* as *canc. in red.* **he** (2)] *ins. above in error.*
10 of] *prec. by* in þe *canc. in red.* **of þe**] of. **21 alogodion**] logodion.

with þe iuse of like. And make of hem pillulis and 3yve
þe seeke. And if he be feble þat he may not be let blode,
ne haue siche stronge purgacion, let his hede be shaue.

[115v]

And make a plastir of syneuei and of vynegre, and medle

5 þerwith castor and euforbe, and ley it on his heed.

A plastir
for þe
same

Anoþir good plastir: Take femygreke and whete
bran, and seþe hem in a litil wiyn. Also let þe heed
be anoyntid with hote oynementis y-made of euforbe, castor,
piretre; or þe iuse of marche and euforbe y-medlyd togedir;

10 or þe iuse of rwe, of carses, and of sauge y-medlyd with

f. 73v

þe oþer. / And if þe greuaunce falle doun in þe chyne,
let him be anoyntid with þe same oynementis vppon þe
cheyne. And þen let him be waisshid with þe watir þat
camemyl, mellilot, anet, sansuke, ben y-soden yn.   And

15 make a plastir of þe iuse of centory, and of netles,
and of saalt, and ley to þe hyndre party of þe heed.
And if he be costiffe, make him a clistir þat is sharpe
and biting, of hocke leeues and betes soden in watir.
And put hony and oyle þerto. And let his fondement be

20 anoyntid with bolles galle. Or make him a suppository of
nytre, dr. ii; of castor, dr. 1/2; of scamone, and hony
þat sufficeþ þerto. Or make a suppository of white sope
þat is harde, and anoynte it with bolles galle and with

[?]

salte.   Blacke soope and white soop ben good for brenyng

---

8 oynementis] *corr. from* onynementis. **18 and betes soden in
watir]** *copied* soden in watir and betes *and marked for reversal.* **19
put]** *ins. above.*

The propirte
and werking
of blacke
soop and
also of
white

[115v]

f. 74v
[123v]

/ or scalding, so þat it lye þer-vppon þre or iiii houres
anoon aftir þe hurting. And þei also ben good for scabbis
and forto opene þe pooris of þe skynne, and it makiþ þe
skynne white.

5 Also in worching of þis sekenes and of alle oþer,
begynne with esy medicyns and aftirwarde with strengir.
And when he greneþ, put a wegge bitwene his teeþ to holde
his mooþe open. And robbe his mooþ with tostid brede
þat is y-wette in þe iuse of myntis. And make him to
10 smelle to a gootis horne þat is y-brent. But alle þes
medycyns shullen be doon in þe lasse apoplexie and not
in þe more, for þat is incurable. And þei muste be dietid
with hoot metis and drinkis. And in passing awey of þis
sikenes, good wyn is good for hem. And vndirstonde /
15 þat a feuer is profitable in þis sikenes, and in þe palesy
also, and þe crampe þat is in replecion of blode. And
þou maist make þat in þis wise: Ley þe seke man bitvixte
two good fyres and ȝyue him to drinke good stale ale.
And let him ete garlike a good quantite and aftirward
20 drinke a gode drauȝte of stronge and fresshe wiyn, so
þat it be warmed. And put þeryn a gode quantite of pepir.
And anoynte al his body with oyle de bay or of lorer
leves, and speciali vndir his arme-pittis and on his
reynes.

18 **him to drinke**] *in l. h. margin.*

Chapter II, The Eyes
Part 1, Ache of the Eyes

Nowe begynneþ þe seconde chaptir of þis boke whiche is deuidid into viii practi[s]es or tretes. Capitulum primum:

[130v]

In a mannes y3en þer fallen meny sikenessis and

5 greuaunces. Sum comen fro wiþynneforþe and sum fro

f. 75 withouten. Fro / wiþynforþe comen greuaunce, ache, myche rennyng of watir, a postem in þe whiyt of þe y3e þat is clepid obtolmye, webbis and cloþes also þat goiþ ouer þe i3e and letteþ a man to see, and hardnes of þe i3e,

10 and cankir of þe i3e. Fro withoute, þe i3en ben y-greued by loking of þe sunne or on a ful-whiyt þing, also by smoke, duste þat falliþ into a mannes i3en, bi wynde, and suche oþer þingis.

Ache of þe i3en comeþ oþerwhiles of smoke or of

15 poudir þat noieþ þe i3en, and oþirwhiles it comeþ of humours þat fallen doun into þe i3en, as of blode, of coler, of fleume, or of malencoly. And if it be of blood,

[131] þes ben þe tokenes: reednes of þe i3en, and hete, and swelling, with moche heuynes boþe of þe i3en and also

20 of þe forehede. And also þe i3en ben moyste and weping.

f. 75v And whan þe liddes ben y-closid, þei felen mo/che sharpenes wiþynforþe, as þoughe þer were grauel in her y3en. And her face is ful of blode.

Of coler, þes ben þe tokenes: redenes of þe y3en

---

2 **viii**] *corr. from* sixe. **practises**] practies. 4 *6-line initial in gold.*

þat is not a cleer redenes as is þat þat comeþ of blode, but a maner brovn-rede. And þei · ben hote and smerting: grete ache and greuaunce wiþouten swelling of þe i3en. But if it be of flevme, þer is more swelling and lasse

5 ache. And þe watir þat flowiþ on ny3tis-tyme fro þe y3en is viscouse as bridlym, and makeþ hem sumwhat blere-y3ed. And her y3eliddis cleuen togedir, and þei felen moche heuynes and greuaunce in her y3en. And if þe ache comeþ of malencoly, þe i3en swellen but litil, ne þei

10 ben not ful hoot ne ful rede. And þe humour þat comeþ fro hem waxit / harde and is of mene colour, not ri3t white ne ri3t brovn. Oþirwhiles þe ache of þe i3en comeþ of þe browis and of sum humour þat is in hem. Of what humour þat it is, þou maist knowe bi þes foreseide tokenes.

15 Also ache of þe y3en comeþ oþirwhiles from þe stomake. And þe ache is grettir aftir mete þen bifore. And if it comeþ of colde humours þat ben in þe stomake, let him caste and brake aftir mete. And vse purgacions þat serven to þe humour þat makiþ þe ache. And oþirwhiles þe

20 greuaunce of þe i3en comeþ of rewme of þe hede. Þan hele þe hede of þat rewme and þe y3en shal be hool.

And forto auoide þis rewme, pillules of diacastor ben good and ben þus y-made: Take of castor, of mirabolani, of eche of hem, / dr. iii; of muske, a greyn

f. 76

[119]

f. 76v

---

1 not] *ins. above.* **8 and greuaunce]** *in l. h. margin.*

and an halfe; of alloes, dr. i; of ase, myrre, euforbe,
of eche, dr. i and xviii greynes; of folii, antimonie,
piretre, liquoris, dragagant, calamus aromaticus, nitrum,
galbanum, squinantum, spike, opopinac, reupont, serapionis,

5 storacis, galengal, ginger, canel, of eueriche, dr. i;
and of greynes, staphine, dauke, fenel, parseli, marche,
siler mounteyn, petrolei, sange-dragon, encense, cardamomi
boþe of þe more and of þe lasse, agarike, mastike, sal
armoniac, zedoare, anisi, of eche of þes, sc. i and ix

10 greynes; of saturey, ysop, camedreos, pileol mounteyn,
origanum, bawme, ozimi, beetis, ditteny, rewe, aristologia
boþe þe longe and þe rovnde, aaron, macematicon, asari,
bdellie, of eche, xviii greynes; epityme, polipodium, /

f. 77 opobalsamum, of eche, xviii greynes; of alipiados,

15 caperis, of eche, xi greynes; of anacardi, sauyn, gencian,
of þe ryndes of mandrake, of eche, xi greynes; of
peusadanum, wormod, of eche, vii greynes; of yreos, xiii
greynes and þe þirde parte of halfe an handful. And
make herof pillulis of þe quantite of a notte. Þese

20 ben gode for þe greuaunce of þe hede, and for þe palesy,
and for þe lyuer, and þe splene, and þe reynes, and for
al colde sekenes. But for þe greuaunce of þe y3en þat
comeþ of rewme, þou shalt put of þes pillulis in wiyn
and put þat in þin noseþrillis. And take poudir of

---

7 **sange-dragon**] savge. dragon. **9 eche**] *prec. by* boþe *canc. in red.*
13 epityme, polipodium] opipolipum. *Other witnesses* epipolipum,
balsamum. *L:* epithymi, polipodii, opobalsami. **16 of** (3)] *ins.*
above.

[131]

f. 77v

piretre, and staphizagre, and mastik and chewe hem in
þi mooþ.   Or mylte hem with wexe and þen leie it on a
lynen / cloþe to þy forehede, for it dissolueþ þe flevme,
and drieþ þe brayn, and clereþ þe si3te.   And anoynte

5 þe forehede with oile of lorer or of piliol, or ellis
make a serid clooþ, and of þe poudre of mastike, and
of olibanum, and citre, and wax y-put þerto and hony.
Or let hem blede on þe cop of þe nose.   Or let him baþe
him, or make a stwe with hoot herbis.   And make him suche

10 a purgacion as Y tolde in þe sekenes of þe hede.

But if þe ache of y3en be of blode, let him blede
at hede veyne of þe arme, or let him be cuppid or garsid
in þe necke-pitte, or bitwene þe two shuldris.   And if
it be of coler, 3yve him a colog[og]e, þat is to sey,

15 a medicyn þat may clense him and purge him of coler,

f. 78

as mirabolani citri, / or oximel y-made with colde herbis,
or an electuarie made with þe iuse of roses and oþir
colde þingis, or pillulis þat ben y-made of þe fyue kyndes
of mirabolani.   And aftir his purgacion, ley þe medicyns

20 to his y3en.

Dieting of suche men shal be as of men þat han þe
feuer tercian.   And let hem absteyne hem fro wiyn and
al fried metis, and rostid metis, and salt metis, and
biting metis, and soure metis.   And let hem be in derke

---

2 a] *ins. above.* **9 him** (2)] *ins. above.* **11 y3en]** *prec. by* hede
canc. in red. **14 him]** *ins. above.* **cologoge]** cologe. **21 men** (2)] *ins.*
above. **22 feuer]** *ins. above.*

placis.   And whan þei slepen, let þeir hedis lye hi3e.
And her metes muste be suche þat may be li3tli defied,
and her drinke smale, þat is, stale and clere, or as

[131v]   smale as watir.

5   Special medicyns for ache of y3en þat comeþ of
f. 78v   hete, as of blode þat is / hote and moyst, or of coler
þat is hote and drye, þei muste be colde forto be
mytigat[i]ues, þat is to sey, to aswage þe violence of
þe ache.   And þey must be colde to be repercussyues,
10   þat is to sey, to smyten a3en fro þe y3e þe humour þat
is cause of þe ache.   And þes two kyndes of colde medicyns
han þei, þat ben, mytigatiues and repercussiues.   But Y
wole not þat þou vse alwei mytiga[ti]ues and repercussiues,
but oþirwhile dissolutiues, þat is to sey, hote medicyns
15   þat mowen dissolue þe mater of þe sekenes ri3t as þe
hete of þe sunne dissolueþ yis or snowe into watir.   Ne
Y wole not þat þou vse euermore dissolutiues, but
oþirwhilis confortatives to comforte þe y3e, for if hote
medicyns eiþir to colde weren y-leide to þe y3e
f. 79   20   contynueliche, þei shulde hurte / þe y3e as moche as þe
ache doiþ.   And so it fareþ of eueriche ache where-þat-
euer it be in a mannes bodi.   And þerfore in þe begynnyng
of þe ache, þou shalt 3eue confortatiues to comforte
þe membre þat akiþ, for but if þe membre be stronge forto

---

7 **be** (1)] *ins. above.* **forto be**] *in r. h. margin.* **8 mytigatiues**]
mytigatues; *prec. by* and *canc. in red.* **13 mytigatiues**] mytigaues. **16**
yis] ies *in l. h. margin with dots indicating it should replace* yis, *which*
is not canc. **snowe**] *prec. by* swo *canc. in red.* **17 þat**] *ins. above.*

worche himsilfe, þe strengþe of þe medicyn shal but litil
auaile: Þe medicyn is but an helper and þe principal
is þe membre þat is seke. And þerfore it nediþ to haue
confortatiues in þe begynnyng þat ben neiþir ful hote ne
5 ful colde. And in þe waxyng of þe sekenes and whan þe
sekenes is most greuous, let him vse medicyns þat ben
confortatiues and dissolutives y-medlid togedir. And in þe

passing / awey of þe sekenes, þou shalt vse dissolutiues.

But þou muste vndirstonde þat of þes medicyns, sum
10 ben symple and sum ben componed. Simple medicyns ben, as
of oon herbe by himsilf, or of oon watir þat is y-made
of oon herbe, or of hony, or of oyle de olif, or of oon
gumme, or of oon spicery by him-silf.

Componed medicens ben made of two þingis, or þre,
15 or of meny þingis y-medlid togederis. And of simple
medicyns, sum ben hote and dissolutiues, and sum ben colde
and mytigatiues and repercussiues. Of hote medicynes þat
ben dissolutiues, sum ben stronge dissolutiues and sum
ben feble dissolutiues.

20 Stronge dissolutiues ben, rede netil, rwe, celidon,
bawme þat is an onyment, / camfer, alloes, aumbir, þe
galle of eueriche beste, euery salt, and euery-þing þat
is ful corisiyf and freting. Þerfore suche stronge
dissolutiues muste be medlid with esy mytigatiues or

---

7 **dissolutives**] *corr. from* dissolatives. 15 **þingis**] *ins. above.*

repercussiues whan þe ache is bowing aweiward. Feble dissolutiues ben, þe 3olke of an egge, þe iuse of myntes, of basilicon, of sansuke, verueyn, endiue,

þe leues of madir, hote crommes of whete brede y-springid

5 with wyne or with rose watir; also þe iuse of fenel, of eufrace, of hayhoue, of licium, þe iuse of sloon, sarcacolle, acacia, muske, þe watir of a vyne, hony, þe blood of a coluir or of an hen or cheken, and lymail of golde. And whan þe ache stondiþ and neiþir waxiþ

10 ne abatiþ, suche muste / be y-medlid with esy repercussiues.

Repercussiues ben also sum ful stronge and sum ben feble. Stronge repercussiues ben y-clepid stupefacris, for þei a-stonyen a membre þoroughe her colde and so þei

15 make a membre to leese boþe his ache and his felyng. And for þeir greet violence, þou shalt not take hem in þe ache of y3en ne in noon oþer ache, but if þe ache be þe more violent and perlouse. And suche percussiues ben þe rynde of mandrake and þe fruyt þerof, and also

20 henbane, and morel, and orpyn, and popy sede, and nameli of þe blacke popi.

Feble repercussiues ben y-clepid mytigatiues, for þei aswagen þe ache and comforten þe membre. And suche ben womanes myl/ke and asse mylke, þe white of an ey,

---

6 hayhoue] *corr. from* hayue. **7 sarcacolle]** *corr. from* sayrcolle. **13 stupefacris]** *corr. from* stupefactis. **15 make]** *in l. h. margin.*

and oile of roses, and of violet, and lynsede. Þes ben
feble repercussiues; and portulake and þe iuse of solatre
and syngrene, þes ben stronge repercussiues.

[131v]   Of componed medicyns, þer ben many þat ben profitable
5   for þe ache of y3en þat comeþ of hete. Oon is þis: Take
watir of roses, and þe white of eggis, and womanes mylke,
and a litil white wiyn. And þerwiþ let him wasshe his
y3en. Anoþir: Seþe fenel rotis, and violet, and popi
sede in watir. And þerwiþ anoynte his y3en. And do
10   psillie in watir of roses and ley þat vppon his y3en
al ny3t in þe maner of a plastir. And ley þis plastir
on his templis: Take roses, anyse, and ceruse þat is
clepid blank plum and white lede, and sandragon, and /
f. 81v   gumme arabike, of eueriche yliche moche, and stampe hem,
15   and tempere hem with watir of roses and white of eggis
y-made into gleir. And leie þis on his forehede and on
his templis. And let it lye þer þre daies.

Anoþir plastir: Take þe iuse of violet, and þe
gleir of eggis, and watir of roses, and barly mele, and
20   make þerof a plastir, and ley on his y3en. Or take þe
iuse of syngreen, and womanes mylke, and þe whyit of an
egge, and þe iuse of endyve if þou wilt, or ellis þe watir
of roses, and medle hem togedir. And wete a cloute þeryn
and ley vppon his y3en.

1-2 þes ben feble repercussiues] *in r. h. margin.* **7-8 And þerwiþ
let him wasshe his y3en]** *copied* and let him þerwiþ wasshe *with
proper ordering indicated by the letters* a, b, c, d, e. **9 y3en]** *prec. by*
hede *canc. in red.*

The Y3en

Also in a grete ache of þe y3en, þou maist wasshe
hem with warme watir þat femygreke and mellilot ben y-
soden yn, if it is so þat þei flowen not, for if þei

f. 82   flowen, þei shalle / not be wasshen with warme watir.

5   But make a strictory and ley to his hede, of encense and
barly mele, or whete mele and gleyr of eggis.   But if
his body be ful moyst and his hede be replete with humours,
make him no strictory, but 3yue him a purgacion acording
to þe humours þat maken þe ache and þe flowing of þe y3en.

10   And whan þe flowing cesyþ or waxiþ lasse þen it was, þen
vse repercussiues and mytigatiues.   And if þe ache be ful
violent, þen vse not only colde þingis, but medle hem
with hote þingis so þat þe hote þingis mowen sumwhat
dissolue þe mater of þe ache, and þe colde þingis mowen

15   aswage þe violence of þe hete of þe ache.   And in þe
ende and in þe declinacion of þe ache, vse dissolutiues.

f. 82v   And whan þou / wilt wasshe a mannes y3en, if his greuaunce
encresiþ, leue it.   And ellis, continue it.   In a rotid
and in an olde greuaunce of þe y3en, it is profitable

20   forto be baþid in a hote baþþe, and aftirward forto drinke
a good drau3t of malmesyn or of sum oþir gode wiyn, and
aftir þat to take a good slepe and a soot.   Also þe iuse

[132v]   of chikenmete þat haþ a rede flour and þe iuse of grapes
þat ben not ripe ben gode.   And þe iuse of planteyn and

3 so] *ins. above.* **15 of þe ache]** *copied* and of þe hete ache *and*
corr. in red. **19 is]** *ins. above.* **21 or]** *ins. above.*

of verueyn y-medlid togedir ben also gode. And y-medlid
with þe gleyr of eggis, it is for ychyng of þe y3en and
forto do awei þe blode þat is in hem. And þe same doiþ
þe crummes of an hote loof y-spreynt with þe watir of
5 roses if þe ache is of hete, and if it is of colde, with
wyin. Also licium y-medlid with womanes mylke or with
white wiyn / and y-leide on þe y3en doiþ awei þe ache,
and þe ychyng, and þe blode. A plastir y-made of þe iuse
of radiche, and of nettil seed y-stampid, and carsede,
10 and mastike, and olibanum, and rye mele, if þey be plastrid
to þe forehede, shal not suffre noon hote humour flowe
at þe yen. And if þe y3en smerte and mowen not suffre
fyer ne li3te, take valerian, and marche, and planteyn,
and syngrene, of eueriche yliche moche, and take þe iuse
15 of hem and medle it with soure whete brede and make
þerof a plastir, not to harde ne to nesshe, and ley it
colde to his y3en. But ley a þynne cloute bitwene þe
plastir and his y3en, and in oon ny3t it shal hele him,
þoughe þe y3en be coverid with blode.

20 A collirie: Take of / amyde, ceruse, gumme arabike,
dragagantum, of eueriche, dr. iii; of opium, sc. i; and
tempere hem with þe white of eggis or with watir of roses.
And see þat alle þe poudris þat ben y-put in colliries
be y-beten as smale as it may ben, and aftirward y-bultid

f. 83

f. 83v
[132]
A collirye

[?]

11 not] *prec. by* d *canc. in red.*

The Y3en

þoroughe a smale lynen clooþ y-doblid or ellis bi a farcer,
for if it be but bostously y-bultid or farcid, þei shal
greue þe y3en. And wasshe þe yen with watir of roses,
or eufrace, or of fenel, or with malmesyn, or whijt wiyn,

5 or þou doo þy colleri into þe y3en. But if þe ache

[132v] of þe y3en come oþirwhiles of colde, as of flevme or
of malencoly, or ellis of þe pose, if it comeþ of þe
pose, hele þe pose as Y shal telle in þe chaptir of þe

f. 84 pose. And if it comeþ / of flevme, purge hit as Y tolde

10 in þe hede-ache and in oþir sikenessis of þe hede. And
if it be of malencoly, purge it. And aftirward let him
be stwid ouer a stewe fyue or seuen tymes, þat is made of
wormod, of betayn, of fenel, of sauge, of þe floris of
tyme, of camemil floures, of mellilot floures, of hockis,

15 and marche. Alle þes muste be soden in wiyn and watir
y-medlid togederis, þe toon halfe wiyn, and þe toþir
halfe watir. And let him holde his y3en and his hede
ouer þe stewe. And aftirward take a lynen cloþe or coton
and wete in þe watir. And anoynte þerwiþ his y3en. And

20 let him be cuppid in þe neþir parti of þe hede bihynde-
forþe or bitwene his shuldir-bladis. Or let him blede

f. 84v on þe veyne of þe elbowe. And sette / an horne al aboute
þe elbowe and cuppe him þer. But vndirstonde þat al þes
blode-lettinggis shullen raþir be y-doon þer-as þe ache

---

2 it] *ins. above.* **5 doo]** *corr. from* put. **6 oþirwhiles]** *in l. h.*
margin. **7 or]** *prec. by* oþerwhile *canc. in red.* **15 þes]** *ins. above.*

comeþ of hete, þen of colde.   Also take rwe and hete
it on an hote tiyl stoon, and make þerof a plastir, and
ley it on his y3en.   Or wete a lynen clooþ in þe iuse
of rwe and of fenel and ley on his y3en.   And wasshe
his y3en in þe euen and in þe morewe in þe watir of lily
rotis or in white wiyn þat spikenard is soden yn.   Or
ellis wasshe hem with white wiyn þat mellilotum, and popi,
and comyn ben soden yn, or with whijt wiyn þat olibanum
and roses ben soden yn, or with whijt wyne þat bras or
golde han ofte ben y-qwenchid yn, or with wiyn þat gynger
and rwe han ben soden yn, or ellis / take peritorie,
and put it in a bagge and make a plastir þerof aftir
þe brede and þe quantite of þe y3e and ley it to colde.
Or make a plastir of barly mele or of bran y-soden in
white wiyn y-put in a bagge and y-leide on þe y3e, for
þis heliþ þe ache þat comeþ of colde.   Or seþe in wiyn
femygreke mele or of lynen-sede, or of mellilotum in a
bagge and ley it on þe y3e.   A colliry: Take of licium,
acacie, amyde, sarc[ac]olle, calamynt, encense, of eueriche,
dr. i; of opium, x greynes.   Tempere it wp with þe
iuse of fenel and of eufrace.   And aftir, drie it þries
or foure siþes in þe sunne.   And tempere it aftir his
drieng in þe same iuse.   And siþ drie it vp and put þerof
in þe y3e in þe morewe and in þe / euene.   And it doiþ

Left margin notes:
5
10 f. 85
[133]
15
20
f. 85v

13 y3e] *corr. from* ye3e. **14 make]** *in r. h. margin.* **15 y-put]** *prec. by* and *canc. in red.* **19 sarcacolle]** sarcolle.

awey hede-ache þat comeþ of colde and heliþ blerid y3en, but it is sumwhat bityng.

Chapter II, Part 2
Ophthalmia

      Obtalmye is a postem in a mannes y3e þat comeþ of corrupte humours þat fallen a-dovn into a mannes y3e. And

5   þis postum is oþirwhiles withyn, and oþirwhiles withouten. And in boþe places, it comeþ of blode, or of coler, or of flevme, or of malencoly. And if þe postum be withyn þe y3e, it is y-drawen abrode, and swelliþ, and akiþ, and þe si3te wexiþ derke, and þe veynes ben fulle. And if it be

10 withouten, it may be soon knowe of whiche humour it is. And if it be of blode, þe y3en watren, and swellen, and wexen rede. And her forehede akiþ and her templis also. If it be of coler, þei felen grete pricking and smer/-

  ting byneþe in þe depnes of þe y3e. And þei han moche

15 hete in her y3en. If it be of flevme, þei ben blere-y3ed, and þei watren white viscous mater. If it be of malencoly, þe y3en watren not moche, but þey ben blerid. And in eueriche of þes, þer is ache, sum more and sum lasse. But oþirwhiles þis sikenes comeþ of þe pose; þen

20 hele þe pose. And if þe body be replete, let him blede in euery cause. And it is profitable to be y-cuppid in þe necke-pitte, or behynde þe hede in þe two hornes þat ioynen to þe necke. And if he be costif, 3eue him a laxe. And also baþing is profitable for him, and gode dieting, as

---

3 *2-line initial in blue.* **22** þe (3)] *ins. above.*

f. 86v

[134]

Y seyde in þe laste chaptir.   And lette / him not waisshe his yȝen with warme watir ne with warme þingis þat ben moyste, for drede of drawing of more mater þerto.   But vse strictories and repercussiues to þe hede in þe

5   beginnyng, as Y tolde before.   And ley þou noon stronge repercussiues in þe begynnyng to þe hede, ne to þe yȝen. But begynne with confortatiues, and mitigatiues, and strictories.   And in þe encresyng of þe sekenes, vse confortatiues and feble dissolatiues.   And whan þe ache

10   and þe sekenes abidiþ stille, neiþir waxyng ne decresing,

[133v]   and in þe passing awei, vse dissolutyues.   And if þe sekenes be of xv daies or of a moneþe, it may liȝtly

f. 87   be helid.   But if it contynue / an hole ȝere or more, vnneþis may it be helid.   For þoughe þe postum be helid

15   and þe ache also, oþirwhiles þer leveþ a litil webbe; and þerof comeþ a clooþ; and þerof a nayl.   Þes þre ben of oo kynde: Þe cloþe is þicker þen þe web, and þe nayl is þicker þen þe clooþ.

[?]
For þe web,
cloþe,
or naile
þat is
curable

For þe web, clooþ, or nayl þat is curable, fasting,

20   chewe clene comyn in þy mooþ, and wringe it þrough a cloote into þe yȝe, and let it be in þe ȝye of þe pacient a forlong wey.   Þen wasshe þe yȝe with watir of eufras meny tymes in þe day.   Þus do þre daies contynuely.   Also drinke þe iuse of ysop and oculus Christi y-temperid with

---

10 abidiþ] *corr. from* stondiþ. **13 contynue**] *prec. by* be *canc. in red.* **17 oo**] *ins. above.* **nayle**] *prec. by* web *canc. in red.* **21 cloote**] *corr. from* clooþ. **be**] *corr. from* stonde.

f. 87v

[134]

A colliri

ale.   And þis wil helpe þis sekenes. / A colliry þer-as
þe obtalmye is hidde withynforþe: Take of roses, dr. iiii;
of acacie,   dr. ii;   of spike,   dr. i;   of opium,   sc. 1/2.
Tempere hem with watir of roses, or of reyne watir, or
5 with þe iuse of planteyn, of violet, of endyue.

A white
coliri

Anoþir þat is a whijt coliry: Take of gumme arabike,
dragagantum, amyde, of eueriche, dr. iiii;   of ceruse,   dr.
i; of opium, sc. i.   Tempere hem with þe white of an ey.

[131]

Anoþir: Take of sarcacolle, dr. iii;   of amyde,
10 gumme   arabike,   draga[ga]ntum,   ana,   dr.   ii;   of cathmie
argente, ceruse, ana, dr. i & 1/2;   of encense, of opium,
sc.   i.   Tempere hem with watir of roses or with þe iuse
of planteyn.

[134]

f. 88   15

Anoþer: Take of dragagantum, sc. i;   of citre, dr. ii;
of sarcacol, dr. iiii;   of / memyth, dr. viii.   Tempere hem
with watir of roses or of reyn.

A colliri

A colliry in þe waxing of þe sekenes to do awei þe
ache: Take of ceruse, dr. ii;   of cathmie, tuchie, gummi
arabike, dragagantum, amide, of eueriche, dr. i;   of acacie,
20 of opium, dr. 1/2.   Tempere hem with reyn watir.

[131]

Anoþir colliry: Take roses, cathmie, gumme arabik,
draga[ga]ntum, amide, ana,   dr.   iiii;   of ceruse,   of coost,
ana,   dr.   ii;   of opium, dr. 1/2.   Tempere hem with reyn
watir.   But aftir þe cesing of þe ache, if þer leue eny

---

9 sarcacolle] ca *ins. above.* **10 dragagantum]** dragantum. **22
dragagantum]** dragantum. **23 ana]** *ins. above.* **24 leue]** *in r. h.
margin.*

[134]

web or wem withouten, ony oþir humour y-hardid, or þe obtalmie be withouten þe y3en, þou must vse colliries þat ben corrisif and freting. But firste, ley þerto mollificatiues to make þe mater neisshe, as femigreke or

f. 88v 5 lyn/sede. If þe soore is 3onge and new, ley þerto esy corosiues. And if þe sore be olde, ley þerto stronge corosiues.

Esy
corosiues

Esy corosiues ben, rwe, eufrace, centrum-galli, filago, licium, mirre, encence, sarcocol, hony, and ceruse, 10 camphore, cathmia, emachites, spike, memyth, ambir, ginger, þe knot of a vyne, acacia, lymaile of golde, muske, and suche oþer.

[134v]

Stronge
corosiues

Strong corosiues ben, þe galle of euery beste and principali of rauenyng briddis and also of a bole, þe 15 fatnes of a qwaal, castor, antimonie, bras y-brent, sandeuer, coperos, calamina, magnes, thuchia, bavme, þe

f. 89 dritte of euery beste y-/brent and namely of a man, eueriche kynde of salte, and sal nitre, sal armoniac, vertigrece, þe inner skynne of an hennes mawe, alyme, 20 lanceola þat groweþ in watir, lymail of bras, comyn, and pepir, aloes, þe sede of spourge, chikenweed, and psilotrum þat is made to doo awey heris. But amonge þe corosiues,

Tuchia
is best
corosif for
þe y3en

thuchia is oon of þe beste for y3en. But þou muste heten him ix siþes in þe fier and quenche him as oftentymes in þe iuse

15 fatnes] *corr. from* fuatnes. **23 y3en**] *corr. from* yen. þou] *ins. above.*

Thre kindis
of tuchia

of soure grapes, or of fenel, or in whijt wiyn. But þer ben

þre kyndes of tuchie: whijt, rede, and blacke, and eueriche

f. 89v

oon of hem is mitigatif, / and repercussif, and corrosif, but

þe white is more repercussif in þe hete and in reednes of þe

5   y3en; þe black is mitigatif; and þe rede is more repercussif.

[135v]
Hov þe grete
malice of
corosiues
shal be
abatid

And meny of þes grete corrosiues muste be wasshen

in diuerse þingis to abaten her malices. Calamina shal

be xx syþes y-qwenchid in þe iuse of fenel, or in a childis

vryn, or in a womanes mylke, or in wiyn of pomgarnad.

Calamina

Cathmia

10   Cathmia shal be ix siþes y-waisshen in gotis mylke, or

in asse mylke, or in a womanes mylke. Alloes shal be

Alloes

ix tymes y-waisshen in þe iuse of fenel. Antimonie and

f. 90
Antimonie

bras y-brente in þe same maner shul/len be y-qwenchid

and y-waisshe, for þey be moste violent corrosiues. And

15   aftir þeyr waisshing, þei mowon be y-put in colliries.

Summe þingis ben y-waisshe to haue more violence

þen þei hadden, as encence y-waisshe in þe iuse of celidon,

and meny oþir þingis þat seruen for oþer sekenessis by

Encense

Lapis lazuli

waisshing lesen moche of her violence, as lapis lazuli,

20   and lapis armenicus, y-wasshen in watir, and spurge sede

Lapis
armenicus

in oyle. And scamonie in þe iuse of planteyn is not so

laxatif as it was tofore, ne aloes, and it be y-waisshen,

is not so sotil and so persyng as it was.

And medicyns ben oþirwhiles y-brente to encresen her

---

2 **tuchie**] *corr. from* tucie. 3 **oon**] *ins. above.*

/ violence, as attrament and calamina. Summe ben brente to
be þe more sotil, as a watir cankre, þat is y-ȝove to men
þat ben etike. Summe þingis ben y-brente for þei shullen
be þe bettir y-poudrid, as syndel; summe to leesen his
5   venemousnes, as a scorpion when it is taken for þe stone.
And grettir medicynes þat ben of grete mater, þoroughe
brenyng, þei wexen þe more violent. Sotil medicyns in
brenyng lesen her violence, and mene medicyns þat ben notte

riȝt sotil ne riȝt grete. But in making colliries þat ben
10   corrisyues, þou muste medle with corrisiues mitigatiues and

confortatiues, as when þei ben y-poudrid, / tempre hem
with watir of roses, or with þe iuse of planteyn, or of
fenel, or of eufrace, or of rewe, or with þe blode
of a lapwynge or of a swalewe. And aftir, drye hem in
15   þe sunne. And do so iii or iiii tymes. And þen poudir it
smale and bolte it þoroughe a smale clooþ. And aftir medle
it with þe iuse of oon of þe foreseide herbis, or with
þe blood of a capon, or of an hare, or of an ramme, or of
a boor. And so do it in þe yȝe. But see þat þy colliries
20   ben not to stronge and violent, for harmyng of þe yȝe.
And if ony suche be in þe yȝe, put in it anoon womanes

mylke. And gader it / oute as clene as þou may. And
aftirwarde ley to þe yȝe mytigatiues and confortatiues,
as dragagantum resolved in coold watir.

50

[?]

Mussilage
of psilie

Eiþir take þe mussilage of psillie þat is þus made:
Take þe seed of psillie and put it in a vessel of colde
watir. And þe watir shal wexe þicke as gely or as gleyr
of eggis. Wringe it þoroughe a clooþ and kepe it. For
5 it is callid mussilage. And in þe same maner þou may make
mussilage of oculus Christi. Boþe ben good mitiga[ti]ues.

[134v]

A colliri

A gode colliry: Take of sarcacolle, encense, gumme
arabike, and of amyde, dr. iii; of licium, mirre, and
ceruse, dr. ii; of alloes, tucie, roses, and of campher,

f. 92   10
[135]

dr. i; of opium, sc. i. And when þou 3euest a / man
colliries, boþe before and aftir, anoynte þe y3en with
watir þat roses or planteyn ben y-soden yn, in greuaunce
þat comeþ of hete; but if it comeþ of colde, with watir of
eufrace or of fenel. In coolde causes, vse medicyns siche
15 as is y-rehersid in þe laste chaptir, and þe colliries of
þis chaptir. But or þan þou 3yue him colliries, make him a
plastir of been mele in a bagge y-soden in wiyn, or of
gynger and a litil hony, or of suche oþer as it is tolde
in þe laste chaptir tofore þis, and also baþing and
20 strictories as it is y-tolde þer.

A colliri

Anoþir colliry: Take alloes, and mirre, and encense,
calamina, ceruse, tuchia, of eueriche, yliche moche; /

f. 92v

of amyde, sumwhat more; of opium, wel lasse. And make
þerof a colliry.

1 **mussilage**] *corr. from* mussailage. **5 same**] *ins. above.* **6
mitigatiues**] mitigaues. **7 gode colliry**] *marked for reversal.* **10 when**]
in l. h. margin. **15 þe (2)**] *prec. and followed by* in *canc. in red.*

Chapter II, Part 3
Web, Cloth, and Nail

Web

Clooþ

Ungula

f. 93

f. 93v

Good and esi mollificatiues

Other sikenessis þer ben of þe y3en. Oon is a web or a wem þat coueriþ þe myddis of þe y3e. And þis is in two maners: Oþirwhilis he is whiyt and þynne, and oþirwhiles he is þicke, as when obtalmye is not cleen y-

5 helid vp but þe rote abydeþ stille. Oþirwhiles þe web is not whijt, but reed eiþir blacke. But when al þe y3e is couerid, þen it is clepid a clooþ. And when it coueriþ þe oon corner of þe y3e, þen it is clepid vngula. And þis greuaunce comeþ of corrupte humours as obtalmie / doiþ.

10 And it shal be helid by corrosyues, confortatiues, repercussiues, mytigatiues, and strictories, and blood-lettinggis, like as obtalmie is y-helid. But if it comeþ of obtalmye or of hurting of þe y3e þat is not wel y-helid, þou maist vsen consolidatiues in þy colliries,

15 as sarcacolle, or alloes, mirre, encense, emachites, sandragon, with þe whijt of an egge, or with þe iuse of planteyn, or with þe iuse of auence. And in þe begynnyng, it is good to vse mollificatiues if it be so þat þe y3en ben not ful moist. And aftir, worche with corrosiues, first

20 with eesy, / and aftir with strengir.

If it be nede of mollificatiues, take womanes mylke, and þe watir þat þe hocke and þe holihocke ben y-soden yn, and lynseed, femygreke, with þe iuse of fenel, and þe watir þat dropeþ of a snayl when it is wel priked.

---

1 *2-line initial in blue.* **10 corrosyues**] *corr. from* corrysyues. **18 be so**] *marked for reversal.*

[?]

Oyle of
notes

And þe beste of al is oyle of notes þat is þus maad:
Take notes and seeþ hem in watir al hool.   And aftirwarde
breke hem, and take oute þe kernels, and stampe hem.
And aftir þat, wringe hem þoroughe a clooþ.   And þat

5 oyle is a noble mollificatif.   And if þe greuaunce be

[135v]

f. 94

of newe, take þe iuse of chekenmete or of rede popi.   And
þat shal sufficen.   Or ellis make a colliri / of mirre,
alloes, licium, with þe iuse of fenel.   Or take licium
and campher and temper hem with þe iuse of fenel.   And

10 if þes freten not awey, take sum strengir freteris, as os
sepie, spume of þe see, calamina, and tucie: Þat is þe
best of hem al.   Or seþe salte in vinegre and poudir it.
And put in þe i3e, for it fretiþ awei þe web.   And so
doiþ þe iuse of celidon and of verueyn, if þe sore be newe.

15 Also take a rede snayl and salte him in a bacyn.   And let
him lye so iii^e daies.   And aftir, set þe bacin a-slont
and sidingli, þat þou may rescyue þe licour into a clene
vessel.   And close it.   And take of þis watir and put in þe
i3e.   And let it be þeryn þre daies; þan do awei þe pece

20 þat it haþ y-freten awei.   And aftir, do oþir licour þat is
eesi in his i3e.

f. 94v

A good
poudir for
þe webbe

A good poudir to fre/ten awei eueriche kynde of web in
a mannes i3e, and þoughe it be olde so þat mollificatiues
goon before: Take of amyde,   of sarcacolle, dr. ii; of

8-9 Or . . . fenel] *in r. h. margin.* **11 þe see**] *corr. from* þese see.
16 set] *corr. from* do.   **a-slont**] *prec. by* to *canc. in red.*

roses, dr. 1/2; of tucie, dr. 1/2. Tempere hem with þe iuse of eufrace or fenel. And aftir, drie þat in þe sonne. And þan do þerof in þe i3e. And if he may not suffre it, medle it with þe blode of an henne, or with þe iuse of

5 eufrace, or plantein, or egrimoyne, or verueyn, or endyue, or filago, or celidon: Þer is no better medicyn for þis greuaunce.

[136]

Regula

f. 95

[?]

And vndirstonde þat þe beste maner to make poudirs smale for þe i3en is to rubben hem with þe iuse of þe

10 foreseide herbis, or on a barbours / wheston, or in a clene-scourid bacyn. Also þe iuse of þe iii-leuyd gras þat haþ white spekis is good for þe web, and also golde or laton y-robbid on a wheston with vynegre til þe vynegre be þicke, and aftirward y-dried is gode. And it drieþ moche

15 þe y3en.

Poudir
of lede

[136v]

Poudir of lede shal þus be made: Take lede and melte it ouer þe fier and stere it with a grene haselne sticke. And it wole turne to blacke povdir, and þat is good for þis greuaunce. Whan þou comfortist þe y3e, comforte him

20 boþe withyn and withoute. And also comforte þe stomake, for þat is profitable for þe y3en. And in drye y3en, vse

f. 95v

moyste corosi/ues; and in moyste y3en, drye corosives; in olde greuaunces, stronge corosiues; in newe, esy corosiues.

[?]

For þe web in þe i3en or pyn: Take eufras and stampe it.

---

5 or (1)] *ins. above.* **10 a (2)**] *ins. above.* **16 melte**] *corr. from* myelte. **17 haselne**] *corr. from* hahelen.

Þen streyne it þoroughe a clooþ and lete it clere. And put
in þe i3e of þe clere duringe þre daies at eue and at
morwe. And he shal be hole. Probatum est.

Chapter II, Part 4
Red Eyes

[137v]   Also a mannes i3en ben oþirwhiles rede or infecte.
5   Redenes comeþ of blode; infeccion comeþ of oþer humours and
of oþer sikenes, as of þe 3elewe yvele, or of stopping
of þe splene, or of heting of þe lyver.   To hele suche
infeccions, firste þou muste hele þe sekenes þat ben cause
f. 96   of hem, and aftir/warde vse colliries þat ben a litil
10   corosif and mundificatif to freten awei and to clensen
þat infeccion and purge þe body of þat humour þat is cause
of þat infeccion. Of blode comeþ redenes, and not þat al
oneli, but oþirwhiles a gobet of fleisshe growing on
þe i3e. And oþirwhiles, for grete plente of blode and
15   feblenes of þe i3e, þe blode lieþ y-congelid on þe i3e and
makeþ þe i3en rede. Oþirwhiles þei ben rede for grete
plente of blode þat is in þe veynes, and oþirwhiles
þoroughe falling or þorou3 smerting, blode falleþ into þe
i3en and makeþ hem rede.
20   If þer growe a pece of fleisshe on þe i3e, let frete
f. 96v   it awei with / stronge corosiues. But let hem not touche
þe y3e. And if it may not be freten awei by corosiues,
þen wiþ a strictory and leting of blode, make þat þe
blode be y-let of his course to þe y3e. And aftirward,

4 *2-line initial in blue.* **12 redenes**] *corr. from* rdenes. **13 a**] *prec.
by* of *canc. in red.* **18 þorou3**] by *in r. h. margin with dots indicating
that it should replace* þorou3.

3yue him colliries þat mown clense and comforte þe y3e, as
Y haue tolde tofore.   And if þer be moche blode in þe
veynes of þe y3e, lete him blede in þe veyne of þe hede in

[138] þe arme, or in þe veyne of þe elbowe, or of þe þombe.   And
5 if þe y3e be kitte in þe whijt of þe y3e,   or if þe whijt be
y-broke, heel it herwith: Take sarcacol, mastike, encense,
sandragon, emachite.   And tempere hem with sangrinary þat
is clepid sheppardis purse,   or planteyn.   But vse here

f. 97 consoli/datiues, þat is to seie, suche þingis þat han
10 vertu to souden a þing þat is y-kitte or broken, as
comfery, and daiesy, and þe myddel comfery, and centory,
and planteyn, and auence, and sandragon, and emachite. And
if þe blode be congelid, þat is to sey, y-hardid and y-made
þicke þoroughe coold, þen consume it, and dissolue it, and
15 departe it fro þe place þat it is yn wiþ þe iuse of verueyn
and of planteyn y-medlid togeder.   And clense þe y3e wiþ
mundificatiues, as with þe iuse of endiue, or with watir of
a vyne, or with comyn and þe iuse of rwe and wiyn y-soden
togeder, or with a croust of a loof y-rostid and y-braied
20 with þe iuse of rwe and with þe foreseid wiyn and y-/

f. 97v plastrid on þe y3e, eiþir fresshe chees þat is newe and not
saltid y-plastrid on þe y3e, eiþir encense and mastike
y-medlid with þe iuse of marche and þe gleyr of an ey,
eiþir ysope y-soden in watir and y-plastrid on þe y3e,

---

4 þombe] *corr. from* wombe. **11 daiesy]** *corr. from* daisy. **16 togeder]** *corr. from* togederis. **19 croust]** *corr. from* croost.

eiþir vertegrese y-put in wiyn and y-soden, and aftir it is cleer, y-put in þe y3en.

For ycching of þe y3en: Draga[ga]ntum is gode in colliries and also bi himselue in colde watir, and psillie
5 and his mussilage, oyle of roses, and þe white of eggis. But be þei ware of clawing.

Moystnes of y3en comeþ of þe hede þat is replete with
f. 98 humours; blereship of y3en / comeþ of cooldnes and of moistenes of þe brayn. And þerfore it behoueþ to purge þe
10 heed and namely of malencoly, as it is tolde in þe sekenes of þe heed. And aftirward, let him baþen him in a baþ y-
[138v] made of lorer leues, and of rw, of egrimoine, and betayn, and fenel, and oþir herbis þat ben comfortable for þe
A confortatif baþ for þe heed and þe y3en brayn. And let his heed be wasshid with þe same watir
15 while it is warme. And 3yue him sumwhat in his nose to make him snesse, as sauge or plemeros y-brusid and y-holde longe in þe nose. And 3eue him þe poudir of piretre, of
f. 98v staphie, and syneuey y-sowid / in a lynen cloþ. And let him holde þis in his mooþ and chewe it ofte. And when þe
20 humour falleþ dovn from his brayn into his mooþ, þen alwei let him spet it oute. And aftir þat he is y-purged, take a woman-is mylke þat fedeþ a knave childe and anoynt his y3en þerwiþ. And aftir þat, make him a colliry confortatif of spike, and folium, and watir of roses, and eufrace, and

3 **Dragagantum**] Dragantum. **8 blereship**] *prec. by* as *canc. in red*.

fenel, and suche oþir confortatifs.

Chapter II, Part 5
Watery Eyes

Weping of y3en comeþ oþirwhiles of enchesons wiþouteforþ, as of smokis, or of wyndes, or duste, or of a stroke. Oþirwhiles it comeþ of withyn, as of ioye, or of sorow, or of angir, or of plente of humours in þe / heed, as of feblenes of þe veynes þat ben in þe y3e. If plente of humours ben þe cause, a purgacion is good for him. And if he haue grete plente of blode, lete him blede in þe veines þat clenseþ þe y3en and þe heed, as þe hede veyne in þe arme, or þe veyne þat is bitwene þe þombe and þe nexte fyngir, or in þe veyne of þe elbow. And make a plastir of encense, mastike, bole, sandragon, þe white of an ey, and a litil wiyn, and a litil vinegir, and ley þat on his forehed. But see þat in noon sikenes of þe y3en, be it of coold or of hete, þou leie noon hote plastir to þe y3en. And if þou leie a colde plastir to þe y3en / þat ben y-disesed by grete hete, let not þe plastir lye ouir-longe vppon þe y3en, lest it take hete and hurte þe y3en. And if weping comeþ of feblenes of þe brayn, þen comfort þe brayn. And in þe begynnyng, make a colliry of ceruse, dragagantum, folium, and roses, of eueriche, yliche moche. And smyþþes watir is good for þis greuaunce, and for þe web, and for þe bries þat ben y-turned inward. Also take of ceruse, gumme arabik, and of encense, dr. ii; of draga[ga]ntum, dr. i; of

f. 99   5

10

[139]

[142]

15

f. 99v

[139]

20

2 *2-line initial in blue.* **8 he**] *ins. above.* **9 in**] *corr. from* of. **10 þombe**] *prec. by* wo *canc. in red.* **24 dragagantum**] dragantum.

opium, dr. 1/2; or ellis, of þe watir of egrimoyne, of
fenel, of verueyn, and of roses, and þerwiþ wasshe daily
þe y3en.

Chapter II, Part 6
Canker of the Eye

For þe canker in þe y3e: If it be of coler, it makeþ

f. 100 5 þe y3e harde, and freteþ awei þe bries, and / makeþ þe y3e
ful hoot. Þan he must be y-helid with a plastre y-made of
litarge and solatre, or with hempe sede and oculus Christi
y-stampid togedir and y-plastrid on þe y3en. If it be of
malencoly, þe y3e is ful hard and ful heuy. Þan make a

10 plastre of been meel and boles galle.

Chapter II, Part 7
Injury to the Cornea

[139v]

Horned
cloþ

For hurting of þat horned cloþ þat is withyn þe white
of þe i3e and þe humours þat ben aboute him, þou must vse
consolidatiues in þy colliries, and not suche þingis þat
maken þe i3en to smerte or yche, but mitigatiues and

15 confortatiues. Neþeles, woman-is mylke is not good here, for
it is to moyste, but þe blood of a coluir or of a chiken is
good here, and þe consolidatiues þat Y tolde in þe sekenes /

f. 100v of þe y3en. Also þe watir þat whete is y-soden yn with
oþir consolidatiues and confortatiues, as roses, eufrace,

20 and suche oþir ben good. Thou muste leye aftirward suche
þingis to þe y3e þat þe wounde be not seen, þat is, þe iuse
of mader, and boras, and þe fatnes of an henne and marye of
her boones. And if þer waxeþ ony postomes, as blaynes, on
þat partie of þe y3e, take apostolicon and medle it over þe

---

4 *2-line initial in blue.* **10 galle**] *corr. from* galles. **11** *2-line initial
in blue.* **17 þe** (2)] *in r. h. margin.* **20 aftirward**] *in l. h. margin.* **23 if**]
prec. by a canc. in red. **as**] *corr. from* or.

fyer with oile and with boles talowe. And wete a lynen
cloute in wiyn, and aftir anoynte it with þis oynment, and
leye to þe yȝe. Or ellis, take þe pouder of gynger, and
alloes cicotryn, and medle hem with hony, and leye vpoon
5   þe yȝen. /

Chapter II, Part 8
Feebleness of the Sight

f. 101   Feblenes of siȝte comeþ in meny maners, as by sekenes
[140]   of þe yȝen, as Y haue tolde before; or of sekenes of þe
heed, and þan it is y-holpe by helyng of þat sikenes; or of
greuaunce of þe stomake, whiche may be amendid by heling of
10   þe stomake. Oþirwhiles þe feblenes of þe iȝe comeþ of
feblenes of her spiritis. And here, þou muste vndirstonde
þat suche spiritis ben smale bodies þat ben in a man-is yȝe.
And þei ben þe instrumentis þat þe siȝte seeþ with; for
suche spiritis resceyuen þe liȝtnes of þo þingis þat a man
15   seeþ. And þerfore whan þey ben feble, nedes þe siȝt muste /
f. 101v   be feble.
[142]   For þis sekenes a pye is gode in þis maner: Pul
her, and take oute hir guttis, and brenne þe remanant in
a newe erþen pot wel-y-stoppid aboue. And make þerof
20   povdir and vse it in þy metis, and drinkis, and colliries.
Þis poudir is also good for þe cardiacle, and for malencoly,
and oþer coold sekenesses, and for þe canker in a mannes
ȝeerd. Also take þe pye, and pul hir, and take oute hir
guttis, and seeþ þe toþir deel in white wiyn til þe wiyn be

---

3 þe (2)] *ins. above.* **6** *2-line initial in blue.* **9 heling]** *prec. by a*
canc. in red. **22 sekenesses]** *corr. from* sekenes.

consumed and þe fleisshe departid from þe bones.   Þan
stampe it al togedir, and put it in a vessel, and let þe
þin renne fro þe þicke þre daies.   Þan take a smale lynen
f. 102   cloute and wete in þat liquor, / and put þerof in þe y3e
  5   boþe withyn and withoute, for it doeþ awei þe deerknes and
þe smerting of þe y3e, and þe redenes, and þe ache, and
comforteþ þe spiritis.   Also, netle seed is good for
derkenes of y3en, and þe watir þat þe seed is soden yn;
[141v]   also þe watir of eufrace, of celidone, of rwe, of egrimoyn,
 10   of fenel, of   rooses, is gode for þe si3te.   Also, seeþ
[142]   turmentil in wiyn and drinke þe wiyn.   Þen ley of þat soden
herbe on þe y3e, and withyn ix daies it shal see.   Also,
take þe iuse of fenel and of hayhoue and set it in þe
sunne iii daies in a brasen vessel.   And aftir do þerof in
 15   þe y3e.   Or medle þe iuse of heyhoue and hony togedir; or
f. 102v   make a plastir of comyn y-pov/drid and whit wiyn and ley it
on his y3e, but ley a clooþ bitwene.   Or take þe iuse of
wormod and of rwe, of boþe yliche moche, and put in þe y3e;
or take þe iuse of rwe and hony and medle hem togedir and
 20   put into þe i3e.   And it shal make þe flowing of watir to
ceesse.   Or take gynger, and þe iuse of fenel, and whijt
wyin, and medle hem togedir.   And drie hem in þe sunne and
do þerof in þe i3e.   Or take þe iuse of celidon, and of
rwe, and of morwetidis dew, and hony, of eueriche, yliche

3 þin] *corr. from* þicke. **10 is]** *prec. by* be *canc. in red.* **11 drinke]**
prec. by ley þe herbe *canc. in red.*

moche. And drie it in þe sunne and aftir do þerof in þe y3e. Also þe watir of þes erbis: of eufrace, celidon, rue, egrimoyne, fenel, and of roses, ben good for feble si3te.

[141v]

[141]

 5

f. 103

A good poudir þat cleriþ þe si3te, and comforteþ þe stomake, and wasteþ corrupte wyndes in a mannes body: Take of louage, anys, ameos, marche, ca/nel, cardamome, origane, anet, carewei, fenel, siler monteyn, comyn, sauge, mynte, calamynte, eufrase, tyme, pepir, ysope, parsely, of eueriche, oz. i; of gynger, liquoris, piliol, notemyg, oz.

 10

ii; of clowis, galenga, and citre, oz. 1/2; and if þou wilt, take a pounde of piliol and put þerto a pounde of sugir. And þou maiest make it in fourme of electuary.

Anoþir poudir for þe same cause: Take of notemyg, ligni aloe, siler monteyn, citre, mastik, reubarbe,

 15

eufrace, carewei, anet, fenel, and maces, dr. ii; of gynger, of long piper, dr. 1/2. Make of þes a poudir and vse it with þy metis in savcis.

[141v]

f. 103v

A colliry for feble si3t: Take houndistonge, gallitricum, rwe, / celidon, eufrace, memythe, egrimoyne,

 20

of eueriche, an handful. Take þe iuse of þes herbes and seeþ it in wiyn. And aftir, put þis poudre y-made of alloes and tute þat is quenchid as Y tolde before þerin; and of sarcacolle, and of þe ryndes of mirabolani, of eueriche of þes, dr. ii; of whijt pepir, camphore, whijt

---

2-3 Also . . . si3te.] *in bottom margin.* **21 y-made]** *in l. h. margin.* **22 and]** *ins. above.* **þerin]** *in l. h. margin.* **23 of (1)]** *ins. above.*

coral and also reed, dr. 1/2 of eueriche; and of citre, of
margery peerles, ana, dr. 1/2. Þis colliry clereþ þe
si3te, and freteþ awei þe web, and staunched þe watryng
of þe i3en, and doeþ awei þe reednes of þe y3en.

Chapter III
Eyelids and Lashes

5   Here beginneþ þe þrid chaptir, þat is not deuided,
and conteineþ but oon practis or title.

[142v]   In a mannes y3eliddis and his bries, þer ben meny
greuauncis, as pimples, ycchyng, clevyng togedre by sum

f. 104   viscouse mater, turnyng of þe bries inward, / wormes in
10   þe i3eliddis, and luys among þe heris.

Pymples and postemes ben oþirwhiles of viscouse mater
y-gaderid togedre in a litil skyn, oþirwhiles in þe maner
of scabbes, oþirwhiles in þe maner of stoones. If it
be in þe first maner, it may be helid with a plastre aftir
15   þe quantite of þe pimple, y-made of swynes galle and been
mele y-leide þerto, or with a plastre of lilye rootis and
of affodille y-stampid togedre. If it be in þe seconde
maner, as a scabbe, make a plastre of lilye root, and bran,
and scabeous, and langdebef. If it be in þe þrid maner,

f. 104v **20** take þe ius of mellilot and a litil of þe poudre of / an
ademant stoon and medle hem togedre ouer þe fier. And ley
it on a pece of leder aftir þe quantite of þe greuaunce.

[143]   For yching, take vynegre and let it stonde þre daies
in a brasen vessel. And þan put þerto a litil hony and

---

2 1/2] *prec. by* ii *canc.* **5-6 Here . . . title.**] *in l. h. margin.* **7** *2-line
initial in gold.* **19 þe**] *ins. above.* **23 ta-**] *followed by* poudir of a reed
wheston *canc. in red.*

iiº pipir-cornes y-poudrid.   And let it stonde a while in þe sunne, and þerwith anoynte his bries.   For viscouse mater þat makeþ þe bries to cleve togedre, waisshe þe yȝen

[142v]   with þe skym of white soop and watir.   And also camphor in

5   watir is good.   If þe heris growen inward toward þe yȝe,

f. 105   pulle hem oute, and wete a nedlis po/ynt in lye and aftir let a drope of þe lye þer-as þe heer stood.   Aftirwarde, waisshe þe yȝen with þe iuse of grapes þat ben not rype. And if þe iȝeliddis be so fleissheli þou may not pulle oute

10   þe heris, robbe hem wel with peritorye leves til þey bleden, and aftir þat pulle oute þe heris by þe root.   And þan anoynte it with gleyr of eyren.   And if it be wintir ceson, resolue þeryn a litil saffron, and þus þou mai do as ofte

[143]   as it is nedeþ.

15   For wormes: Take þe iuse of camedreos and anoynte þe bries; or plastre þe herbes on þe yȝen; or take alloes and rubbe it with white wiyn on a wheston and do þerof in þe yȝen.

For luys: Take þe watir þat lupynes ben y-soden

f. 105v 20   yn.   If þei be / heuy and grete, leye a plastre of peritorie on hem, or þe rote of marche, or þe leues a litil y-soden. For cleving of þe skyn in þe corner of þe bryes: Take sauge and bren it, and medle it with mastike and olibanum, and springe it þeron.   Or take serapinum and dissolue it

in wiyn, and it shal soude þe place.   For swelling of þe
bries: Leye goottis mylke on hem, or hony and sal armoniac
togedre. Or ley þerto mollificatiues þat Y spake of before.

Chapter IV, The Ears
Part 1, Earache

[?]   Here beginneþ þe fourþe chaptir of þis boke, þat
    5 conteineþ sixe titles or practises.

[145]   In a mannes eren þer ben meny greuauncis, as ache,
postem, flowing of blode, flowing of qwiter, wormes,
ringing in þe eeris, falling of sum-þing into þe eeris,
f. 106   and deefnes. Ache comeþ of meny causes: of postem, / of
    10 smyting, of wiynde withyn þe eeris, of grete hete or of
grete coolde, or of sum-þing þat is y-fallen into þe eeris,
or of sum corrupt humour þat is in þe eeris. And if it
comeþ of sum corrupt humour, þen þer is moche heuynes in þe
eere, and nameli if it be of coold.   If it comeþ of
    15 corrupte wyinde, þer is ringing in þe eere withoute grete
heuynes.   Oþirwhiles it comeþ of þe brayn, and þen it
dureþ contynuely.   Oþirwhiles it comeþ of þe stomake, and
þen it contynueþ not contynuelli. Of clene moystenes ne of
clene drines, þer comeþ no greet ache. But when þe ache is
    20 of heet, þe eere is hoot and reed, and þe ache is sharp.
f. 106v   And / if it be of eny hoot corrup humour, it is with
pricking, and with hoot smoke, and with a swiffte pouse,
and litil sleep, and in his sleep, he shal dreem of reed
þingis.   And if þat corrup humour is of þe brayn, his

4-5 Here . . . practises.] *in bottom margin.* **6** *2-line initial in gold.*
11 is] *ins. above.*

foreheed and his chekis wolen be reed; and he is þrustful;
and his heed akiþ. Coold þingis comforten him and hoot
þingis ercresen his greuaunce. If þe ache be of coold, þe
eere is pale and þe ache is but eesy. And if þat colde be

5 of a corrup humour, þe ache is with moche heuynes, and in
colde wederis þe ache is moost greuous. And if þis humour

[145v] be of þe brayn, þe foreheed is pale and heuy and akeþ a

f. 107 litil. And if it comeþ of / þe stomake, þen þe stomake is
y-greued by sum colde and haþ but litil talent to mete.

10 And comenly þe ache of þe eeris comeþ not of coold, but if
it be with sum postem, ne of grete heet, but if it be with
a feuer. And if þer is a postem withinforþ, þe ache is
greuous withinforþ. And if þe postem be outeward, þen þe
eere is swolwe withouten. And if þe eere akeþ and þes

15 forseide tokenes foloweþ not, loke in þe ӡeere if þou may
see if eny-þing is falle þeryn þat makeþ it so ake.

Ache þat comeþ of hete is a corrupte humour by þe
encheson þerof. Let him be purgid with suche þingis þat
purgen coller and purgen also blode. And aftir þat he is

f. 107v **20** purgid, worche as þou / shuldest if þer were no corrupte
humour, þat is to sey, stuwe his eeris ouer a watir þat
hockes ben soden yn, and also violet, planteyn, roses,
wormod, verueyn, and smale chaf of barliche or of oten.
And aftir þat, bringe him to bed and put in his eeris þe

17 þe] *ins. above.*

66

iuse of an oynon and woman-is mylke, or þe iuse of senegren
with oile of roses, or þe oile of violet with þe iuse of
coliandre, or ellis aftir his stufe, let him haue a sleep
and swete wel.   And þat shal do awei þe ache.   And

5 vndirstonde þat alle þe medicynes þat shullen be doon in þe
3eris muste be warme and smalle y-grounde.   And stronge

f. 108 medicynes / shullen not abiden in þe 3eris, lest þei drawen
to myche mater to þe eeris, ne no-þinge shal be doon in þe

[146v] 3eere but it be with oile or with sum oþir fatnes, þat

10 mowe come li3tly oute a3en; ne no medicyn shal be doon in
þe 3eere but if þe heed be y-stufed and þe heed y-purged
before, and þis y-vndirstonde þer-as þe sekenes is oolde.
And suche stufes or fumigacions shullen be of suche þingis
þat be contrarie to þe sekenes.   And if þe sekenes be of

15 oolde, þei shulen be colde.   And þe best maner for þe

[146] stufyng for þe eeren is, þat a man lye in his bed and ley /

f. 108v his eere ouer þe potte þat þe herbis ben y-soden yn, and
holde it so stille til þe herbis waxen coolde, and þen lye
doune in his bed and take a gode swete.   And þis shal be

20 doon in postems of þe eere, and in oþer sikeness of long
contynuance þat a man haþ longe tyme had.   And aftir þis
disposicion, ley þe medicyns in þe eere.   And if þe ache be
of hete as Y seide before, take a drope or ii° of letuse

[145v] and medle it with as moche of oyle of roses or of violett.

14 of] *ins. above.* 15 best] *in r. h. margin.*

Or seeþ in oyle of roses: acacie, violet, licium, and two
greynes of mastike. And þen clense it and put a drope
þerof in þe ȝere with coton, or wolle, or flexe. Or take

f. 109   þe iuse of syngrene, and of letuse, / and womanes mylke,

5   and seeþ hem togedre. And put þerto campher, þe sede of
planteyn, and a litil saffron. And streyne it and þan put
þerof in þe eere, and stoppe it. And if þe ache be stronge
and greuous, take acacie, and þe seed of popy, and of
planteyn, and medle hem with oile of roses, and womanes

10   mylke, and þe white of an ey, and a litil opium dissolued
in vynegre. Þen streyne it þoroughe a clooþ and put þerof
in þe eere. Or medle oile of roses and of violet togedre,
and put þerof in þe eere. And anoynte þe eere withouten
with þe iuse of coolde herbis, as it is tolde in þe hede-

15   ache þat comeþ of hete.

        Dieting of hem þat han þis sekenes shal be as of hem
þat han þe feuer tercian, saffe it maste be more laxe.

f. 109v   But / if þe ache come of colde, let him haue purgacions
as it longeþ to þe humour þat is cause of þe ache. And

20   aftirward make him a stufe of þes herbis y-soden in watir:
fenel, verueyn, wormod, weilde sauge, mynte, bavme, sauge;
and put a litil wiyn to hem. And make him vse þis stufe
þre nyȝtis contynuely, and euermore stop a mannes eris
aftir his stufyng. And iii nyȝtis aftirward, put in his

---

6 planteyn] *corr. from* plantyn. **14 is]** *ins. above.*

68

eeris oile of lorer, and woman-is mylke, and gleyr of eyren
y-medlid togedre.   And if it comeþ of þe stomake, let him
vse suche þingis þat comforten þe stomake.   Þese þingis ben
comyn, and þei ben also good for alle greuauncis of þe eris

f. 110   5   þat comeþ of colde.   And / also for þe same cause is oyle
of lorer, and of notes, and of bitter almondis, and of rwe,
riʒt gode.   And þe beste stufe is of grene been stelis or
of beenes hemsilfe y-medlid with comyn.   And aftir þe
stufe, put in þe eere oile y-made of bitter almandes.

[?]   10   A special medicyn: Take rwe, and oynons, and a litil
oyle, and medle hem togedre.   Þen roste hem in a caule
leef and plastre it withouten þe ere.   Or stampe wormod
or mugworte with oyle of rwe or of piliol and a litil wiyn.
Þen roste it in a caule leef vndir þe axes and ley it to þe

15   eere.   And in colde causes, take þe iuse of garlike, and
[146]   leke, and fenel, and rwe, and betony, and netles, and of
f. 110v   onouns, and chiboillis, / and þe iuse of yue, and mastike,
and womanes mylke, of eueriche, yliche moche.   And stampe
hem togedre and put alle in an holowe oynen.   And roste it

20   in axes.   Þen take it oute and wringe it þoroughe a clooþ
and put þerof in þe eere.   And it shal heel þe ache and þe
rennyng of þe eris.   Dieting of þis sykenes shal be as
in a feuer cotidian.

Chapter IV, Part 2
Apostem of the Ear

The postem of þe eris if it be of colde or of hete,

---

10 oynons] *corr. from* onons. 12 withouten] withouten with. þe]
prec. by clay *canc. in red.* 24 *2-line initial in blue.*

þou maist knowe by þe tokenes þat Y shewid in þe laste
chaptir tofore. And in heling of þis postem, þou shalt not
worche with repercussiues, but with mytigatiues; if it be
of hete, with maturatiues to make it to wexe repe. And if

5 þe postem be of hete, make a plastre of oile of roses, and

f. 111 of violettis, and þe rote of hoc/kis and betis y-medlid
togedre. Or take þe fatnes of a calfe, and þe grece of an
henne and of a gandir, and medle þerwiþ violettis, and
roses, and a litil waxe. And make of þis an oynement and

10 anoynte þe eris withoute with þe same. Or take hockes, and
bottir, and oyle of violettis or of roses. Or make an
oynement of gandres grece and henne-is grece and þe merie
of an herte. And if þe ache be greuous, take oile of
roses, and opium, and wexe, and medle hem togedre, and put

15 þerof in þe ʒeere; or ellis þe iuse of solatre, and oile of
roses, and þe white of an ey y-medlid togedre, and put
þerof in þe eere, dippid in a wike or in coton. Or take þe
grece of an eyron, and of an eel, and þe talowe of a goot

f. 111v bucke, and put / hem in an holowe oynen vndir hoot axen.

20 Þen wrenge it þoroughe a clooþ and put þerof a drope or
ii° in þe eeres. Þis is good for ache, and hete, and
defaute of heryng, and forto turne þe postem to quyter.
But if it comeþ of colde, vse þe oynementis þat Y tolde in
þe laste chaptir. And anoynte þe ere withoute with bottir

---

4 to (1)] *ins. above.* **18 of** (1)] *ins. above.*

or fatnes of bestis.   Þen ley þerto oþir maturatiues þat
maken postomes ripe forto breke.   And also crommes of brede
y-soden in wiyn and y-plastrid ben good.   And if egrimonye
be medlid with-al, it is þe bettir.

5   Good maturatif: Take grece, and oile, and hockis, and

[?]

f. 112

[146v]

10

betis, and egrimoyne, and make of hem a plastre and ley to
þe eere.   Also take þe iuse of shepperdis / ȝeerd, and þat
is good for postomes in þe eeres.   And þe iuse of syngrene
y-medlid with oile of roses ceesiþ þe ache of eeris and
helpeþ men þat ben deef.   But when þe postem is y-broke
and þe quytour flowiþ oute at þe eere, þou muste vse
mundificatyues to clense þe eere of quitour.   But
vndirstonde þat quitour of þe eris comeþ oþirwhiles of
breking of a postem, and oþirwhiles it comeþ of sum festre

15   of þe eere, and oþirwhiles it comeþ of sum oþir sikenes of
þe heed.   But wherof-so it comeþ, þou must vse
mundificatiues to clense þe eren.   And if it comeþ of þe
heed, vse þen þe medicynes þat purgen þe heed of suche
corrup humours.

f. 112v **20**   Good mundificatiues ben, myrre, nitre, and / hony

Mundificatives

y-medlid togedre; or alym, and myrre, and vinegre; or
olibanum y-resolued in þe iuse of sheppardis purse; or
salte y-medlid with woman-is mylke; or nitre, alym, and
hony; or comyn, castor, cost, y-medlid with vynegre; or

2 breke] *in l. h. margin.* **And**] *prec. by* ripe *canc. in red.* **5
maturatif**] *corr. from* maturatiues. **8 postomes**] *corr. from* postoms.
17 it] *ins. above.*

eueriche of þes by himsilf. And if þes þingis clensen not
þe eere, þen it semeþ þat þe quitour comeþ of sum festre.
And þan þe hede muste be ofte y-shaue and he must be cuppid
in þe necke, or y-sooken with watir lechis to drye þe place
5 aboute þe eris and to make þe flux ceese. Þen make a
stronge medicyn to go to þe rote of þe eere. And if it
ceseþ not, þen it is tyme to leue werke, lest þoroughe
violence of medicyns, þe eere or þe heed fal into a gret/-

f. 113   tir greuaunce. Þe root of a white vyne and a blacke wielde
10 vyne is þe best medicyn to clense þe ere of quiter and of
suche filþe, and it is also a good medicyn for deefnes.
And also þe iuse of a like, and of centorie, and of þe mawe
of an hare: not þe skynne, but þat þat is withinforþe, and
vynegre y-medlid togedre, clensen þe eere of longe
15 quitering. Also þe iuse of þe rote of radiche, and
cardamomum, and nitre, and drye fyges y-clensid and y-soden
in þe iuse of rwe or of radiche, and y-do þre daies into þe
ere, is good medicyn to make þe eris cleen of suche filþe.

[147]   But vndirstonde þat aftir þou hast put suche þingis into a
20 mannes ere, aftir oon houre is y-passid, þou must make him /

f. 113v   to snese, þat þe medicyn come clene oute, for drede of more
harme.

Chapter IV, Part 3
Flowing of Blood at the Ears

Flowing of blode at a mannes eris, oþirwhiles it
comeþ of smyting, oþirwhiles it comeþ fro withinforþe,

---

3 y-shaue] *corr. from* shaue. **6 it]** *ins. above.* **7 is]** *ins. above.* **to
leue]** *ins. above.* **13 of]** *ins. above.* **15 and]** *corr. from* or. **23** *2-line
initial in blue.*

72

and þat may be in ii⁰ maners, for oþirwhilis it haþ a
certeyn tyme of his flowing, as þe þridde day or þe iiii^e
day, eiþir more or lasse. And þis flowing is not good to
be y-staunchid, and namely if it comeþ of an-oþer sikenes,

5   and principaly in þe day þat it shulde flow.   Anoþir
flowing þer is þat is not at certeyn cours of flowing, but
comeþ oþirwhiles raþir, oþirwhiles latter.   And þat comeþ
oþirwhiles of plente of blode and of breking of sum veynes,
f. 114   or ellis of sum postem þat is y-broken / or þan he be
10   fulliche ripe. And wheþir it be oon or oþer, it muste be
helid by mundificatiues þat mown clense þe eere of þe blood
þat is withyn, and with consolidatiues þat moun soude þe
place þat is broken.   And it is good to menge with hem
special medicynes þat seruen to lete blood.   And be war þat

15   noon coolde medicyn, ne ful sharpe, ne biting entre into þe
eere.

A medicyn forto clense þe eere: Take þe iuse of leke
and of vynegre and medle hem togedre, or with wiyn þat
galles ben y-soden yn, and þe iuse of radiche togedre.

20   And aftir, take þe iuse of sheppardis purse and encense and
medle hem togedre, and put into þe eere, or þe iuse of
netles and sandragon y-medlid togedre, or encense and
f. 114v   womanes / mylke y-medlid togedre. Consolidatiues shullen
be y-leide boþe withyn and withoute, and mundificatiues

9 is] *ins. above.* **13 it is good to]** *in r. h. margin.*

withyn þat wolen make noon echyng. And euermore aftir þe
breking of a postem in þe eere, make a colliry with þe iuse
of leke and encense smale-y-beten and medlid togedre, or
oile of rooses and mastike. And if it make þe ere to hote,

5   medle þerwith woman-is mylke. And þis shal clense awei þe
quitering and kepe þe eere from festring. And wite wel þat

[?]   þer is no medisyn so good to clense þe eres as is a stufe
in þe maner þat Y told tofore.

Chapter IV, Part 4
Worms in the Ears

[147]   Also wormes in a mannes eeren comen in two maners:

10   Oon is y-gendrid withynforþe of corrupcion of þe eers,

f. 115   anoþir fro / wiþouten, þat crepen into þe eris. And wheþir
þei comen in o maner or in þe toþer, þei shal be slayn by
medicynes þat ben bitter. For suche wormes: Take oile of
lorer, and put it in þe eere, and stoppe it an hour

15   togedre, and if þer be a worme þeryn, þou shalt see him in
þe ere þer-as þe oile was. Þen, take þe iuse of wormod,
and of calamynte, and of bitter almondis, and put al in a
caule leef vndir asshes. Þen wringe oute þe oile and put
þerof in þe eere, or seeþ mirre and alloes in wiyn and put

20   þerof a drope into þe ere, or with a pipe þou may souke
oute þe worme. Or take þe iuse of radiche or of neep and
put into þe ere, for þes ii⁰ sleen creping wormes þat is

f. 115v   in þe ere. Also / þe iuse of wormod, of centory, of
horehone, of elleborus niger, sleeþ wormes in þe 3eere and

---

4 **it**] *ins. above.* 9 *2-line initial in blue.* 12 **þei** (1)] *corr. from* þe.
comen] *prec. by* þe *canc. in red.* **þei** (2)] *in r. h. margin.* 15 **him**] *prec.*
by cast *canc. in red.* 17 **put**] *prec. by* cast *canc. in red.* 20 **þe**] *ins.*
above. 22 **creping**] *prec. by* cle *canc. in red.* 24 **in þe 3eere**] *in l. h.*
margin.

[147v]   in þe wombe. A gode medicyn: Take a ripe appil and a wel-
smelling and warme him bi þe fyer, þat he be smelling. And
þen leye him to þe ere al ny3t. And ley þat ende þat growe
on þe tree of þe appil to þe ere as ny3he as þou may, and

5   on þe morwe þou shalt fynde þe worme in þe myddil of þe
appil. It may be knowen if wormes be in þe eere by iching,
and tincling, and mouyng withyn þe eere. An attir-coppe is
y-slayn þat is in þe ere with olde oile of notes, or with
syneuey, or piliol, or eleborus niger, or euforbe, or with

10   þe iuse of radiche y-medlid with oile. And þe iuse of

f. 116   chesteyn sleeþ also euery kynde of wormes in þe / eere, and
so doeþ þe iuse of centorye, þe iuse of lupines, þe iuse of
wielde gourdis. And aftir a worme is slayn or y-take oute
of þe ere, þen take mundificatyues to clense þe ere, and

15   consolidatiues to hele vp þe ere withinforþe. If a flee be

[?]   in þe ere, put a litil wolle in þe ere and he shal com to
þe wol.

Chapter IV, Part 5
Ringing in the Ears

[147v]   Ringing in a mannes eris, or oþer noise liche blowing
of hornes, comeþ in diuerse maneris: Oþirwhiles, of a

20   grete wyndi mater þat is in þe eere and moveþ vp and dovn
and al abouten withinforþe and may not oute for his
boistesnes, and þerfore þer is a contynuel ringing and
noyse in þe eeris; oþirwhiles, it comeþ of a viscouse

[147v]   corrupte humour þat stoppeþ þe eere withinforþe, and þan

---

2 **bi**] *corr. from* in. **14 mundificatyues**] *corr. from* mundicatyues.
16 to] *ins. above.* **18** *2-line initial in blue.* **22 boistesnes**] *corr. from*
boistnes.

Rynging or Sowning in þe Eris

f. 116v þer is moche gre/uaunce in þe eres. And if it comeþ of

[?] hete, it comeþ with bitternes of þe mooþ, and heuynes of þe

ri3t eere, and reednes and hete. And if it comeþ of colde,

it is with contrary signes and heuynes of þe lifte eere.

5 Oþirwhiles, it comeþ of feblenes of þe ere, and þan þe

[147v] ringing is withoute þes signes forseide. Of ringing þat is

of wyndi mater enclosid or of stopping þoroughe a viscouse

humour, þer is oon maner cure, saaf if it be of a corrupte

humour: 3yue him firste a purgacion þat accordeþ to þe

10 humour. If it is of hete, purge þe colere. If it is of

f. 117 colde, purge malen/coly. And make him to snese, and

aftirward make a stufe of been stalkis, and anise or comyn

y-soode wiþ hem, or of cleen benes y-soode by hemsilf.

And if it be of hete, seeþ wormod with hem, and anoon aftir

Hou

oile

of almondis

shal be

made

15 his stufe, put a drope in his ere of oyle þat is made of

bitter almondis. And þat is y-made in þis wise: Take

bitter almondes and stampe hem, and put hem in a closid

vessel vndir hote asshes. And aftir, wringe oute þe oile

of hem þoroughe a lynen cloþe. Or make a stufe of þes

20 seedis y-sooden in watir: þe seed of fenel, of parseli,

of anyse, of carewei, of dauke. And if þou wilt, put þerto

f. 117v lauendre and tyme. But if þe stop/ping be of colde, make a

colliry of mirre and castor. Or take þe iuse of radiche,

or of leke, or of oile of roses, or womanes mylke. Or take

6 ringing is withoute] *copied* is withoute ringing *and marked for reversal.* **is]** *prec. by* ere *canc. in red.* **8 is]** *ins. above.* **cure]** *prec. by* of *canc. in red.*

sum of þe oiles þat Y haue spake of in þe aking of þe eres.
And if it be of feblenes of þe eres, take þe iuse of
wormod, and medle it with warme vynegre, and put it in þe
ere. A good oynement for þe eris in al maner of greuaun-is

5 þat comen of colde: Take peletre of Spayne, and of castor,
dr. i; of mirre, of nitre, of long pepir, of rwe, dr. ii; of
euforbe, dr. i. Poudre al þes and medle hem with þe iuse
of radiche or of leke, of þe quantite of iiii oz. And see

f. 118 þat in medi/cynes of þe eris, þou do noþing withinforþe þat

10 is sharpe and biting but his malice be repressid and abatid

[148] by sum oþer þing þat is a mitigacion (not þe iuse of
radiche) þat is oon þe beste for greuaunce of þe erys.

Chapter IV, Part 6
Deafness

Deefnes of þe eris comeþ in meny maneris, boþe of þe
enchesons withouteforþe, as of smyting, and of þe enchesons

15 withinforþe. And þat may be in two maneris, as by þes
sikenesse of þe hede: litarg[i]e or frenesie, or by his
awne greuaunce wiþouten eny oþir greuaunce. And þat may bi
in ii° maneris: Oon is withyn bi þes sikenes þat Y haue
tolde herebefore; anoþir is bi stopping withoute bi a

20 wherte or growing of flesshe in þe hole of þe ere. If

f. 118v def/nes comeþ of a sekenes of þe hede, it is y-helid by þe
heling of þe selue sekenes. If it comeþ of eny of þes
forseide greuauncis, it is helid as þei ben. If it comeþ
of whertis or of þe flesshe growing, it shal be helid by

1 **spake**] *in l. h. margin.* 3 **and** (1)] *ins. above.* 13 *2-line initial in blue.* 16 **litargie**] litarge. **or** (1)] *corr. from* and. 17 **awne**] *in r. h. margin.* **bi**] *ins. above.* 19 **herebefore**] *in r. h. margin.* 23 **greuauncis**] *prec. by* sekenesses *canc. in red.*

corosiues þat shullen freten hem awei. If it comeþ of yuel
dispocicion of þe ere withinforþe, it haþ propir medicyns.

[148v] Neuerþeles, þe medicynes of oþer greuaunce of þe eris
helpiþ, if it may be helid, for þou shalt vndirstonde þat
5 olde sekenes of þe eris, and namely defnes, ben vncurable,
but defnes þat is newe and oþirwhilis grettir þen
oþirwhilis, may ben y-holpe. Defnes þer is also, þer-as a

f. 119 mannes heryng is bynome him, / is incurable but if it be
helid in þe begynnyng at þe taking þerof. And of what
10 encheson defenes comeþ, it mai be y-knowe by þat þat is
seide tofore. And if it be of eny corrupt humour, 3yue him
purgacions aftir þe kynde of þat humour. And make him to
snese, and aftirward make a stufe of been stelis and of
anise. And þen put in his eere þe iuse of radiche. Or
15 seeþ lorer leues and spikenard in wiyn, and let þe smoke
þerof come into þe ere þorou3he a pipe. Or put ampte eiren
in oyle and let hem roten þeryn and do þerof in þe eris.
And þe same maner þou mayst do with þe iuse of synegrene
and of oynons y-put in oile of lorer. Or take þe bowes of
20 green asshes and leye on þe fyer, and take of þe watir þat

f. 119v com/eþ at þe endes of hem þe quantite of a sponeful and
halfe, and put þerto ii° sponful of oile or of bottir, and
oon sponful of þe iuse of synegrene, and ii° sponful of
hony, and a sponful of womanes mylke þat norisseþ a man

---

4 helpiþ] *in l. h. margin.* 7 þer is also] *copied* also þat is *corr. and
marked for reversal.* 16 put] *prec. by* do *canc. in red.*

childe. And medle alle togedre. Þen put a drope or ii°
in þe ere and stoppe it. Or take þe ius of syngrene and þe
fatnesse of an eel yliche moche, and put þerof in þe eere,
or þe cleen grees þat dropeþ from a rosted eel, or castor,

5 or gumme of yuy and mirre y-medlid with þe iuse of radiche,
of rwe, or wormod, or of yuy. And if it comeþ of hete,
aftir purgacions and stufes, put þe iuse of syngrene in þe

f. 120   ere y-med/lid with þe fatnes of an eel. Þer-as defnes is
olde, take synegrene and put it in an erþen vessel y-closid

10 twelue monþes vndir þe erþe. And at þe ȝere-is ende, take
þe moistnes þat cleueþ by þe pottis side and do þerof in þe
deef ere. Oþer þingis þat Y tolde in þe ache of þe eris
ben good for defnes, and also þe iuse of houndestonge and
of saueyn ben good, boþe for oynementis and stufes of þe

15 eris, for þei open wel þe poores þat ben in þe eris, and
y-stoppid with corrupt humours.

Chapter V, The Nose
Part 1, The Pose

[?]   Here beginneþe þe fiueþe chaptir of þis boke þat
conteniþ foure titlis or practiues.

[150v]   In a man-is nose þer ben meny greuauncis, as þe pose,

20 stynche of þe nose-þirles, and flowing of blode at þe nose;
and withouten, þer is a greuaunce y-clepid gutta rosacea.

f. 120v   Oþer greuauncis þer ben also / of þe nose, as cancre, and
flesshe þat stoppeþ þe noseþirles, as noli me tangere. Of
an vnkyndeli humour and corrup þat is aboute þe brayn is þe

---

4 cleen] *corr. from* cleer. **5 or**] *ins. above.* **10 ȝere-is**] *prec. by* e
canc. in red. **17-18 Here . . . practiues.**] *in bottom margin.* **19** *2-line
initial in gold.*

[151] pose engendrid, for þat humour stoppeþ þe ouer-parte of þe

nose and letteþ a man of his smelling.   And as sum

men   seyen   þe   pose   is   a   stopping   of   þe   nose-þirles

þoroughe   a   revme,   for   as   þei   seien,   þe   revme   falleþ

5   oþirwhilis   dovne   into   þe   nose   and   makeþ   þe   pose.

Oþirwhiles   it   falleþ   into   þe   chekis,   and   makeþ   hem   swellen

and   aken.   Oþirwhilis,   it   falleþ   dovne   to   þe   rote   of   þe

teeþ,   and   þen   it   makeþ   hem   ake   and   rote.   Oþirwhilis,   it

falleþ   to   þe   rote   of   þe   tunge,   and   þen   it   makeþ   hir

f. 121   10   swelle   /   and   to   be   ouer-laxe,   and   bringeþ   hir   into   a

palesie,   and   makeþ   a   man   to   leesen   his   speche.   Oþirwhilis,

it   falleþ   dovn   to   þe   brest,   and   makeþ   þe   breste   stri3te.

Oþirwhilis,   it   falleþ   dovne   to   þe   li3te,   or   to   þe   stomake,

or   to   þe   reines,   or   into   a   mannes   guttis.   And   but   if   þe

15   membre   be   þe   more   mi3ti   to   put   it   awei   fro   him,   it   wole

make   þer   a   posteme.   Oþirwhilis,   it   falleþ   doune   amonge   þe

veynes   and   guttis   in   diuerse   placis   of   þe   bodi.   And

oþirwhilis,   it   roteþ   and   heteþ   in   þe   veynes   and   makeþ   a   man

to   falle   into   a   feuer.   Alle   þes   greuauncis   comen   of   revme,

20   and   þerfore   it   is   ful   nedeful   for a   man   to   kepe   him   from   þe

f. 121v   greuaunce   of   revme,   lest   he   falle   in/to   þes   forseide

sekenessis   and   greuauncis.   In   þe   pose,   a   man   haþ   moche

greuaunce   and   ache   in   his   forhede   and   in   his   i3en,   and

sneseþ   ofte,   and   smelliþ   febeliche.   And   if   it   comeþ   of

9 hir] *in l. h. margin.*

hete, a man shal feel sharpnes and grete hete in his
noseþirles. And if it comeþ of colde, he shal fele colde
þeryn. Neþeles, of salte humour þat flowiþ þoroughe þe
nose, þer comeþ smerting and sharpnes, and syþþe þis

5 greuaunce comeþ of þe hede. In þe begynnyng, ȝyue him a
purgacion and forbidde him to wasshe his hede and his fete.
And ȝyue no medicines, wheþir he be with a feuer or
withouten. And ley no dissolutiues þerto in þe beginnyng,

f. 122 ne sharp þingis, as stronge / wiyn; ne suche þingis þat

10 dissoluen more þen consumen and wasten, as þingis þat moche
pepir is yn; ne soure þingis, for þei wolen make þe mater
falle doune to þe breste and make him to chache a coughe.

[151v] And alle metis and drinkes þat he takeþ muste be hote. And
lete him be war of moche eting and drinking, and of late

15 soopers, and speciali of late drinking, and of moche slepe,

Late sopers
and drinkis
and moche
slepe
norisshen
revme

for þer is no-þing þat encreseþ and norissheþ revme more
þen late soopers, and drinkinggis, and moche slepe. And
also be war of moche liȝt, and moche smoke. And be war of
bleding, lest þe mater of þat revme be drawe into þe veynes

20 and be cause of more. Ne ȝyue him no laxatif to make him /

f. 122v a fluxe, leste þe mater falle dovne to þe breste or to þe
stomake and be cause of sum postem or of sum oþir
greuaunce. But if þe pose com of colde, and be not a ful
grete colde, make him a fumigacion of lignum aloes, and

---

10 and] *corr. from* as. 11 þe] *ins. above.* 13 And (1)] *corr. from*
þe. 20 Ne] *prec. by* ha *canc. in red.*

encense, and calamus aromaticus, and of lapdanum.   And
aftir, make him a stufe of lignum aloes, and of storax, and
of lap-danum.   And aftir his stufe, lett him drinke a litil
drau3te of good wiyn, or make a stufe of lorer leves and of
5   auence, or of roses.   And aftir þat, anoynte his hede with
hote oiles, as of lorer or of rwe.   Or þou may make him a
stufe of hote herbes and wel-smelling, as puliol, mynte,

f. 123   camamille, betayn, origane, / and suche oþir.   And make him
a fumigacion with hote sedis, as of fenel, anys, carewei,
10   whete bran, and suche oþer.   And if þou hast hem not alle,
take hem þat þou fyndest.   But þe beste stufe of al is y-
made of olibanum y-soden in wiyn, with roses, auence, and
fenel.   And aftir, make a plastre of affodille rotis y-
braied with wiyn and oile togedir, and y-warmed, and leied
15   on þe hede.   Good pillulis: Take of mirre, of olibanum, of
lapdanum, ana, dr. v; of opium, of henbane, of
houndistonge, and of radiche, ana, dr. iii.   And tempere
hem with watir of roses.   And make pillulis of hem of þe
quantite of a been.   And when he goeþ to bed, 3yue him fyue
20   of hem at oones.   Oþer good pillulis, when þe mater floweþ

f. 123v   from þe / heed to þe breste: Take of storax, mirre, opium,
ana, id est, yliche moche.   And tempere hem with dispumed
hony.   And make of hem pillulis of þe quantite of a pees,

[152]   and 3yue of hem ii⁰ or iiiᵉ when a man goeþ to bed.   But

3 litil] *ins. above.* **22 id est]** *ins. above.*

if it comeþ of hete, make him a stufe of watir þat mirre, camemille, and vynegre ben y-soden yn. Make þy stufe in þis wise: Do of þat watir on an hoot gloyng stoon and let þe fume þerof go vp into his nose. And anoynte þe forhede

5 with oile of violet and bottir y-medlid togedir. And if it be nede, purge þe heed of þe humour þat greueþ. And þen ley plastris þerto þat opium is medlid with, for it is good

f. 124   wheþir it comeþ of heet / or of colde. Reume þat comeþ of hete þat haþ longe be contynued in þe heed, it is ful harde

10 if it be euer helid. And it is profitable in þes ii⁰ causes to hele þe heed with herbis þat ben conuenient and acording to þe dissese, and not shaue þe heed, but dodden it. And þan þe heris and þe oynementis þat comen amonge hem wolen lye togedir in þe maner of an emplastir.

Chapter V, Part 2
Stinking of the Nostrils

15   Stynking of noseþirlis comeþ oþerwhilis of humours þat fallen doune fro þe heed to þe poores of þe noseþirlis and lyen þer and stynken. Oþerwhilis, it comeþ of strei3tnes of þe noseþirlis, for corrupte humours lyen withinforþe and movn not come oute for strei3tnes of noseþirlis.

f. 124v 20 Oþerwhilis it comeþ of bleynes and boc/ches withinforþe, for þei ben not wel y-clensid. If it be of strei3tnes of noseþirlis, it is incurable. If it comeþ of a bocche or of a byle withinforþe, it shal be helid þoroughe heling of a bocche. But if it be of þe heed, and þe nose be hool and

7 is(1)] *ins. above.* 9 be] *ins. above.* 14 emplastir] *prec. by a canc. in red.* 15 *2-line initial in blue.*

sounde, purge firste þe heed.   And if he haue heet and
pricking in his nose, put þeryn oyle of roses and of
violet, or oon of hem, and make him to snese.   And if he
haþ no pose, let him waisshe his heed with watir of roses
5   and violet, and þe rynde of popy is soden yn.   And þen
plastir þe herbes on his hede.   If it be of þe pose, heel
þe pose.   And if it is of cold, and withoute aking and
pricking, and he haue no pose, make him to snese wiþ þe
f. 125   poudir of piretre, and of canel, and of castore, / and of
10   seneuey, of eueriche, yliche moche.   And if þe nose may not
suffre þes sharpe poudirs, þou muste vse esy desiccatiues
to drye vp þe nose, as poudir of roses, or of beenes, or of
canel.   Mastike y-chewid is ful gode also, and to ben y-
cupped or y-horned in þe necke-pitt.

Chapter V, Part 3
Nosebleed

[?]   15   Flowing of blode at a mannes nose comeþ in many
maneris and of diuerse causes.   Oþerwhilis it comeþ for
sharpnes and kenship of þe blood þat persiþ þe veynes,
oþerwhilis for sotilte of þe blood, and oþerwhiles for
[152v]   grete abundance of blood.   If it be on þe firste maner, þes
20   ben þe tokenes: Þe blood is hote, and cleer, and rede, and
biteþ þe nose in his flowing.   If it be of þe seconde
maner, þe blood is þinne, and moche flowing where-euer it
f. 125v   stondeþ.   And if it be of / þe þridde maner, þer comeþ
moche blode oute at þe nose, and þe veynes ben ful neisshe

3 he] *ins. above.*   **4 waisshe]** *corr. from* wasshe.   **8 he]** *ins. above.*
11 vse] *prec. by* ta *canc. in red.*   **15** *2-line initial in blue.*

and ful of blood. But of whiche maner þat it be, it may be
in ii⁰ maneris: in sikenes or oute of sekenes.   And it
may be in sekenes in ii⁰ maneris: eiþir hauing a certeyn
tyme for his flowing, as þe seconde day or þe þridde; eiþir
5 comyng vncerteynliche, oþerwhilis raþe oþerwhilis latter.
And wheþir it be in oon maner or in oþer, if it liȝteþ a
man of his oþer sekenes, it is not good to staunche it.   If
a man be þe febler aftir his bleding and he haue tokenes of
lijff, it is good to staunche it, but not sodenli, but if a
f. 126 10 man be moche y-feblid by his bleding. / And whiche of alle
þes maneris nose-bleding be, it may be of þe lyuer, or of
þe spleen, or of þe emeroides.   And suche bleding is
profitable.   But if it comeþ of þe lyver, þes ben þe
tokenes: greuaunce of þe riȝt side, reednes of þe vryn and
15 bleding of þe riȝt nose-þirle.   And if it be of þe spleen,
þe spleen swelleþ and þe lifte side is y-greued.   And þe
lift nose-þirle blediþ.   And if in þe nose-bleding þe lyuer
or þe liȝt swelleþ, or if aftir þe staunching of þe blood
[153]   þe body is infecte with ȝelow spottis, it is a token of
20 deeþ.   If it is of moche blood, þou muste worche with ii⁰
maner medicynes: sum to make þe blood þicke, as a coolis
f. 126v   of an / olde henne, and harde ȝolkis of eggis, and oþer
þingis þat Y wole speke of in þe fluxe of þe wombe.   It
behoueþ also to haue medicynes þat ben strictory to leye to

3 be] *ins. above.* 4 eiþir] *corr. from* oþer. 8 tokenes] *corr. from*
tokens. 18 aftir] *in r. h. margin.* þe (3)] *ins. above.* 24 medicynes]
corr. from medicy.

þe forheed and also þe nose, to staunche þe blood. And if
þer flowiþ moche blood, it shal not be sodenly y-stauchid
by stronge strictories, but by easy strictories, as sugir
roset, and syrip of roses, and suche oþer esy þingis y-
5   leyde to þe forhede and to þe nose. And if a man blede
moche for grete plente of blood, and he haue no feuer
tercian, ne noon suche sharp sekenes, let him blede at þe

f. 127   heed veyne of þe arme on þe same / syde þat his nose
blediþ. And his dieting shal be with smale ale and suche
10   metis þat makiþ litil blode, as herbes and frutis. And

[153v]   leye consolidatiues withouten-forþe, for þe grete plente of
blood brekiþ þe veynes. But if it comeþ of sotilnes of
blood, let him ete suche metis þat makeþ þe blood þicke, as
riys, and harde ȝolkes of eggis, and oþer metis þat Y shal
15   speke of in þe fluxe of þe wombe. Meny þingis þer ben þat
staunchen blood, as coral, emachites, and sangrinarie þat

[153]   is sheppardis purse. Also a plastir y-made of barly mele,
sandragon, and encense, and þe white of an ey y-medlid
togedir; or a lynen clooþ y-wette in colde watir and y-

f. 127v 20 leide to þe forhede or to þe / þrote. Also smelle of
stinking þingis is good, as swynes dritte, and þe heris of
an hare y-brent, or oþer heris, or of hornes y-brent. And
if it be of þe lyver, make a plastir for þe lyuer of þe
rynde of elme y-poudrid, and of sandragon, and boole, and

---

3 **by** (1)] *prec. by* ne *canc. in black.* 4 **oþer**] *prec. by of canc. in*
red. 7 **tercian**] *prec. by of canc. in red.* 9 **shal**] *in r. h. margin.* 10 **þat**
makiþ litil blode] *in r. h. margin.* 17 **sheppardis**] shappardis. 22 **of**]
ins. above. 23 **it**] if. 24 **boole**] *corr. from* bole.

mastike y-medlid with þe iuse of synegrene, or of verueyn,
or of planteyn. And put þerto spodie and roses. And if it
comeþ of þe spleen, do þerto medicynes þat Y shal speke of
[153v] in þe sekenes of þe spleen. And let his priuey membre be
5   y-put in a disshe with vynegre. Or take rede netlis and
salt y-stampid togedir and put þe iuse in his nose, or
f. 128 ellis þe poudir of þe same netlis y-brent, / or þe poudir
of þe shellis of eggis y-brent. Or ellis take sangrinary
and bruse it and make him to holde þat in his hande. And
10 þat shal staunche his blood. Or put vnsleckid lyme and
coperos or attrament vppon þe veyne, and it shal staunche
þe blood. And so wolen an hote yren y-leyde þerto where-
euer it be. And þoughe it be good to staunche blood at þe
nose, it is ful profitable oþerwhilis to make þe nose to
15 blede, as in þe frenesy and in þe hede-ache. And þat þou
may do if þou put a branche of saueyn in þe nose-þirl or
þe leef of mylfoil.

Chapter V, Part 4
Gutta Rosacea

[156]   Gutta rosacea is an infeccion of þe nose withoutenforþ
of moche reednes. And oþerwhilis, it is a token þat a man is
20 disposid to be a mesel. And it comeþ oþerwhilis of
f. 128v blo/de, and oþerwhilis of coler. And it is not þe morfu,
but it is clepid a rosi goute. And if it comeþ of blood,
þes ben þe tokenes: iching of þe nose and lyking in þe
yching, and breking vp of pemples þat soone turnen to

---

9 bruse] *followed by* sed *canc. in red.* **þat**] *corr. from* þe. **10
vnsleckid**] *corr. from* vnslekid. **12 an**] *in r. h. margin.* **yren**] *corr. from*
eyren. **15 þat**] *ins. above.* **16 nose-þirl**] *corr. from* nose-þirles. **18** *2-
line initial in blue.* **19 man is**] mannes. **21 is**] *ins. above.* **þe**] *ins.
above.*

quytour. If it comeþ of coler, þer is iching and pricking
in þe nose and pymples þat ben þeron quiteriþ not but
litil. And þe place of þe greuaunce is harde in þe
handling. And if it is of blood eiþir in þe necke or in þe
5 cop of þe nose, he muste blede or be y-cuppid vndir þe chyn.
Wheþir it be of blood or of coler, make him a purgacion.
But firste, to defie þe mater, 3yue him to drinke of þe

[157]   syrip of fumiter and oximel y-medlid togedir, of boþe
f. 129   iliche moche. / Aftir þis, make him a stufe of colde
10 herbis, as of fumiter, scabious, and suche oþer. And aftir
his purgacion, lete him blede, to drawe awey þe blood from
his visage. And aftir, make a stufe of watir þat wormod,
and hockis, and violettis, and þe smale chaf of barly and
otis been y-soden yn. And aftir, anoynte him with þis
15 oynement: Take barly mele, and femigreke, and as moche of
madir, and of planteyn y-poudrid, and medle hem with þe
iuse of oynons and hony dispumed. Of cancre of nose and

[?]   of noli me tangere, Y wol speke withinforþe.

Chapter VI, The Mouth
Part 1, Cracked Lips

Here beginneþ þe sixte chaptir of þis boke þat conteneþ
20 iiº titles or practi[s]es. Capitulum viᵐ:
In a man-is mouþe þer ben meny greuauncis, as cleving
of lippis, stenking of mooþ wiþinforþe, ache, and oþer

f. 129v   greuaunce / of þe teeþ, and sekenes of þe tunge. Cleving
[156v]   of lippis is in meny maneris, as of pimples y-broke, or of

---

19-20 *in bottom margin*. **20 practises**] practies. **21** *4-line initial in gold.*

smyting, eiþir of an yvel humour and a corrupt þat cleviþ
to þe lippis, or of colde, or of wiynde, or of cancre.   But
if it be of smyting, it shal be helid as oþer woundis.   And
if it be eny of þes oþer maneris, it may ben y-helid with
5   an oynement y-made of oile of violet or of roses, and waxe
y-medlid togederis; or with an oynement y-made of þe iuse
of sorel and of oile and wexe togedir; or with wexe and
henbane sede soden in oile.   Also þe poudir of portulake
heliþ and hideþ þe cleving of mesel lippis, if portulak be
f. 130   10   y-brent.   For cleving of þe lip/pis or of þe tunge and for
bledders withyn þe mooþ, make an oynement of þe poudir of
licium, and amyde, and penides y-medlid with þe watir of
roses.   And anoynte þerwith þe same greuaunces.   A-noþir
for þe same greuauncis, and for cleuyng of þe roof of þe
15   mooþ: Take dragagant, and resolue it in colde watir, and
clense it, and medle þerwith þe poudir of amyde.   And
þerwith anoynte þe soor with a feþir.   And if þe greuaunce
be of moist pemplis, anoynte it with cleen hony, or with þe
poudir of benes y-brent and hony, or with þe poudir of
20   portulake and hony y-medlid.   Also þe iuse of centory, and
of wormod, and of aristologie þe rounde is good þerfore.
f. 130v   Also for cleving of þe lippis and of / tittis, melte wex,
and oile of violet or oile de olyf togedir.   And put þerto
þe poudir of mastike and of olibanum togedir.   And þerwith

1 eiþir] *in l. h. margin.*   4 if] *corr. from* of.

anoynte þe soor. Or take poudir of roses and medle it with
gumme resolued in watir. Or medle sandris and þe poudir of
roses, and gumme, and ceruse, with watir of roses, and
anoynte þe sore lippis. For cleuing of þe lippis þoroughe
5 cold or þorou3 contageous wiynde, anoynte hem with hony.
And þen strawe þeruppon þe povdir of colofoyne. And if þe
lippis swellen, make an oynement of þe iuse of pasnep leues
and of litarge y-medlid togedir, and þerwith anoynte his
lippis.

Chapter VI, Part 2
Stinking of the Mouth

10 Stynking of þe mouþ comeþ operwhilis of corrupcion of
þe gummes and of þe teeþ; oþerwhilis it comeþ of þe
stomake; oþer/whilis it comeþ of þe li3te. If it comeþ of
þe teeþ and of þe gummes, frote and rubbe þy gummes with þi
fyngir and þy mouþe wil stynke. If it comeþ of þy stomake,
15 þe mouþe stynkeþ whilis a man is fasting. And al þe while
his mouþe is open, me shal smelle þe stynche. If it comeþ
of þe li3te, me shal smelle þe stynche þou3he þe mouþe be
closid. If it comeþ of þe teþe and of þe gummes, if þer be
eny roted flesshe, let freten it awei and þen hele it vp.
20 If þer be no roten flesshe, let þe mouþe be wasshe with
wiyn þat birche or myntis ben y-soden yn. And let þe
gummes be wel rubbid with a sharpe lynen clooþ vnto þey
bleden. And let him ete / origanum, mynte, and peletre,
til þey be wel chewid. And let him rubbe wel his teeþ with

[158v]

f. 131

f. 131v

---

10 *2-line initial in blue.* þe] *ins. above.* 15 þe (1)] *corr. from* þy.
22 þey] þy.

þes herbis y-chuwid and also his gummes. And þis is good
also if þe flesshe of þe gummes beþ y-rotid. And let him
drinke euery euentid wiyn þat ysope, or canel, or spike, or
quibibis ben y-soden yn.   And let him absteyne him from
5   grete metis and yuel-y-sauorid, and from moiste metis as

[159]   mylke and suche oþer.   And aftir euery mele, let him
waisshe wel his mooþ and rubbe wel his gummes and his teeþ
so þat no corrupte mater abyde amonge þe teeþ. And let him
vse þis poudir: Take of pepir, oz. i; and of myntis, as
10   moche; and of sal gemme, as moche. And make him to chewe
þis poudir a good while in his mooþ, and þen swolle it

f. 132   dovn.   But if þis com/eþ of þe stomake, it comeþ of a
corrupte fleume þat is in þe stomake.   And þan þe stomake
muste be y-purgid of fleume, as Y shal telle in þe sekenes
15   of þe stomake. And make him to absteyne him from al maner
fisshe, and flesshe, and herbis þat maken moche flevme in a
mannes body.   And let him oftesiþes waisshe wel his moþe
and rub wel his teeþ, as euery day oones or ii.   And
oþirwhile with a sharpe lynen clooþ, rubbe hem þat þe blode
20   renne oute of hem.   Þen make him to chewe swete-smelling
þingis.   Neuerþeles, moche chewing of spicis apperiþ þe
sauour of þe mooþ, for þei dissoluen moche þe corrupcion of
þe gummes and make þe mooþe stinke more þen he did. And

f. 132v   let him vse þes pillules þat ben good for / alle maner

---

1 **is]** *prec. by* doing *canc. in red.* 2 **beþ]** *corr. from* be. 7 **waisshe]**
corr. from wasshe. 8 **no]** *ins. above.* 11 **swolle]** *prec. by* sol *canc. in*
red. 17 **waisshe]** *corr. from* wasshe. 18 **as]** *ins. above.* 24 **pillules]**
pullules.

styngkingis of þe mooþ: Take of clowes, notemyggis, canel,
and of macis, dr. viii; of rede sandris, dr. x; of
quibibis, dr. vii; of cardamomum, dr. v; of lignum aloes,
oz. i; of gallia muscata, dr. v. Tempere hem with þe iuse

5   of myntis and make pillules of þe quantite of a fygge. And
let him to haue ii° of hem vndir his eiþir sidis of his
tonge at oones. Also, take good aloes and poudir hem and
tempere hem with þe iuse of wormod. And 3yue him iiie
sponeful at morwe and as moche at evene. And anoon aftir,

10   let him take as meny sponeful of hony. And let him do so
eueri day til he be easid. By þis maner meny men han ben
helid.   And if it comeþ of roten teeþ, let him rubbe wel

f. 133   his te/eþ with þe poudir of hertis horne y-brent. And if
it comeþ of þe heed, it is holsum to eten hote spicis and

15   wel-smelling. And if it comeþ of þe li3te, þen heel þe
li3t. And if þe stenche is not destroied by alle þes
maneris of medicynes, þen hele it with pillulis y-holden
in þe mooþ of swete-smellyng spices.

Chapter VII, The Teeth
Part 1, Toothache

[?]   Here beginneþ þe seueneþe chaptir of þis boke, þat
20   conteneþ þre titlis or pract[is]es. Capitulum viim:

[159]   In a mannes teeþ ben diuerse greuauncis: ache,
wormes, stynking, rotenes. Ache comeþ in diuerse maneris:

[159v]   Oþerwhilis, it comeþ of þe hede and of þe humour of þe heed
þat falleþ doun into þe teeþ, and þan comenli þe ouer-teeþ

19-20 *in bottom margin.* **20 practises]** practes; *corr. from* prates
to practes. **21** *4-line initial in gold.* **23 hede]** *prec. by* stomake of
canc. *in red.* **24 teeþ]** *prec. by* heed *canc. in red.*

f. 133v   aken. Oþerwhilis, it com/eþ of þe stomake, and þen þe
neþir teeþ aken. Oþerwhilis, it comeþ of ii° hote metis
þat a man etiþ, or of ii° colde, or of a sodeyn changing
fro hote metis to colde, or of ri3t sovre metis, or ri3t

5   keen, or of corrupte metis þat cleuen bitwene þe teeþ, for
þe teeþ ben not þicke y-nowe sette, but a-twyny.
Oþerwhilis, þe ache comeþ of corrup humours þat ben at þe
rote of þe teeþ. And if it comeþ of hete of þe heed, þe
chekes ben to-swollen, and reed, and hoot. In ache þat

10   comeþ of cold, þer is palenes of þe cheke and colde of þe
teeþ. And if it comeþ of moistnes, þer is swelling and
softenes of þe cheke, and if it comeþ of drines, þer is

f. 134   hardenes and litil swelling with þe ache. And / so if þe
cheke be swarte rede, þe ache is ful kene. And if it is of

15   flevme, þei ben ful whijt and þe ache is with heuynes. Of
blood comeþ reednes and swelling of þe chekis. Of
malencoly comeþ swart 3elewnes of þe chekis, with litille
swelling, and grete heuynes in þe ache. And if it comeþ of
þe heed, it may be knowe by greuaunce of þe heed. If it

20   comeþ of a keen humour amonge þe teeþ, it makeþ wormes in
þe teeþ, eiþir it makeþ þe teeþ holewe. And if it comeþ of
þe heed and þer be no rewme, let him blede on þe heed veine
of þe arme. And if þe body be ful of blood, let him blede

f. 134v   at / þe veyne þat is vndir þe tunge. And þat is good for

---

10 þer] þat. **14 swarte]** *prec. by* harde *canc. in red.* **þe]** *prec. by*
and *canc. in red.*

þis greuaunce, and for þe breest, and to make a man to haue
a cleer voice. But if it comeþ of colde, let him not blede
at no veyne, but let him be cuppid in þe necke-pitte. And
if it comeþ of rewme, make þat þe humours flowen not to þe
5   teeþ, and if it comeþ of hete, with fumigacions of roses y-
soden in watir, eiþir oþer colde herbes þat movn let þe
humours of her course. And if þe revme is of colde, make a
fumigacion of encense. And in boþe causes, a fumigacion of
henbane and of leke seed is good. And if it comeþ of þe
10 stomake, let him chewe portulake or solatre with vynegir, /
and purge þe stomake of corrupcion. A strictorye to ley
vppon þe templis to staunche þe flowing of þe humour þat
comeþ from þe heed, shal be made of mastike, of bole, of
sandragon, and þe white of an egge. And it is good to leye
15 colde plastris to þe chynne with a quantite of myntis y-
medlid þerwith. But if þe ache be ful greet, leie a
plastir withouten of henbane or of opium. And medle
galbanum, mirre, and opium togedir, and ley to þe tooþ or
in þe tooþ, or mirre with vynegir, eiþir henbane bi
20 himsilf. But if it be of revme, ley þerto no vynegir, and
namely if þe ache be on þe side, but make a plastir of
roses, and of watir lilies, and henbane with peri/tory or
comyn. And if al þis helpiþ not, it semeþ þat þe ache
comeþ of sum worme, or þat þe teeþ ben y-persid bi sum

f. 135

[160]
f. 135v

13 shal] *prec. by* it *canc. in red.*

corrupte humour, eiþir y-rotid. And if it be with swelling of þe cheke, it is a token of a postem of þe gummes. And if þe ache be greuous withouten swelling, it is token of a worme. For þe toþe-ache: Take galbanum, and of gumme

[?] 5 edere, and poudir of gallis, and povdir of gynger, and grinde hem togedir. And þen make of hem ballis of þe quantite of a filbert, and swe al in a cloute. And þen wete it in vynegir and ley to þe tooþ. Or take ix leues of sauge, and ix croppis of rede netle, and ix pipir cornes in

10 þe same maner.

Chapter VII, Part 2
Worms in the Teeth

[160] For in þe beginnyng of wormes in þe teeþ, þe ache is ful kene, and þan it may ben y-helid with þe smoke of

f. 136 henbane. But aftirward it is ful harde to / destroy þe worme. And þerfore þe toeþ moste be drawen oute. And

15 þeras þe ache is colde, it is perilouse to drawe oute a tooþ. In ache þat comeþ of blood, it sufficiþ to blede. And if it comeþ of coler, let him be purgid with a colo[go]ge and haue fumigacions of colde herbis, and namely of henbane. And if it comeþ of flevme þat falleþ dovn from

20 þe heed, let him of his course bi strictories. And if it comeþ of þe stomake, let þe stomake be purgid. And þan make a litil bagge of þe quantite of þi lytil fyngir, and ful it with þis poudir: Take peritre, pipir, castor, staphi, euforbe, and make poudir of hem. And put hem as Y

8 **take**] *ins. above.* **14-15 And . . . colde**] *in r. h. margin.* **17 it**] *ins. above.* **18 cologoge**] colage.

haue seide in a bagge. Þen seeþ þe bagge in vynegir. And
f. 136v þen ley / þe bagge bitwene his teeþ and make him gnawe
faste þeron. And if þe humours comen from þe heed to þe
teeþ, make him a gargarisme to gnawen on of wiyn þat ysope

5 is soden yn, and also piretre, and euforbe, and pipir. And
make a plastir of amoniac and of poudir of brenston y-knede
by þe fyer, and þen al warme ley to þe place þat akeþ. And
if it comeþ of revme, make him a fumigacion of þe smoke of
encense and of clowes poudrid and mengid togedir. And

10 among al herbis origanum is best for ache of teeþ þat comeþ
of colde, for þe wiyn þat origanum or mentastre ben soden
yn is good to be holden in þe mooþ, and þe herbis to ben y-
f. 137 plastrid withou/ten; also a plastir y-made of hony and of
salte, eiþir of hony and of storace. A strictory to lye

15 on þe templis: Take þe poudir of encense, of mastike, and
of spike, y-medlid with þe white of an egge. Medicines
special for þe toþe-ache: Oon is, take þe watir þat is
distillid of þe rede netlis, and wete a cloute þeryn and
ley to þe soor cheke. Or take þe iuse of netlis and medle

20 þerwith halfe so moche of rede wiyn. And wete þen a cloute
þerin and ley to þe cheke. Or take piretre and seeþ it in
vynegir and chewe it a good while in þy mooþ. Þen spet it
oute. And do so ofte til þou be amendid. In þe same maner
þou maist chewe iiii^e or v greynes, or of staffie, or of

1 þe] *prec. by* al *canc. in red.* **And**] *ins. above.* **2 make**] ma. **7
fyer**] *prec. by* fyngir *canc. in red.* **12 be holden**] beholden. **14 lye**]
corr. from leye. **16 an**] *ins. above.* **17 Oon is**] *ins. above.* **24 or v**] *in
r. h. margin.* **of** (1)] *ins. above.*

f. 137v

[160v]

mastike, or of galbanum. And alwei spit oute þe fleume,
and take of þy medicyn ofte/tymes and spit it oute alwei
til þou be wel purgid. Also stampe polipodie and medle it
with salte, and make þerof a plastir and leye to þe cheke.

5 Or do of þe iuse in noseþirlis. Or take þe poudir of gynger,
and of pipir, and of piretre, and of cost, and rub wel þe
teeþ þerwith. Or take þe iuse of garlik and poudre of
pepir and medle togedir, and put þerof in þe ȝeere of þe
hole cheke. And also alym, and salte, and columbine, and

10 verueyn, and origanum, and mynte, y-stampid togedir is
gode, and þe poudre of hem y-leide to þe tooþ. And þe iuse
of carsis y-put in þe eris ceesen þe ache of þe teeþ. Þe
same doen þe rotis of netlis y-soden in vynegir, and þe

f. 138   rotis y-plastrid to þe cheke. And þe same doeþ þe ro/tes

15 of pentafilon and of camedreos. If þe ache ceesiþ not by
alle þes medicines, þen worche with stupefactiues, as with
henbane and opium. And if þei ceesen not þe ache, drawe
oute þe tooþ.

Chapter VII, Part 3
Rotting of the Teeth

Rotenes of teeþ comeþ of þe same enchesons þat þe
20 toeþ-ache comeþ. And þei ben y-saued from roting by þingis
þat comforten þe teeþ, as to rub hem with þe poudir of
canel and with mastik, eiþir with þe poudir of origanum, or
of myntis, or of nitre. But it is not good to rubbe þe

[161]   teeþ with riȝt-hote spicis, for þei wol make hem to root þe

---

15 ache] *ins. above.* **16 þes]** *ins. above.* **19** *2-line initial in blue.*

f. 138v

raþir. And also mirre, and egrimoyne, and verveyn, and
gallis þat enke is made of, and olibanum, kepen þe teeþ
from rotyng, / and comforten hem moche. To drye þe teeþ
aftir mete with a drye lynen clooþ is profitable, for þat
5 shal clense hem, þat no mete cleue not, ne no corrupcion
amonge þe teeþ to make hem roten.

Chapter VIII, The Tongue and Throat
Part 1, The Tongue

[?]

[164v]

Here beginneþ þe viii chaptre of þis boke, which
contenieþ but ii° titlis.

A man-is tonge haþ two seruicis. Oon is to taast with
10 a mannes metis and drinkis; anoþir is to speke. And
þoroughe diuerse greuauncis þat comen of corrupte humours,
a mannes tunge is oþerwhiles indisposid, þat a man may
neiþir speke ne taast. Greuauncis of þe tunge ben
postemes, and bledders, eiþir stopping of hir snewis

f. 139

þorou3 / corrupte humours þat maken þe tonge laxe, and
fallen into a palesye. And if þer be a postem eiþir a
blayne ouer þe tonge, if it be of blood, þe tonge is to-
swolle, and reed, and hoot, and nesshe, and aking. And if
it is of coler, þe tonge is ful hoot, and cytryn, þat is to
20 sey, a derke reed. Þe ache is more sharpe þan of blood,
and þe swalme ne þe sooftnes is not so moche as of blood.
But if it is of fleume, þe tonge is colde, and swelling,
and nesshe, and of white colour. Of malencoly, comeþ
cooldnes, and swarte 3elov colour. And þe tunge swelliþ

1 also] *corr. from* þerfore. 2 kepen] *prec. by* for þe *canc. in red.* 8
ii° titlis] *corr. from* oo ii° chaptres. 9 *5-line initial in gold.* A] I. a
cued in margin. 12 indisposid] *prec. by* v *canc. in red.* 15 tonge] *ins.*
above.

not, but is sumwhat y-drawe togedir. Þese ben þe tokenes
by þe whiche þou may knowe what humour is þe cause of þe

f. 139v palesie of þe tunge. And if þe blei/nes of þe tunge
be blacke eiþir grene, it is a token þat þe tunge is

5 y-cancrid. For postoms and bleynes þat comen of colde, lete
him vse hote gargarisme to chewe in his mooþ and to make
him snese; and hoot fumigacions for þe heed, as with anet,
mellilote, camomille, and sansuke, y-soden. And let his
heed be anoyntid with hote oynementis þat moun dissolue þe

10 materis. But if it be of hete, lete him vse fumigacions,
gargarisms, and oynementis, and emplastris on his heed of
colde þingis, as Y tolde in þe sekenes of þe heed. And let
him bleed in boþe þe veynes vndir þe tunge, and þen wasshe
his mooþ with colde þingis. And anoynte þe tunge as Y tol/-

f. 140 15 de in cleuing of þe lippis hou þe bleines of þe mooþ shulde
be helid. And if þe complexion of þe tunge be colde, vse
suche þingis as Y wol telle in þe palesy of þe tunge. And
if þe posteme is harde, make him a gargarisme of mylke, and

[165] of watir þat drie figes and fenel ben y-soden yn. And if

20 it be of colde, wasshe it with watir of camomille, and make
a gargarisme of syneuey and of hony. For pimples þat ben
of heet, let him holde þe iuse of sycomour eiþir of
weybrode vndir his tunge, or þe iuse of solatre, and medle
þat with rede sandris and watir þat sumac, eiþir balaustia,

5 **y-cancrid**] *corr. from* cancrid. 6 **and**] *ins. above.* 7 **him**] *in l. h.
margin.* 12 **heed**] *prec. by* þingis *underd.* 22 **sycomour**] *prec. by*
licoris *canc. in red.*

eiþir mirre, eiþir roses, ben y-soden yn.

f. 140v

[165v]

     A poudir for postemes of þe tunge: Take of dispu/med hony, oz. sex; of þe iuse of erþe appel and of þe milke of a fyge tree, oz. ii; and seeþ hem on an esy fyer. Þen medle

5 with hem þis poudir: Take tartarum of whijt wiyn, and synevei, of eiþir, oz. i; of white pepir, and of sugir, oz. 1/2; of borace, oz. ii; of olibanum, and os sepie, dr. ii. Poudir al þes and medle hem with þe oþer forseide þingis, and þerwith anoynte þe soor withyn þe mooþ. If þe tunge

[?] 10 haue þe palesy þoroughe sum corrupte humour þat stoppiþ þe senewis, of what humour þat it be, þou maist knowe by þe

[165] tokenes þat Y haue told tofore. And if it be of blood, let him blede at þe veynes þat ben vndir þe tunge. And aftir þat, let him holde castor vndir his tunge, or þe iuse of /

f. 141 15 wilde caul. And vndirstonde þat caul seed comfortiþ moche

[?] þe tunge and þe þrote. And þe token þerof is, for þe ny3tengale aftir þat he haþ ete suche seedis, he syngeþ merely. Aftirwarde, let him waisshe his mooþ with oxymel, and pepir, and syneuey, and ysope, and origanum. And þen

20 let him chewe drie piretre or mastike, or staphie and mastike togedir. And let him rubbe his tunge with þe poudir of piretre, and of pipir, and of staphie, and of synevei, of castor, of gynger, of sal gemme, of sal nitre, or of sal armoniake. And if þou wilt, þou may put þerto

18 waisshe] *corr. from* wasshe.

clowes, notemygis, galengal, cardamomum, spike, and suche

oþer þingis. And of þes þou may make a gargarisme.   Eiþir

f. 141v   þus: Take origanum, piretre, / gynger, pepir white and

[165]   black and also long, canel, ysope, nigelle, sansuke, cost,

5   of eche, yliche moche. Tempere hem with oximel. And herwith

þou may also rub þe gummes on boþe sidis, and þe tunge

aboue and byneþe.

[?]   A syrip þerfore: Take auence, and þe flovres of

borage, anthos, drie sauge, calamynte, origanum, baies of

10   lorer, pionie, lauendre, þe herbe of þe palesy, of carses,

ana, oz. i; of quibibis, of reed sandris, of roses, of

melisse, of amomum, ana, oz. 1/2. Stampe hem smale and

seeþ in iiii pyntis of clene watir vntil half be wastid.

Þen streyne it and put it ouer þe fier, and let seeþ with

15   an esy fier.   Þen put þerto ii° povnd of sugir or ellis of

hony.

f. 142   An oy/nement for þe palesi of þe tunge: Take þe iuse

of sauge, oz. i; of wormod, of maioran, and of marche, ana,

oz. i; of baies: of lorer, of iuniper; of castor, oz. i;

20   of marciaton, and of oile of lorer, oz. ii; of reed wexe, a

quartron. Medle hem togedir and þerwith anoynte þe tunge.

[165]   A stufe for þe same cause: Take mug-wede or worte,

myntis, horhovne, origanum, calament, carses; of þe herbe

of þe palesi if þe palesi be of colde eiþir of plente of

---

17 palesi of þe] *in r. h. margin.* **22 wede or]** *ins. above.*

humours aboute þe tunge. Þo þat han þis sekenes must leue
al maner fleumatike metis, and oþer metis þat ben yuel to
defien; and vse sage in her metis, and leeke, and oynons,
and leve stronge wyne and drinke smale wiyn; and baþe not

f. 142v **5** moche, na/mely when þei ben replet. A gargarisme for þe
same: Take origanum, piretre, pepir white and also longe,
ginger, canel, ysop, nigel, sangsuke, coost, ana, yliche
moche. Poudir hem and tempere hem with sape, þat is, swete
vinegir, and make it vp wiþ oximel.

Chapter VIII, Part 2
Quinsy

10 Squynacy is a postem of þe þrote þat lettiþ a man boþe

[177] forto speke and forto chewe his mete. And it wole
strangelen a man but if it be holpen. And if þe postem be
of blode, þes ben þe tokenes: fulness of þe veynes;

[177v] reednes of þe visage, and swelling, and hete; a great

15 pouse, and a stronge, and a swifte. If it be of coler,
þes ben þe tokenes: greet anguisshe, grete hete, and þurste,

f. 143 and bitternes of þe mooþ, and moche flevme / and smoke in
wesaund. Þe pouse is voide, but he is stronge and swifte.
Of viscouse fleume, þer is not so grete ache as is of þe

20 oþer humours. But þer is a swalme, and þe place of þe sore
is nesshe, and þe mooþ vnsauery. And if it be of salte
flevme, þe mooþ is ful salte and ri3t bitter. And þe place
aboute þe sore, sumwhat is rede and hoot. But of whiche of
þes humours þe squynacy be, he muste blede sumwhat on þe

---

10 *2-line initial in blue.* **16** þes ben] *marked for reversal.* **20**
oþer] *prec. by* hi *canc. in red.*

[178]

f. 143v 5

heed veyne of þe arme, and aftir þat on þe veyne of þe tunge, and aftir þat on þe grete too, to drawe awei þe blood from þe postem. And if it be of flevme, let him vse a flevmagoge to purgen him of fleume, if he may resceyue it for greuaunce. / But algatis lete him blede as his state axiþ. If he be yonge and strong of complexion, let him blede þe more.

Diameron

10

Diameron is good for þe squinacy and for greuaunce of þe mooþ. Take mores, and of sicomoris, i libra; of hony, libra 1/2; of sape, oz. iii. Seeþ þes togedir in a tynen vessel til it be þicke and cleuing. With þis and with þe iuse of planteyn, make him a gargarisme. But see wel þat þou ley noon colde plastris withouteforþ in þis sekenese, lest þei letten him of breþing and swolewing. Anoynte his

Be war of col plastris

15

þrote with deute, and ley þeron wol þat is y-shoren of a shepe vnwasshe.

[181]

f. 114

Deute is þus y-made

20

Deute is þus made: Take of þe rotis of bismalue, þat is, þe holihock, ii° / pound; of lynen seed, of femigreke, half a pound; of squille, half a pound. Clense hem wel and stampe hem. Þen put hem in viii pounde of clene renning watir and let hem lye so iiii° daies. And þen seeþ it by a softe fier til it be þicke. Þan wringe it and put þerto a litil hoot watir. And wringe wel þat þe iuse com oute clene. And if þou hast ii pounde of iuse, put þerto iiii

14 swolewing] swelling. *Add 30338* swelling. *L*: transglutiendi. 15 is] *ins. above.* 20 stampe] *prec. by* þen *canc. in red.* 22 þicke] þenke. *Add 30338* þick. *L*: ad spissitudinem.

pounde of oile and þen let it seeþ til þe iuse be consumed.
þen put þerto a pounde of waxe and medle hem wel togedir.
And þen put þerto of turmentyne, of galbanum, of gumme of
yve, oz.ii; and þen half a pounde of rosyn, and as moche of

f. 144v

5 colofyne. And aftir þat, set it from þe fier and kepe it
close. Þis deute is good for greuaunce of þe / breste þat
comeþ of colde, and for þe postem of þe li3te, and for
membris þat ben y-coldid and y-dried, and forto make

[178v]

postemes and bochis ripe forto breke. And vndirstonde þat

Regula pro
spiritualibus

10 þo þat han greuaunce in her þrote, eiþir in her breest,
eiþir in her spirituel membris, þat is to sey, in þo
membris þat ben above þe mydrif, as þe herte and þe li3te,
shullen be ny3e an hoote fier, þat þe eyr þat þey resceyven
in drawing breeþ be hoot, for al colde þingis be noiful for

15 postemes.

A plastir
for al maner
postemes

A plastir to ley withouten to make þe postem ripe, and
it is gode for euery postem boþe withyn a mannes body and
withoute: Take þe rote of malue and bismalue, and lilie

f. 145

rotis, and seeþ hem in watir. Þen stampe hem with fre/sse
20 grece and bottir, and put þerto meel of lynseed and
femigreke, and snalis, and stampe hem togederis. And 3yue
him a gargarisme of vynegir þat barliche haþ leyen yn, and
watir þat balaustia, or sumac, or roses, or gallis, or
lentes, ben y-soden yn. But if a postem be of flevme,

---

2 **hem**] *prec. by* it *canc. in red.* **11 spirituel**] *corr. from* spituel. **18
lilie**] *corr. from* lilies.

A gargarisme

aftir his blood-letting and his purgacions, make him a
gargarisme of saap of a notte tre, and anet, and memyth,
eiþir of þe watir of þe rynde of a notte tree is soden yn
or a mylbery tree, or þe iuse of solatre is soden yn, with
5 licium or with alloes. And if his mooþ smerte or be ful
hote, make him a gargarisme of mylke þat is warme as it
comeþ from mylking. And aftir þat þou may vse strenger

f. 145v   gargarismes, as with / sape of a notte tre, with piretre,
or oximel. And make a plastir and ley to þe þrote withoute

[?]   10 of gandris dritte. And þat shal do it good, and þis
plastir also wole drawe oute of a wounde booþ yren and
þornes. Or make a plastir of galbanum and of picche. Or
hete galbanum bi himsilf and ley withouten to þe soore, and

[178v]   it wole breke þe postem. And so wole a plastir y-made of
15 whete or of soure dowe y-medlid with þe iuse of oynons.
Whan þe mater of þe postem is defied, þe riping þerof is
knowe by þe nesshenes þerof, and also abating of þe hete

[179]   and of þe ache. Take þerfore to ripe it, of dragagantum,
dr. v; of oyle of almondis and of violet, quantum sufficit;

f. 146   20 of watir þat barliche haþ a while / leyn yn, of liquoris, of
hockis, of þe iuse of gourdes, and of planteyn, of eueriche,
yliche moche; and of watir þat cassia fistula haþ be y-
soden yn. Medle alle þes togederis and let him vse it in
þe maner of a gargarisme. Or take watir þat figgis ben y-

---

3 eiþir] *ins. above.* 11 oute] *in l. h. margin.* 22 cassia] *corr. from*
cassi.

soden yn and medle it with asse mylke or gotis mylke.
And if al þis helpeþ not þat þe postem breke, bruse it þen
with þin hande til it breke. And whan it is broken, ȝyue
him þe ȝelkis of eyren y-soden with amyde, and
5 drag[ag]natum, and oile of violet; or with þe iuse of
planteyn, and watir þat barliche and liquoris ben y-soden
yn; or fygis and cassia fistula y-doon þerto and y-medlid

f. 146v   with oile of violettis; or with / þe iuse of planteyn
and watir þat barliche and liquoris ben y-soden yn. An
10 oynement to opene a postem of wesaunde: Take of white
wexe and of oile of violet, dr. xii; of bottir, dr. viii.
Stampe hem togedir and make vp þin oynement. And let

Unguentum   hem þat han þis sekenes ben y-norisshid with bran y-
clensid with watir, and with oile of almondis, and oile
15 of violet, and with penides, and hockes, and arage, and
betis, and gourdes. And let anoynte her wesaunt with oile
of violet, and with drag[ag]antum, and with þe gleyr of
eyren.

Chapter IX, The Upper Chest
Part 1, Hoarseness

[?]   Here beginneþ þe ixᵉ chaptre and it is deuidid
20 in þre titles or pract[is]es.
[183]   Hosnes comeþ in iiº maneris: Oon is of humours
f. 147   þat been in þe vessellis þat ben / cause of þe voice,
þat is to sey, in þe liȝte, or in þe breest, or in þe
þrote-bolle. Oþerwhilis, it comeþ of sekenes of þe heed,

---

2 þis] *in r. h. margin.* **5 dragagantum]** dragantum. **12 let]** *in l. h.*
margin. **17 dragagantum]** dragantum. **19 ixᵉ]** *corr. from* xᵇᵉ. **21** *5-*
line initial in gold.

as apoplexie, and epilencie, or falling dovne of þe pose into þe spirituel membris. Oþerwhiles it comeþ of feblenes, and nameliche of suche men þat drinken moche watir, and þe coldenes of þe watir streyneþ her breest,

5 and hurteþ her li3te and þe þrote, þat ben þe instrumentis of þe voys. And if it comeþ of blood, þes ben þe tokenes: a moyst coughe, and reednes of visage, swelling and fulness of veynes, swetnes of þe mooþ, and withholding of blood þat was wont to be voided by þe nose or at

f. 147v 10 sum oþer place, or defaute of blood-let/ting in suche men þat ben wonte forto blede. Of habundance and plente of flevme þat is aboute þe li3te and þe breste, þes ben þe tokenes: a moyst coughe, and vnsauerynes of þe mooþ, and colde, and moche spitting, pale colour,

15 and moche greuaunce on ny3tes, and moche slevþe. Of feblenes, þes ben þe tokenes: feblenes of al þe body, and leenship þat comeþ of moche fasting beforne, eiþir of fluxe, or oþer þingis þat maken a mannes body leen. Hoosnes þat comeþ of drines of þe brest, comeþ on two

20 maneris: Eiþir it comeþ of duste, or of smoke, or sum suche þing þat comeþ from withouten into þe breest; /

f. 148 eiþir of þe drynes of þe placis þat a mannes breeþ passeþ þoroughe, and þat drines comeþ of wynde, eiþir of vse of salte metis and soure. And þe tokenes herof

---

8 fulness] *corr. from* fulling.

ben a drye coughe, and drynes of þe mooþ, and pricking
withinforþe. If þe hoosnes be of blood, let him blede
at þe heed veyne of þe arme aftir þat his astate axeþ,
and let him be purgid with a cologoge. And let him

5   vse an electuary y-made of diapenidion, and diarris,
but þe ii° partis muste be of diapenidion, and þe iii°
parte of diarris. And let him vse þes pillulis: Take
þe seed of melone, of gourdes, of portulake, cytonies;
þe iuse of liquoris; of amyde; of gumme arabike; of

10 dragagantum; of penides; of eueriche, yliche moche. /

f. 148v   Tempere hem with þe sirip of violet and with þe iuse of
hockes, and ley hem vndir his tunge. But if it be of
flevme, purge him with a fleumag[og]e. And aftir þat
ʒyue him a gargarisme of oximel, and þe clensing of piretre

15 y-soden in meeþ. And make him a stufe of þe watir þat
yreos, and ysope, and sauery, and sauge, and fenel, and
horshel, and spike, and femigreke, and lynseed y-rostid,
and calament, and pynes, ben y-soden yn. And let him vse
þe forseide pillulis. Anoþer gargarisme for þe same:

A gargarisme
20 Take piretre, pepir, calamynte, puliol monteyn, origanum,
gynger, and make a gargarisme of hem. And if a man haþ

[183v]   not had þis greuaunce but a litil while, let his heed
f. 149   be stufen ouer warme watir þat puliol mon/teyn and roses
ben y-soden yn. And let his heed be wel couerid from

---

13 **fleumagoge**] fleumage.   20 **monteyn**] *in l. h. margin.*
origanum] *corr. from* organeum.

chaching of colde. And let him ete diapenidion with
ptisane. (Ptisane is watir þat barliche is soden yn.)

Tisan

And in þe euening, let him ete an egge and orpement þeryn.
And let him anoynten his breste, and þe nolle of his heed,

Unguentum

5 and þe þrote-bolle with deute, eiþir with marciaton,
or sum oþer suche oynement. And seeþ drie fygis and
piretre in swete wyn and 3yue him þat wyn for a gargarisme.
Or take rede netles croppes and stampe hem with þe 3olkes
of eggis, and make an harde cake þerof on an hote tiyl

10 stoon, and let him ete þerof. Or let him ete figis y-
rostid and y-strawid with poudir of gynger. If þe coughe
come of moistnes, let him vse þis electuarie y-made of

f. 149v

com/yn y-rostid, oz. i; of syneuey, oz. ii; of pepir,
of calamynt, of piretre, ana, oz. ii. But if þe hoosnes

15 come of drines, þou maist knowe by þe fore-seide tokenes,
and by moche wagging and litil spetting or noon. And
þat þat he spettiþ is bitter or salte. And he haþ an
hoot coughe, and a drie, and a greuous, and his þrote-
bolle is sore. In þis greuaunce, þou shalt 3yue him

20 no purgacion, but þou shalt vse mollificatiues to make þat
nesshe þat is hardid, and lenetiues to make þat smoþe þat
was roughe, and sharpe, and harde, þorou3 drynes. And
it is good for him to take þe colde dia[dra]gagantum,
and diapa[pa]uer, with sugir of violet or with diapenidion.

---

14 calamynt] *prec. by* oz. iii of canel *canc. in red.* **22 roughe]** *prec.*
by smoþe *canc. in red.* **23 diadragagantum]** diagagantum. **24**
diapapauer] diapauer.

f. 150

And let him holde vndir his tunge þe seed of citonies, and /
pscillie, and dragagant. And 3yue him a sirip of violet
y-medlid with watir of gourdes, not of þe sedis þat is in
þe grete gourdes, but of þe herbe þat Y clepid gourdis in

A sirip

5 al þis treatis. And lete him drinke watir þat draga[ga]nt,
and gumme arabike, and liquoris, and colde seedis ben
y-soden yn. And medle amyde, and dragagant, and gumme

Dragagantum

arabike, and þe sede of citonye, and hockis. Stampe
þes togedir and medle hem with ptisane þat is y-made
10 of dragagant infuse. And of þes make pillulis. Let
him holde ii⁰ vndir his tunge on eiþir side oon.
Dragagantum is a gumme, but dragagantum is infuse whan

[?]
See hou gumme
arabike and
dragagantum
shal be f. 150v
resoluid in
þe later
ende of þe
bok

dragagantum is resolued in cold watir or ellis in ptisane.
So gumme arabike tempriþ enkis. Anoynte his breste and
15 his þrote-bolle with bot/tir þat is not saltid, and ley
a plastir on his breest of hockis y-soden in botir or

A
lectuare

in oyle. A good electuare: Take of dragagantum, of
gumme arabike, amyde, of þe seed of citonies, of gourdes,
of mellone, of portulake, dr. iiii; of saffron, dr. i; of
20 penydes, dr. vi; mellis, quantum sufficit. Anoþir: Take
of dragagantum, dr. v; of gumme arabike, of amyde, of

Anoþir
electuare

almondis, of gourdis, dr.; of penides, dr. xxx; mellis,
quantum sufficit. Anoþir: Take of ceterake, meiden-
here, ysope, sauge, barliche y-clensid, liquoris, and

---

1 holde] *in l. h. margin.* **9 is]** *ins. above.* **10 dragagant]** *corr. from*
dragant. **12 a]** *ins. above.* **13 cold]** *ins. above.* **20 mellis, quantum**
sufficit] *in l. h. margin.* **21 dragagantum]** *corr. from* dragantum.

Anoþir
electuarie

f. 151

þe iuse þerof as moche as þe likeþ.   Seeþ hem in watir
or in wiyn and 3eue þe seeke to drinke.   His dieting
muste be colde and moyste, as of clensing of bran, and
of gotis mylke, or shepis mylke, / þe colis of an hen

5   or of a cheke.   And let him vse penides, and amyde, and
applis y-rostid, and bottir with al maner of mete.   And
he muste leve al salt mete, and rostid, and fried, and
sharpe, and excesse of eting and drinking, and namely
late, he muste eschewe, and also taking of colde, and

10   moche waking, and fasting, and angir, and moche speking
and crieng.

Chapter IX, Part 2
Stricture of the Breast

Streitnes of þe breste comeþ oþerwhilis of drienes.
And þe tokenes þerof ben leenschip, pale colour, þurste,
and hoot coughe and a drie, and moche waking.   This nedeþ

15   no purgacion, but he muste be helid as he þat haþ hoosnes

[184]

f. 151v

of drines of þe breest.   Sum han streitnes of þe breest of
humours þat stoppen her breste.   And þat / may be knowe by
moche spetting, and cou3hing, and suche oþer tokens.   And
þat shal be helid as hoosens þat comeþ of humours of þe

20   breest.   And he muste vse diarris, diaprassium,
diacalamentum, and diatrion[piperon].   And his breste
muste be anoynted with marciaton and oile of lorer.   And
oþerwhile let him have a fumigacion of orpement.   And let
him stufe him with horshel.   And make him to drinke wiyn

---

3 be] *ins. above.* **3-4 as of clensing of bran, and of gotis mylke]**
and clensing of brayn as of gotis mylke. **10 and fasting]** *in r. h.*
margin. **12** *2-line initial in blue.* **21 diatrionpiperion]** diatrion. **23**
him] *ins. above.*

þat calament is soden yn. Diapenidion is good for euery greuaunce of þe li3te, and for þe coughe, and for hoosnes, and streitnes of þe breste þat comeþ of drynes, and for þe ptisike; and is þus made: Take of penides, oz. ii & 1/2;

f. 152   5   of / blanchid almondes, of white popi seed, dr. ii & sc. i; of canel, of clowes, of ginger, of þe iuse of liquoris, of dragagantum, of gumme arabike, of amyde, seed of gourdes, of melone y-clensid, ana, dr. i; of camfer, þe þrid parte of a sc.; of þe sirip of violet, quantum sufficit. And make it

10   in þis maner: Take oz. iii of violet and seþe hem in a pounde of watir til þe vertu of þe herbis be in watir. Þen take þat watir and put þerto þe foreseide sedis y-stampid and þy penides. And if þer houeþ ony-þing of þe sedis aboue þe watir, stamp it and cast to þe toþir. And medle hem wel

15   togedir þat no-þing þerof appere. And aftir þat, put þy poudirs þerto and stire al wel togedir, til it be wel y-medlid. And let þe seeke vse þis on even and on morewe with

f. 153   tysan and with wyne if he haþ cold. / Diadraga[ga]ntum þat is colde is good for þe breste and for þe mooþ in al hote

20   causes. But whan a man vseþ it, he muste holde it in

his mooþ til it be dissolued. And it is þus made: Take of dragagantum, dr. ii; of gumme arabike, oz. i & dr. ii; of amyde, oz. i & 1/2; of liquoris, dr. ii; of penides, oz. iii; of gourdes sedes, of melone, ana, dr. ii; of

---

4 is] it. **6 of (2)]** *followed by* ca *canc. in red.* **13 and þy]** *corr. from* with. **13-14 And if . . . toþir]** *in bottom margin.* **15 þing]** þig. **18 he]** *ins. above; f. 152v is marked in red* Al þis is voide hederto. **Diadragagantum]** diadragantum. **þat is]** *in r. h. margin.* **22 dragagantum]** *corr. from* dragantum.

f. 153v 5

campher, dr. 1/2; of þe sirip of violet, quantum sufficit. Diadraga[ga]ntum þat is hote is good for colde coughes þat comen of flevme, and for men þat mowen not spitten, and for hem þat mowen not breþen, and for þe postem of þe li3te and of þe side. And it is good for þe / stomake and makeþ good digestion. And it is þus y-made: Take of dragagantum þat haþ be þre daies infuse in clene colde watir, oz. iii; of ysope, oz. i & dr. ii; of canel, oz. i; of gynger, dr. ii; of liquoris and of his iuse, dr. i & xv

10 greynes. And make it in þis wise: Clense þy dragagantum and with sufficient hony seeþ it til it be þicke. And þen take it fro þe fier. And whan it is colde, put yn þy poudris and medle al wel togedir. Anoþir hote diadragagantum: Take of hony, viii pounde; of dragagantum,

15 oz. iiii; of gumme arabike, oz. iii; of liquoris eiþir of his iuse, dr. ii; of spike, dr. i; of clowes, oz. i. And make þis in like wise as þe toþir. /

Chapter IX, Part 3
The Cough

f. 154

An-oþer sikenes þer is in a man-is breest þat is þe coughe. And þe mater of þis sekenes is þe wiynde þat a

20 man breþiþ to delyuere him of sum corrupcion þat is withyn him. Oþirwhiles it is a sekenes bi himsilf; oþirwhiles it follewiþ anoþir sekenes. And if it is a sekenes bi himsilf, it comeþ of humours þat fallen down fro þe heed into þe breest and into þe li3t, eiþir of fumes, eiþir

2 **Diadragagantum**] diadragantum. **6 is**] *ins. above.* **7 colde**] *in l. h. margin.* **18** *2-line initial in blue.* **24 eiþir** (2)] *corr. from* oþir.

of humours þat comen into þe brest from þe stomake, or
from þe lyver, or fro sum oþir place þat is byneþe þe
mydrif. Eiþir it comeþ of sum corrupte humours þat ben
y-turned into postemes in þe breest or in þe liȝte. Thes

f. 154v 5 couȝhis / þat comen of humours, eiþir þei comen of hote
humours, as of coler eiþir blood, eiþir þei comen of
colde humours, as þynne flevme eiþir of viscouse flevme
þat is þicke as bridlym. Ther is anoþir maner coughe

[187] þat is drie, and it may com by þre enchesons, as for
10 rownes of þe þrote, eiþir of þe brest, and þe liȝte, and
þe þrote, eiþir of viscouse mater þat is in þe liȝte,
and þe liȝte wolde delyuer him of þat mater and may not.
But þe mater þerof is þynne and is mevid vp by þe couȝhe,
and is y-sparplid abrode, and wexeþ drye or it comeþ to
15 þe mooþ, and þat makeþ it drie. The coȝhe þat comeþ of

f. 155 drines and sharp/nes of þe þrote is y-helid as is hoosnes
þat comeþ of rouȝnes of þe þrote. And þe couȝhe þat comeþ
of drynes of þe complexion of þe þrote is y-helid with
moyste medicines þat ben molli[fica]tif and lenetif, of
20 þe whiche medicines Y spake in þe chaptir of hoosnes.
And if þe couȝhe comeþ of an-oþer sekenes, it is helid
if þe same sekenes be y-helid. That coughe þat comeþ
of hete, and of rouȝnes, and greuaunce of þe þrote, and
moche þirst, and grete liking to drawe breeþ of colde eyre;

19 mollificatif] mollitif. **21 comeþ**] *ins. above.* **sekenes**] *in r. h. margin.*

if his visage be rede, and his veynes ful of blode, and his mooþ swete, it is a token þat þe cou3he comeþ of blood. But if þe mooþ be / bitter, and þe visage derke reed, and þe breþing ful hote and ful drie, it is a tokene of coler. If it be of blood, lete him blede at þe veyne of þe arme þat is y-callid basilica, eiþir at þe veyne þat is vndir þe tunge. And if he haþ moche blood, let him be garsid aboute þe shuldres. And wheþir it be of blood or of colre, let him be purgid with a colog[og]e, for þe same þat purgeþ coler purgiþ blood. And aftir þat, 3yue him simple medicines in dieting to abate his hete, eiþir his drines, eiþir boþe if it nedeþ. And let him vse þe colde diapa[pa]uer þat is þus y-made: Take þe iuse of liquoris, of dragagantum, of gumme arabike, ana, dr. x; of white po/py seed, and of penides, ana, dr. xx; and of almondis y-blanchid, dr. x; and of amyde, and of þe sede of cytonie, and of portulake, ana, dr. v; and of þe seed of gourdis, and of melone, and of letuse, and of hockis, ana, dr. iiii. Tempere hem with þe sirip of violet eiþir with sape, þat is, swete vynegir y-made of swete wiyn. And let him vse electuaries with þe sirip of violet eiþir with þe watir þat watir-lilies eiþir her leves ben y-soden yn, and dragagantum, and gumme arabike, and

f. 155v

5

10

f. 156   15

Diapa[pa]ver
þat
is cold

20

Sape is
vinegir
y-made of
swete wyn

9 cologoge] cologe. **13 diapapauer]** diapauer.

liquoris, and þe seed of citonies. A good sirip for
hem: Take inubes, plumbes, and violet, and þe iuse of

Sirip   gourdes, of portulake, and seed of scariole, and gumme
arabike, and dragagantum, and sugur. And seeþ hem in

5   watir, and aftir þat clense it. And þen put þerto /

f. 156v   þe musculage of psillie and þe seed of citonies. Anoþir
for hem: Take violet, liquoris, þe sede of hockis and her

Sirip   flovres, and seeþ hem in watir, and put þerin gumme
arabike, and dragagantum, and swete plumes, and penides,

10   and sugir, and make vp þy sirip. In al maner siripis, or

[?]   watres, or oþir licour þat gumme arabike or dragagantum
shal be put yn, resolue hem in þe same sirip or licour when
it is colde, for þei wolle moche and bettir be dissolued

[187v]   in a colde liquor þan in an hote. Anoþir sirip for þe

15   coughe and for þe stiche and ache in þe side, and it is

Sirip   þus y-made: Take of þe rote of fenel, of marche, and of
liquoris, ana, dr. x; of meiden-here, þe sede of citonies,

f. 157   of dragagantum, and of / hockes, ana, dr. iiii; of cleen
barly, dr. v; xxx inubes; of reysens y-made cleen dr. i;

20   of figis, a pounde; of watir, iiii pounde. Seeþ hem
togedir, and aftir it is soden, put þerto a pounde of
penides. Anoþir sirip of inubes: Take an hundrid inubes,

[187]   of reysens y-made cleen, and of liquoris, dr. xx; of
meiden-here, of violet, and of þe seed of hockis, dr. x; of

---

1 þe seed of] *in r. h. margin.* **8** þerin] *ins. above.* **20** iiii] *corr.
from* a. hem] *ins. above.* **23** cleen] *followed by* dr. i of sugir, a
pounde *canc. in red.* and] *ins. above.*

þe seed of citonies, of melone, of letuse, of popy, of
dragagantum, of barly y-clensid, dr. vi; of watir, x
pounde; of penides, eiþir of sugir, eiþir of sape, iiii

[187v] pounde. And make vp þi sirip. Good pillulis for þe
5 couȝhe: Take of mirre, dr. vii; of encense, dr. v; of
marche, of henbane, dr. iiii; of þe rote of houndestonge,

Pillulis dr. iiii. Make vp þy pillulis with watir of roses of þe
f. 157v quanti/te of a fygge, and ȝyue him twies a wike oon of hem
wiþ watir of roses. And let him holde it vndir his tunge
10 til it be dissoluid.

An oynement forto anoynte þe breste with: Medle
Oynement white wexe, and oyle of violet, and bottir togedir.

An oynement Anoþir: Take þe iuse of colde herbes, and þe leues of þe
watir-lilie, and medle hem with wexe, and oile, and bottir.
15 Anoþir is made of watir-lilie leues, and þe white of an ey,
Anoþir and woman-is mylke, and oile of violet, and bottir, and
oynement wexe. Anoþir: Take oile of violet, popilion, deute, þe
musculage of silly, and þe iuse of letuse, of eueriche,
yliche moche. And medle hem togedir, and þerwith anoynte
f. 158v 20 an olde lam/bes skyn on þat side þat was nexte þe fleisshe,
and ley þe same side to þe breste, for it is good for
alle greuauncis of þe brest þat comen of hete. And it
behoueþ þat þe hote humours þat comen fro þe heed into
þe breest be defied, lest þei fallen dovne to þe lungis

20 *f. 158 marked in red* vacat. **fleisshe**] *prec. by* skyn *canc. in red.*
21 is] *ins. above.*

and letten a man from his breþing. Also it behoueþ to see
wheþir þe mater be þicke, or þynne, or viscouse. And if þe
brest be hote, and he fele a sharpe smoke come þoroughe his
breste and his þrote, and be also þirstful, and spet litil,
5   and his colour be swarte ȝelewe, or cytryn, þat is swarte
reed, and his mooþ is salte, þat it is a token þat it is a

f. 159   þinne humour þat is cause of his / sekenes. And he may be
made þicke with þe sirip of inubes.

A colde couȝhe comeþ of a colde humour, as of flevme.
10   And þe tokenes þerof ben, litil þirste, no comforte of hote
þingis, litil greuaunce.   Malencolies and flevmatike metis
doon him harme and greuance; and if he spettiþ moche, he
feleþ moche colde withinforþe, and haþ no þirste ne fume
comyng vp þorouȝhe his breest and his þrote. Þe flevme þat
15   is cause of his coughe is grete and viscouse, and þerfore it
behoueþ to make it more sotel þat it may þe more esely come
awey with couȝing, eiþir in sum oþir wise as Y shal tel her-
aftir.   For þis colde couȝhe, firste þou muste defie þe mater

f. 159v   with / oximel squillitike.   But adde þerto fenel seed, and
20   marche seed, and horehovne, and tyme, and epityme. And aftir

[188]   xiiii dayes, purge him with a flevmagoge or with a malagoge.
And aftir þat, make a stufe of hote herbis and wel-smelling.
And make him to wasshe his breste with watir þat sauge is
soden yn, eiþir souþerenwode. And make him an hote aromatike

---

5 **ȝelewe**] and ȝelewe; *L*: lividus vel citrinus. **8 made**] *ins. above.*
10 no] *ins. above.* **15 þerfore**] *in. r. h. margin.*

Pillulis

f. 160

f. 160v

drinke y-medlid with a litil watir þat liquoris and sene ben y-soden yn. And ones in þe weke lete him take þes pillulis: Take ysope, mirre, and drie figgis, in euen porcion, and medle hem with hony. And make vp þi pillulis. And

5 anoynte his breste with oile of violet and of piliole y-medlid togederis. And let him vsen dyapenidion and diadragagantum / y-medlid togedir. His dieting must be moyst and hote, of gynger, of saffron, of galengale, of comyn, of ysope, of sauery, and of myntis, and of good wyne

10 y-warmed. These medicines and dietingis is of þe couȝhe þat comeþ of malencoly, and þat þou may knowe by swarte ȝelewe colour of þe man, and if his spitting is litil and þicke, and if his couȝhe greueþ him more whan þe norþen wynde blowiþ þan in oþir wyndes, and in harueste more þen

15 in oþir tymes of þe ȝere. But if it comeþ of flevme, þe tokenes wole be open þat we han ofte spoken of, and his couȝhe is ful greuous on nyȝtis and in wyntir. And þe mater of his couȝhe muste be defied with oximel of radiche and oximel duretike y-medlid togedir. And aftir, let him

20 stufe him in / hote herbis and wel-smelling. And þen lete him vse hote electuaries, as diacinimum, diapagamum, diacalamentum, diaperetron, and suche oþer. And let him vse þe salte þat Y spake of in þe sekenes of þe hede. And make him a sirip of ysop, of horehoune, of calamynte,

2 þes] *corr. from* þis. 20 in] *followed by* with *canc. in red.*

and of hony. Also let him haue a fumigacion of calamus aromaticus, of terebentyne, of orpyment, and þe kidney and þe fatnes of a goot y-caste vppon hote coles. And let him

holde his mooþ ouer þe smoke. Fyggis and ysope y-soden
5 togedir comforten moche þe li3te, and mirre and lynseed y-soden with purid hony. A good oximel is y-made of ysope,

sauerei, white hore/hone, origanum, parseli, fenel, liquoris, pynes, drie fyggis.   Seeþ al þes in vynegir til þei goon dovne to þe botme.   And þen clense it and put
10 þerto þin hony. Also orpiment y-stampid smale and y-eten with a rere eg is good.   And aftir let him vse sum lenetif, as dragagantum.   And let him vse bottir to his mete.   And

if þe cou3he be of viscouse fleume, 3yue him a sirip y-made

with horehoune, and þe i rote of fenel, and of radiche, of
15 marche, and anese.   Also suche viscouse flevme is dissolued in a mannes brest with calamus aromaticus, or with orpiment and terebentine, and Y haue told tofore.   A good electuarie: Take of lynsede y-rostid, of almondis, of

pines, of eueriche, dr. x; of liquoris, dr. x; of / fenel,
20 of ysope, of gynger, ana, dr. iiii; of pepir, dr. ii; of hony, quantum sufficit.   Anoþir: Take of spody, dr. vii;

of bole, of notemige, ana, dr. i; of long pipir, dr. iii; of sugir, dr. xxx; of hony and of bottir, quantum sufficit. Oon sponeful her-of is ful good for a drie cou3he. To men

3 hote coles] *marked for reversal.*

þat ben ful lene and moche y-feblid by þe cou3he, þou shalt not make a fumigacion of orpiment, but to ceesse þe fluxe of humours þat fallen doune into her brestis, þou shalte make hem a fumigacion of encense. Also take a pyne appil þat

5 haþ moche gumme and seeþ it in watir. Þen clense it and put þerto a litil hony. And let þe seke drinke herof a-morewtide and at euen, þe quantite of an eg-shelful with

f. 162 warme watir, so þat þre / parties be of watir and þe iiii

[189] parte, of þis drinke. Diapiretrum is good for þe coughe

10 and for al greuauncis of þe breest þat comen of colde. And

Diapiretrum it is good for þe splene, and for þe reynes, and for þe stoon, and for þe strangury. And it is þus y-made: Take of newe piretre þat is y-made clene, dr. xxv; of canel, of spike, of anise, of fenel, of squinantum, ana, dr. vi; of

15 hony, quantum sufficit. Let þe seke take þerof bi þe morwe and at euen, dr. iiii.

Chapter X, The Lungs
Part 1, Apostem

[?] Here beginneþ þe x chaptir þat conteneþ v titlis or pract[is]es.

In a mannes li3te þer ben meny greuaunces, as

20 postomes, and gadering togedir of corrup humours þoughe þer

[189v] ben no postem. The postem of þe li3te is y-clepid

f. 162v periplemonie, but þer is / an-oþer posteme of þe mydrif and of þe sides vndir þe ribbis þat is y-clepid pluresie. And þes postomes acorden moche togedir boþe in tokenes and also

17-18 *in bottom margin.* **18 practises**] practes. **19** *5-line initial in gøld.*

in þe causes þat þei comen of. And by oon maner medicynes
þei ben y-helid. And þe tokenes of boþe greuauncis ben,
greuauncis of þe brest and of þe side, coughe, and a sharpe
feuer. And oþirwhilis þer foloweþ þes sikenessis, spitting
5 of blood, and spitting of glat, and of qwiter. And aftir
þat comeþ tisike and oþir sikenessis þat comen of plente of
humours in þe li3te or aboute it, as hardnes to drawe breþe
and to breþen also. In þe holewnes of þe li3te þer may be
þre humours þat maken hir seke and letten hir of hir
10 kyndeli worching. And þo humours ben / fleume, coler, and
malencolie. Of fleume, þes ben þe tokenes: hardenes and
greuaunce to breþen, and oþirwhilis a cou3he and hoosnes,
and þe greuaunce is more on ny3t þen on day-tyme, and in
wyntir more þen in sommer, and moche greuaunce aftir þat a
15 man haþ y-ete, and moche spetting and diuerse, aftir þe
diuersite of flevmes; for of þe kyndeliche fleume, þe
spitting is watri and white, þyn and vnsauery, and li3tli
comeþ vp by a reching and spitting. Of glasi fleume, comeþ
spitting of grete gobettis and harde-y-gaderid, and pale
20 and vnsaueri. And it is greuous in þe spitting, in-so-
moche þat it makiþ a noyse withinforþe and semeþ as þou3he
it cleuid within to þe breste or to þe sides. Of flevme
þat is y-/clepid salte, þe spitting is white, and þicke,
and salte, and esy forto spitte. Of kene fleume and egir,

Marginal notes:

Tokenes of ii⁰ maner of postems

In þe holewnes of þe li3t   f. 163 þer may be þre humours

Of fleume þe tokenes

Kindeliche fleume

Glasi fleume

Salt fleume   f. 163v

15 and diuerse] *in r. h. margin.*

comeþ þin spitting and vndefied, and moist and soure. Of
coler, þe tokenes ben, hardnes of breþing, hoosnes, a drie

couȝhe, þirste, bitternes of þe mooþ, drines of þe tunge,
an hote breþing, and hir þirste is more y-kelid bi colde

5 eyr þen by eny drinke.   Þe breste is hote and it feliþ hete
comyng vp from þe depenes of þe breste.   And þei han more
greuaunce a-day þen a-nyȝte, and in sommer þen in wyntir.
And if it is of coler þat is cytryn, þe spitting is citrin

and þicke, and comeþ gobet-mele.   Of rede coler, þat is,

10 reed or of þe colour þat ȝolkis of eggis ben, þe spitting

is citrin or grene, and defied grene when / it begynneþ to
ben y-bred.   It is esy in spitting.   Of malencolie, þe

tokenes ben, greuaunce in breþing, a coghe, and grete
greuaunce in spitting, and litil þei spitten, and þat is

15 ȝelew and sovre, or blacke and soure, and her greuaunce is

grettir in heruest þen in wintir.   And in olde men þer is
moche colde aboute her breste þat comeþ as hem semeþ from
þe depnes of her breest.   And her breest is colde and þe
coloure of her breste is ȝelewe or blacke.   Oþirwhilis, þe

20 veynes þat ben aboute þe liȝte ben ful of humours, and
þristiþ þe liȝt togedir, and makeþ a man narow-y-breþid.

If þat replecion be of eny oþir humour þen of blode, þou
maist knowe by þes foreseide tokenes.   And if it be of

blode, þes ben þe tokenes: re/dines of þe visage, fulnes

of þe veynes, and swetnes of þe mooþ, and oþir tokenes of blood þat Y haue oftesiþes y-spoken of. And þe sekerist token to knowe wheþir þe liȝte be ful of humours is

A siker
token to
knowe if
þe liȝt be
combrid
with humours

5 spitting, not eueri spitting, but spitting þat comeþ with coughing, for oute of þe hede þer comeþ humours þoroughe iiº holes into þe mooþ whan a man drawiþ breeþ, and enforsiþ him to spitte. Anoþir spitting comeþ from a

Spetting
from þe
chekis

mannes chekis and his þrote, with a-forsyng to spitte withoute drawing breeþ. Also from þe breest þer comeþ

Spetting
from þe
liȝt,
from
þe   f. 165
mydrif,
and fro
þe sidis,
and þe
stomake

10 spitting, with a reching and breþing. Oute of þe liȝte þer comeþ spitting with couȝhing. And also from þe mydrif and þe sidis it com/eþ with a stronge coughe. And from þe stomake comeþ spitting bi his aune acorde. And if þes humours lien longe in þe liȝte, þei maken þer a posteme þat

15 is y-clepid peripleumonie. And of whiche humour he comeþ,

Þe briding
of a postem

þou maist knowe by þe tokenes aforseide. And oþir special

The
tokenes
of
peripleumoni

tokenes þer ben of peripleumonie, as a contynuel feuer, and a coughe, and a grete greuaunce in þe breste, and namely in þe lifte side vndir þe lifte pappe, and vndir þe shuldir-

20 blade boþe behinde and before vp to þe shuldir, and heuynes of þe yȝen, and swelling of þe veynes, and redenes in þe myddel of þe chekis. And þes same ben þe tokenes of

The
tokenes
of pluresy
          f. 165v

pluresy, saf in þe pluresie þer is moche ache and greuaunce aboute þe si/dis and aboute þe ribbis. And þe coughe comeþ

---

15 is] *ins. above.* **16 aforseide]** *corr. from* forseide. **16-17 special tokenes]** *marked for reversal.*

from þe side. But þer ben two maneris of pluresie, very
and not very. Very pluresie is in þe mydrif, and he may be
in two maneris: eiþir aboue, eiþir beneþe. Not very is in
oon of þe sides eiþir vndir þe ribbis. And þes two han

5   oon maner tokenes, saaf þat þei ben more greuous in very
pluresie þan in þe toþir. And also in pluresie of þe
sidis, a man may fele oþirwhiles withoutenforþe þe postem
and þe boche, but of þe mydrif, he shal not so. And whan
þer is but an esy cou3he, and with oon coughing or two,

10 a man deliueriþ him of glet, þat it is a good token.
But whan þe cou3he is trauelous, and litil deliuerance
is of corrupte mater, it is a token þat þe mater of þe

greuaunce is yuel to defie and to deliueren oute / fro
withyn þoroughe coughing or spitting. A good experience to

15 wite wheþir þer be a posteme in þe li3te: Let him spitten

Experiens bi
þe whiche
a postem in
þe li3te is
knowen

on coles. And if it stinkeþ, þer is a postem in þe li3te.
Anoþer: Let him spitten on watir, and if it houeþ
abouen altogedir, þan þe li3te is hool. But if sum þerof
houeþ abouen and sum þerof goeþ to þe grounde, it is

20 a token þat þer is a postem in þe li3te. But in case
þe corrupte spitting is holden vp bi þat, þat is good:

þat it may not go to þe grounde. Pluresie þat is in þe
neþir party of þe midrif is not so perilous as þat þat is
abouen, ne in þe lifte side as in þe ri3t side. But if þe

10 þat] *ins. above.* **22** þe (2)] *in r. h. margin.* **23** **perilous**] *corr.
from* perlous.

li3te haue replecion of humours and no postem, if it be of blood and if it be of ony oþir humour, let him haue a

f. 166v

purgacion / acording to þe humour. And vse suche medicines as it is tolde in hoosnes and streitnes of þe breste and in

5 þe coughe, for al þes sekenessis acorden moche, boþe in medicines, and in dietingis, and in tokenes, and enchesons þat þei comen of. But if þer be a postem, wheþir it be in þe li3t, in þe midrif, or in þe sidis, withdrawe not his mete, but fede him with comfortable metis, as with coliis,

10 and almonde mylke, and ptisan þat drie figgis and draga[ga]ntum and liquoris, and reisens ben y-soden yn. But if her greuaunce be of flevme, let hem not ete figis. And if þei ben costif, 3yue hem no ptisane, but 3yue hem

f. 167

crummes of brede and þe clensing of bran / y-soden with

15 almond mylke, and peres y-rostid, and chesteynes, and penydes, and blacke plumbes. But be þei ware of soure metis. Electuaries þat ben good for þes postemes ben diapenidion, and diadraga[ga]ntum, and sugir of violet, and sugur of roses. Good siripis ben þe sirip of inubes,

Sirip

20 or of roses, or of violet. Or take of barliche y-clensid, of reisens, of violet, of inubes, þe sede of mellone, of govrdes, of amide, of dragagantum, of liquoris, of rede ciceres, of blacke plumbes, þe sede of citonies, þe rote of fenel, of parseli, of marche, of anet, of ameos, of

---

8 **þe** (2)] *ins. above.* 9 **coliis**] *corr. from* coolis. 11 **diadragagantum**] diadragantum. 18 **diadragagantum**] diadragantum. 19 **þe sirip of inubes**] *copied* inubes þe sirip of *and marked for reversal.*

carewei, of dauke, of pastnepe, of pynes, of penides, ana,

f. 167v

[?]

vi dr. And make herof a sirip, / þat is to sey, seþe al þes in watir vntil þe vertu of hem be in þe watir. Þen streyne it and put þerto sugur or hony, þat is to sey, þe v parte

5 of þy licoure muste be of sugur or of hony. And þen set it ouer þe fier til it seeþ a litil while sooftli. And take white of þre or iiii eggis and swenge hem wel, and put þerto. And alwei squoyme it til al be clere. Þen take it dovne, and streyne it cleen þat noon dreggis remayn þeryn.

10 And þen put it in a close vessel. Anoþir: Take of barliche y-clensid, of reisens, of drie figgis, of sugur,

[193v]

of þe rote and of þe iuse of liquoris, of damasenes, of violet, of þe sede of þe iiii colde herbis, of ysope, of

A sirip

þe rote of fenel, of parsely, ana dr. iii. And with a

15 pounde of sugir, maken of hem a sirip for þe pluresie,

f. 168

and / hete of þe breste, and for drie coughis, and for þe ptisike in þe begynnyng. Take also of violet, of dragagantum, of þe sede of citonies, of barliche y-clensid, of þe sede of hockis and of gourdes, ana, dr. vi; of

20 inubes, xx. Seþe hem in iiii pounde of watir. And when it is y-soden, put þerto a pounde of sugur. A plastir: Take

A plastir

þe rote of holy-hocke, and þe leues of hockis, and þe rote of fenel, and lynsede, and drie figgis, and oyle, of eueriche, yliche moche, id est, a quartir of a pounde.

---

5 **it**] *ins. above.* 7 **swenge**] *corr. from* swengid. **hem**] *in l. h. margin.* 8 **sqyoyme**] *corr. from* swyme. 10 **it**] *ins. above.* 12 **damasenes**] *corr. from* damascenes. 13 **þe (2)**] *ins. above.* 15 **þe**] *ins. above.* 24 **quartir**] *corr. from* quartron.

And firste stampe hem and þen seþe hem. And ley hem hote to þe sore side. But anoynte bifore with deute, or popilion and oile of violet y-medlid togedir. And oftetymes renewe þi plastir. Anoþir: Take þe rote of bismalue, and / þe leues

5 of malues, and lynsede, and femigreke, and drie figgis, of eueriche, oz. i. Stampe hem and put to hem oile of roses or of violet, or of comen oyle de olijf. And make a plastir and lei to his side. But firste anoynte þe sore place as Y seide tofore. And þou maist put þerto datis and

10 reysens, and barly mele. And it is þe beste plastir, for it is mitigatif and maturatif. In al greuaunces þat comen of colde, let þe breste and þe side be anoynted with deute. And if þe greueuance comeþ of hete, medle with deute þe oile of roses or of violet. And þen ley þeron wolle þat is

15 y-shore of an vnwasshen shepe, so þat al þe wolle may chache moistnes. And al warme ley it to þe breste or side. And whan þe pos/tem is broken and þe quiter begynneþ to cese, let him vse siripis þat ben mundificatiues, and electuaries also, as þe sirip of inibes, and diapenidion,

20 and diadragagantum, and diacodion, þat is, diapa[pa]uer. But let him not vse diacodion but if þe boche heliþ not as faste as it shulde. And þan in pluresie, let him vse diadragagantum with a quantite of mirre and of sandragon y-do þerto in þe making. In peripleumonie, let him vse

[194]

f. 168v

Anoþir
plastir

f. 170

diapenidion with mirre and sandragon. And in al þy medicines, þou muste consider his hete þat is seke, and of his feuer. And þeraftir, þou muste ordeyne þy medicyns in hete and in colde. And if he haue a

f. 170v

5 kene feuer, let his dieting be sotil, and litil, and of souþing þingis as broþþes. If þe feuer be esy, þen he may vse grettir metis. And if / he be feble and þe mater of colde and þe feuer is esy, he may vse a colis of an hen or of a capon with þe clensing of bran. And let him kepe his

10 handes, and his armes, and his fete from colde. Neþeles, if he chache a coughe, 3yue him ptisan of whete. Clensing of bran is, whan bran is caste in cleen watir and aftir þat, is clensid þoroughe a clooþ. Þis clensing of bran is a good mundificatif, and so it is good for postemes þat ben

15 withyn a man. And for-as-moche þat it is not generatif of moche blood, it is gode for men þat han þe feueris.

[?]

Chapter X, Part 2
Spitting of Blood

[194v]

Spitting of blode, if it comeþ with cowghing, it comeþ fro þe li3te eiþir fro þe mydrif. If it comeþ withouten coughe, it comeþ from as meny places as / oþer spitting doeþ.

f. 169

20 Also it comeþ from oþer parties of a mannes body, of brusyng of veynes, as from þe stomake. And þat greueþ a man byneþe his mydrif, and makeþ volaten his mete, and makiþ him to haue yuel digestion, eiþir comeþ from þe lyuer, and þan þe greuaunce is in þe ri3t side. And if it comeþ of þe splene,

12 **is** (2)] *ins. above.* 17 *2-line initial in blue.* **blode**] *corr. from* blove. 21 **a man**] *in r. h. margin.*

þen it is in þe lifte side.   If it comeþ of þe hede, þe
hede is heuy and al a man-is wittis ben y-feblid þerby.
And if it comeþ of veynes of þe brayn, by ny3t her
greuaunce is more þan on þe day.   And it comeþ whan a man

5   draweþ breeþ and arecheþ strongeliche to spit.   From þe

f. 169v   li3t it com/eþ with coughing and from þe mydrif with a
stronge coughe.   And it is sum-what fomy.   But whan it comeþ
from þe breest, it is not fomy.

Bleding þat comeþ of breking of veynes, comeþ in to

10   maneris, as from withinforþe, eiþir from suche encheson
withouten-forþe: from within, as for grete plente of blode
þat brekiþ þe veynes, eiþir of sotilte, eiþir of sharpnes
and keneship of þe blode þat makiþ hem to breken also.   From
withoutenforþe, veynes ben broken þoroughe smyting, eiþir

15   leping, eiþir falling, eiþir þoroughe moche crienge and
suche oþir þingis.   Spitting of blode þat comeþ in a greuous

[?]   sekenes and li3teþ a man of his sekenes, is a token

f. 172   of his / heel.   And if it heuyeþ a man moche, it is a token
þat he shal sone dye, ne he shal not be y-staunchid.   But

20   if a man haþ suche greuous sekenes, it is good to staunche
it, but discretly, as Y seide in þe nose-bledyng.   And if
it comeþ of stopping of sum oþer places, let him vse
medicynes to make þo placis flowe.   And if it comeþ of
a stroke, let þat be helid by surgery.   But be þei war

---

3 by] *prec. by* and *underd.* 9 in to] into. 18 And] *corr. from* eiþir.
19 shal not] *corr. from* may not. 20 suche] *prec. by* so *canc. in red.*

Thes þingis
chausen þe
spiritis
and drawe
hem outward

from wraþ, and compenyng with women, and waking, and
fasting, and from soure metis, and salte, and kene, and
from chaching of grete hete, and from baþing, and moche
trauel, and also moche þou3t, and moche besines, for al þes

f. 172v 5 þingis heten þe spiritis, and maken hem drawen / outewarde
with þe blode, and brekiþ þe veynes of þe whiche breche

[194v] comeþ spitting of blode. And if spetting of blode comeþ
of grete plente of blode, diete þe pacient with suche metis
þat gendreþ litil blode, as herbes and fruytis. And if it

10 comeþ of keneship of þe blode, 3yue him siripis and
electuaries, þat is to sey, suche þingis þat mowon abate þe
keneschip of þe blode and turnen it into anoþer kynde. And
if it comeþ of sotilte of þe blode, 3yue him suche metis and
drinkis þat wolen make þicke blode, as Y tolde in þe bleding

15 of þe nose and Y wole telle more in þe chaptir of þe fluxe.

A good sirip for spitting of blode wherof-euer

f. 171 it comeþ: Take ypoquistidos, / chymole, bole armoniac,

[195] acacie, coral white and rede, þe poudir of onyfacie, mummie,
mynte, psidie, galles, balaustia, gumme arabike, dragagantum,

20 symphite, corigiole, þe sede of planteyn, roris ciriaci,
sumac, pentaphilon, radiche, sandragon, of eueriche of
þes, oz. i. Seþe hem in reyn watir til þe þirde parte of
þe watir be wastid. Þen clense it and put þerto iii
poundes of sugir. And 3yue þe pacient þis sirip with þe

---

7 **if**] *ins. above.* 15 **þe** (3)] *ins. above.* 19 **balaustia**] *corr. from*
balaustiantia. **dragagantum**] *corr. from* dragantum. 21 **pentaphilon**]
pantaphilon. 22 **parte**] *in r. h. margin.*

iuse of planteyn.   And þe sirip þat is make of planteyn
is ri3t good also.

A confeccion þat soudeþ and a-swagiþ þe bledyng: Take
ypoquistidos, acacie, balaustia, of eueriche, dr. ii; of
5 galles, as moche; of opium and of citre, dr. vi. Tempere
hem with reyn watir and 3yue him to drinke with reyn watir.

f. 171v   Also take of / spodie, dr. iiii; of þe sede of gourdes
and of portulake, bole, carabe, of eueriche, dr. iii.
Tempere hem with þe watir of shepardis 3erde.

10 A lectuarie þat clenseþ þe breste withinforþe of
blode: Take of amide, dr. v; of been mele, of þe sede of
melone and of hockis, ana, dr. vi; of barliche y-clensid,
dr. x; of gumme arabike and of dragagantum, ana, dr. iii;
of þe sede of citonies and of borage, ana, dr. v. Bete
15 hem to poudir and put to of hony, quantum sufficit.

[?]   Also for blode þat is congelid and lieþ acoldid in
a mannes breste: Take tansey and stampe it with vynegre
and wringe it and 3yue him to drinke þat is dissesid.

[195] Forto stanche spitting of blode: Take of wormode, of
20 anyse, of dauke, ana, dr. iiii; of storace, of opium,
f. 173   of mir/re, of nitre, of anet, ana, dr. iii; of canel, of
castore, ana, dr. ii; of hony, quantum sufficit. And 3yue
him þis a-morewetide and on þe euen þe quantite of a walle-
notte with watir þat planteyn is soden yn, and þat muste be

13 dragagantum] *corr. from* dragantum. **23 him þis**] *marked for
reversal.* **23-24 walle-notte**] *marked for reversal in error.*

warme.   Dieting of hem shal be fisshe rostid fresshe, and
rise, and hard eggis, and crabbis of þe see ben medicinable
and good mete for þis sikenes, and chesteynes y-soden and
y-fried with 3olkis of eyren, and whete mele y-soden

5   with mylke. A gargarisme of vynegre and salt is god.

Chapter X, Part 3
Spitting of Gleet

Spitting of glat and of quitere comeþ of infeccion
of þe li3t, as whan corrupte blode haþ y-leyen in þe
li3te and is rotid, eiþir corrupte humours han y-fallen
doune from þe hede and ben y-turned to suche glat.

10   Eiþirwhilis suche spetting comeþ of infeccion of þe

f. 173v   mydrif, eiþirwhilis / of a postem of þe lyuer and corrupte
humours in him.   Oþirwhilis it comeþ with a feuer, and
oþirwhilis withoute a feuer.   Tokenes herof ben: spetting

[195v]   þat is corrupte, as quitere, leneship of þe body, smalship

15   of þe necke, greueuance in breþing, swelling of þe y3en.
If þey han a feuer, let hem be dietid as þilke þat han
pluresie eiþir peripleumonie.   And if it comeþ of hete,
3yue him diapenidion, and þe colde diadraga[ga]ntum, and
diapa[pa]uer, and þe sirip þat was y-tolde in þe colde

20   coughe, and þe anoyntingis.   And if þe spittinge stynkeþ,

Tokenes
of deeþ   and þe heris of his hede fallen awey, and þe nailes of his
fyngris shrinken and waxen narowe at þe endes, it is a
token of deþe.   And if þis greuaunce comeþ of colde, þe

f. 174   spetting is corrupte, as / quytere, and white eiþir swarte

---

5 A gargarisme . . . is god.] *in r. h. margin.* **6** *2-line initial in blue.*
18 diadragagantum] diadragantum. **19 diapapauer]** diapauer. **20 þe**
(1)] *ins. above.* **24 is]** *prec. by* stynkeþ *canc. in red.*

ȝelewe. The cure herof is as of þe colde coughe. And ȝyue him medicynes to restreyne þe humours and to clense his breste as it is tolde before.

A plastir for hem to ley on her breste byneþen: 5 Take spica celtica, and apium ranarum, and anet, and seþe hem in wiyn and in oile. Also centorie y-soden in oile of carses and y-plastrid aboue is good.

A lectuarie for an olde coughe and for spetting of glat: Take piretre, bitter almondes, lauriole, and radiche, 10 of eueriche, yli[che] moche; of hony, quantum sufficit. Tempere hem togederis and ȝyue him on morwe-tide and on euen, þe quantite of a walis-not. Anoþir: Take of femigreke, and lynsede y-rostid, and of carewei, yliche moche; of hony, / quantum sufficit. Anoþir: Take of horehone and of orobus, 15 ana, dr. iii; of citre, mirre, gynger, ysope, long piper, anise, yliche moche; of hony, quantum sufficit. Anoþir: Take of calament, of parsely, of sileos, dr. vi; of marche, and of ameos, ana, dr. i; of ysope, dr. viii; of pepir, dr. iii; of hony, quantum sufficit. Horshel y-povdrid and y- 20 medlid with hony is good. ȝiue him þerof at euen and at morewe þe quantite of a walis-not. Aristologia rotunda y-soden in watir is good for þe coughe.

Pillulis for hem þat han þis greuaunce of rewme falling dovne to þe breste: Take of galbanum, mirre, storace,

Electuarie

f. 174v

A sirip

[196]

---

6 hem] *corr. from* þe. 10 yliche moche] ylimoche. 12 Take] *in r. h. margin.* 19-22 Horshel y-povdrid ... þe coughe] *in l. h. margin.* 24 to] *corr. from* into.

olibanum, dragagantum, yliche moche.   Medle hem togedir
with an hote pestil and make þy pillulis of þe quantite
of a fich.   And 3yue him þerof v or vi at ones.   Eueriche
crabbe of þe see is good for þis sekenes.   If þei han þe

f. 175   5   feueris, 3yue it hem with tisane. If / þei han no feueris,
3yue it hem with wiyn.   And undirstonde þat if þilke þat han
peripleumonie be not clene y-purgid withyn xiiii daies
eiþir xx aftir þe breking of þe postem, þei shullen falle
into þis greuaunce.   And þan but if þei ben helid withyn

   10   xl daies eiþir y-purgid, þei shullen fal into a tisike.

Chapter X, Part 4
Phthisis

Tisike is a destruccion of þe kyndely moistnes of
a mannes body.   But þer ben ii° maneris of tisike: Oon
is a very tisike and þe toþir is not a very tisike.   Verry
tisike is a destroing of þe kyndeliche moistnes of a mannes

   15   body þoroughe sekenes and corrupcion of þe li3te.   But þe
f. 175v   tisike þat is not very comeþ not / of þe li3te, but of sum
oþer encheson. Very tisike comeþ in meny maneris. Oon is
of a postem of þe li3te þat was not wel y-helid. Anoþer is
of humours þat ben kene, as salte fleume and coller þat

   20   falliþ adovne from þe hede into þe li3te and appeireþ
hir. But þe þridde maner is of humours þat comen from
oþir places and appeireþ þe li3te, as of squinacie,
eiþir of pluresie, eiþir of greuaunce of þe lyuer, eiþir of
þe splene, eiþir of sum oþer place.   Tisike also þat is not

4 han] *in l. h. margin.* **8 þei]** þe. **11** *2-line initial in blue.*

very is in þre maneris.   Þe firste is with grete hete
withoutenforþe on a mannes body.   And þat is helid as þe

f. 176   feuer etike.   Þe toþir / is of grete dryenes and colde.
And þat is y-helid   as spetting of glat þat comeþ of drienes
5   and of colde. Þe þrid maner comeþ of moche flevme þat is
in a mannes bodi, and þat is y-helid as þe fluxe of a
mannis wombe.   Of verry tisike þat Y wole speke of nowe, þe

[196v]   tokenes ben contynuel hete, in sum more, as in hem þat han
a feuer þerwiþ, and in sum laas, as in hem þat han no
10   feuer; thirste, and drienes of þe tunge, small[n]es of þe
necke, and leneship of al þe body, costifnes of þe wombe,
corrupcion of þe nailes, holewenes of þe y3en, and ache
of þe lift shuldir-blad vp to þe shuldir.   And comenly

f. 176v   al suche men be disposid / to þis sekenes þat ben leen
15   of bodi, and ben strei3te aboute þe breest, and han hi3e
shuldres.   Tokenes of deeþ in þis sekenes ben: falling of
heres, feueris, streynyng togider and corrupcion of þe
endes of her nailes, falling dovne of her browes, a simple
fluxe of her wombe. Suche men shullen speke and dye, and
20   die spekeng. Also let hem spetten in a basyn and on morewe
cast þerto hoot watir and stire it, and if þer goeþ bi þe
grounde þicke dros, he is incurable.   Or if his breþe
stenkiþ in his sekenes, and was before wel smelling, he
is incurable.   Also very tisik haþ þis tokene: a contynuel

8 tokenes] *corr. from* tokens. **10 smallnes**] smalles. **14 al**] *ins. above.* **19 speke**] *prec. by* die *canc. in red.* **20 die spekeng**] *marked for reversal.*

f. 177 coughe.   And if it comeþ of hete, his / spetting is citryn,
eiþir ʒelewe as safron, eiþir grene.   And þe body febleþ
euery day moche and openly.   It must be helid as þe coughe
þat comeþ of hete.   But if it comeþ of colde, þe spitting

5 is white eiþir ʒelewe, and it shal be helid as þe cold
couʒ.   But whan ptisike comeþ of a wounde of þe liʒte, þou
muste ʒyue him mundificatiues and consolidatiues.   And þou
muste be war lest þe quitere abide stille in þe brest.   And
if þat hapneþ, and he may not spit wel and delyuer him of

10 þat corrupcion, ʒyue him hony þat ysope and violettis ben
y-soden yn.   A gode electuarie for þis greuaunce: Take of

f. 177v reysyns þat ben cleen, xx. dr; / of hocke sede, dr. iii; of
þe leues of watir-lilies, of crabbis of þe see, of

Electuarye shepardes ʒerde, of planteyn, ana, dr. v; of liquoris, oz.

15 i.   Seþe al þis in þre pounde of watir and caste þerto
a pounde of sape or ii° pounde of sugir, and make þerof a
sirip.   Aftirward, take of gumme arabike, of dragagantum,
of þe sede of citonies, ana, dr. viii; of amide,
of þe sede of portulake, dr. vii.   Poudir al þes and medle

20 hem with þe forseide sirip and ʒyue it in þe maner of an
electuarie.   It is gode for peripleumonie, and pluresi,
and for a febil stomake.   And aftir þat þe postemes ben
broken and ben not wel y-clensid, þis sirip and þis
electuarie ben good.   And whan þe mater wexeþ harde, it is

13 of crabbis of þe see] *in l. h. margin.*

f. 178   good to ȝy/ue hem hote medicines þat moun hete hem
withinforþe, and clense hem and make hem to haue a couȝhe.
And suche ben þe sede of orobus, and of aristologia rotunda
and longa, and of longe pipir, canel, anese, cost, cassia
5   fistula, and spike.   But þou shalt not vse þese if he
haue a stronge feuer, but whan þe mater is fleumatike.
And if he be costif, purge him with esy clisters þat
ben y-made of mollificatiues, for a stronge fluxe is
perilous in þis sekenes.   And if he haue oon, staunche it
10   as sone as þou may, but do it discretly, for drede of
more peril.   And if þat wounde of þe liȝte drie to slouli,
[197]   wheþir þe wounde be of an hurting or of a boche, þou
f. 178v   muste ȝy/ue him subtilatiues to maken þe mater sotil,
þat it may þe raþir com oute and þe wounde þe raþir be
15   drie.   And if it be with a rewme, ȝyue him bole armoniac
with þe iuse of planteyn, or with dragagantum, or liquoris,
for it drieþ and regendriþ þe fleisshe.

    A gode medicyn to soude veynes þat ben broke in
þe liȝte or in þe breste: Take of bole, of amide, ana, dr.
20   iii; of crabbes of þe see y-brent, of þe seed of purslane,
ana, dr. x.   Povdir al þis and medle it with þe iuse of
planteyn, and make rounde balles þerof.   And ȝyue him at
ones þe quantite of oon exage with þe iuse of purslane or
f. 179   of gourdes.   Anoþir þat is good for / bleynes, and woundes

1 hote medicines] *marked for reversal.*

of þe li3te, and clenseþ him and soudeþ þe woundis: Take
of balaustia and of roses, ana, dr. iii; of sandragon, of
amide, of encense, ana, dr. i; of carabe, of safron, ana,
dr. 1/2.   Tempere hem with þe iuse of citonies, and make

5   þerof rounde balles.   And 3yue herof oon exage with colde
watir.   Neþeles, take hede þat he shal not vse þes drie
medicines but þe mater be y-clensid.   And þat þou may
knowe if þat he spettiþ no glette ne gobetis of þe li3te,
for þer may no wounde be helid and dried but if he be y-

10   clensid.   And þan he may vse in his medicines roses, and

f. 179v   balaustia, dragagantum, mastike, / carabe, bole, sandragon,
mirre, emachites, þe sede   of planteyn, and suche oþer.

A gode electuari for hem þat han þis sekenes with

Electuarie   a feuer: Take of þe sede of gourdes and of melone,

15   ana, oz. i; of letuse, violetis, liquoris and his iuse, of
þe sede of popi, of amide, of dragagantum, oz. ii.   Medle
hem with watir þat liquoris is y-soden yn and dragagantum
haþ be resolued yn.   Let him take of þis electuary a-
moreutide and at euen, for it restoriþ his kyndeli moistnes

20   and saueþ it, þat it be not destroied þoroughe vnkynde
hete of þe feuer.   Take of rosis, dr. i; of spodie and of

f. 180   þe iuse of liquoris, ana, dr. v; of amide, of portula/ke,
of endiue, dr. iii; of þe sedis of gourdis and of melone,
of sandris, ana, dr. ii.   Tempere it with þe iuse of psilly

---

6 þat] *ins. above.*   **19 restoriþ]** *corr. from* restorid.

and with þe sirip of violet.   And vndirstonde þat sirips
and electuaries for men þat han þe ptisike shullen not be
made ouer þe fier as oþer electuaries ben, but þei shullen
be y-made in a tynen vessel and þat shal be sette in a

Regula **5** caudron of seþing watir ouer þe fier, for if it were made
ouer þe fier, þe spicis shullen lese moche of her kynde
and þe smoke of þe fier wolde medle with þe medicines, and
þat shulde aftirward noye þe breste ful moche.

Profitable þingis þat clensen þe breest ben:

f. 180v 10 gargarismes y-/made of whey of gotis mylke, and watir
þat liquoris is soden yn, and barliche, eiþir barliche
y-soden with liquoris and with radiche.   Also seþe
crabbes of þe see til þe fisshe departe from þe bones,
and siþ take þe collis of þat fisshe and medle it with

15 barliche and make a gargarisme þerof. And let him swolewe
sumwhat þerof into his stomake, for it restoreþ þe
kyndeliche moistnes of a man-is body. And as toching þis
poynt of tisike, medicines of etike ben profitable and
good.   And whan tisike haþ a feuer with him, þou must see

20 wheþir it is y-com of hete or of colde.   And þeraftir, þou
f. 181 must ordeyne þi medicines as it is y-tolde / in þe chaptir
of hosnes and of þe cou3he.   And medicines þat weren y-
tolde þer ben good here, for al sikeness-is of þe breste
acorden in medicines and enchesons.   And if þe pacient be

14 it] *ins. above.*

feble and his feuer violent, take of cassia fistula, dr. v;
of drie violet floures, dr. vii; of reisyns y-clensid, dr.
xx; innibes, xx; sebesten, xxx. Seþe al þis in iiii pounde

[197v]   of watir til it come til half a pounde. And þen put þerto

5   xx dr. of hempe sede. And let clense it and 3yue him þerof
to drinke. Dieting of hem þat han þe tisike of wounde of
þe li3te shal be of colde þingis, and moiste, and
conglutinatif, as of newe whete brede and wiyn if he haþ no

f. 181v   feuer, or ellis meþe þat liquo/ris is soden yn and

10   dragagantum resolued yn. But if tisike come of humours,
her dieting muste be of freisshe-watir fisshe, and nameli
scalid fisshe, as pike, perche, roche, and breem; and
fruyt, and drie siripis. And if it comeþ of rewme, þe
humours musten be abatid bi sum strictories of her cours,

15   as it is tolde tofore suffiently. But alle phicisiens
accorde not her-yn, þat woundes of þe li3t ben incurable,
for þei mowon not ben y-helid withoute clensing, and þei
moun not be clensid withoute cou3hing, and þe coughe wole
drawe abrode and make him febler þan he was, and so þat þat

f. 182   20   shulde helpe, doiþ harme. And þerfore þei mo/tne nedis be
incurable. Diarodon abbatis is good for þe tisike, and for

Diarodon   etike, and for þe cardiacle, and for 3elewe yuel, and meny
abbatis
oþir sekenessis: Take white sandris and rede, ana, dr. ii
& 1/2; of gum arabike, dragagantum, spodie, ana, dr. ii; of

11 watir] *in l. h. margin.*

asarum, spike, mastike, cardamomum, citre, zilobalsamum,
clowes, gallie muscate, anise, fenel seed, canel, þe iuse
of liquoris, reubarbe, þe seed of basilicon, berberis,
scariole, purslane, gourde, melone, ana, dr. i;
5 margaritis, þe bon þat is in an herte-is herte, ana, dr.
i & 1/2; ginger, of roses, ana, oz. i & dr. iii; of
camphore, vii greynes; of muske, iii greynes & 1/2. Medle
hem togedir and let him drinke on morwetid and at euen þis

f. 182v poudir / with þe sirip of roses. But medle þerwith rose-
10 watir or colde watir.

A sirip for peripleumonie, and pluresie, and tisike,
and etike: Take iiii pounde of watir and do þerin oz. 1/2
of violet; of liquoris, of white popy, ana, dr. 1/2; of
þe sede of citonies, of melone, of gourdes, of purselane,
15 of gumme arabike, of dragagantum, ana, dr. iii.   Stampe
al þes and do in a bagge in þe forseide iiii pounde of
watir.   Siþ clense þe watir and put þerto ii pounde of
sugir, and þen make vp þi sirip.   Triasandri is good also
for þe tisike, and for þe stomake, and for þe ȝelew yuel.
20 Let him vse þerof at morwetid and at middai þe quantite
of an hasil-not in colde watir.

Chapter X, Part 5
Difficulty in Breathing

[198]   A man haþ defaute in breþing, sum in drawing breeþ,
f. 183   sum in letting oute hir breeþ, / sum in boþe; sum in
breþing to faste.   Alle þese greuauncis comen of þe

---

16 bagge] *followed by* and put in þe watir of roses *canc. in red.* **17
ii]** *corr. from* iiii. **22** *2-line initial in blue.*

same enchesons þat streitnes of þe breste and þe coughe comen, and in þe same maner þei ben y-helid as þei ben.

[198v] Neþelis, þer ben oþer special medicines for þis sikenes, as if it be of grete humours þat stoppen þe breest, 3yue

5 him subtilitiues and dissolutiues, as oximel squillitike eiþir simple, eiþir ysope soden in hony. Eiþir make a sirip of þes þingis: Take of horehoune, dr. xx; of

Sirip liquoris, dr. x; of marche, of radiche, of fenel sede, of anise, of calamynt, of ysope, of meiden here, ana, dr.

10 v; of femigreke, of lynsed, ana, dr. iii; of cleen reysens, an hundrid drammes; of figis, xx; of penides, oz. vi; aqua, quantum sufficit. Make herof a sirip and let him

f. 183v vse smale wiyn / and cleer.

A good emplastir to ley on her brestis: Take

15 lilie rotis, and malues, and bismalues, and betis, and

A plastir drie figis, and reysens, and almondis, and pynes y-clensid. Stampe hem with wiyn and siþ do þerto mele and grece.

Good pillulis also herfore: Take of mirre, storacis,

Good pillulis galbanum, castore, pepir, ana, dr. v; of opium, sc. iiii.

20 Tempre hem vp with tisane þat dragagantum is resloued in. And 3yue him þerof x or xi. Baume is gode for þis greuaunce, and sc. i of gencian y-poudrid and y-ete with an

Baume and gencian y-poudird ben good
ey and with wiyn it is profitable. And so is a sc. of orpiment y-ete with an ey. And oþir þingis þat ben seid

---

5 **subtilitiues**] *corr. from* subtilatiues.

in þe couȝhe, ben good here.   And aftir þe diuersite of þe
enchesons of þe sekenessis, so ordeyne þy medicines, as it

f. 184   is seid / in oþer greuaunces of þe breest.

Chapter XI, The Heart
Part 1, The Cardiacle

[?]   Here beginneþ þe xi chaptir of þis boke, and conteyneþ

5   but ii° titles.

     A man-is herte, þat is þe principal membre of a
mannes body, haþ a sikenes þat is clepid þe cardiacle.

[199]   And þat may be on ii° maneris: Oon is of humours þat
ben enclosid withyn þe vttir skynnes of þe herte, and

10   þo maken þe herte to tremble and to quake. Anoþer
cardiacle þer is þat is of þe spiritis þat ben withyn
þe herte, and þat is y-clepid sincopis. But þe first maner
cardiacle comeþ oþerwhilis of suche humours þat makeþ a man
to haue a feuer, and oþirwhilis he comeþ withouten a

15   feuer, and oþirwhilis þe feuer is sharpe, and oþirwhilis

f. 184v   esy. But / what maner feuer euer it be, it makeþ a man to
haue an hote swote, and his kyndely hete draweþ outeward
from þe herte and from withinforþe, and brekiþ oute at
þe pores þat ben withoutenforþ in þe skyn. Oþirwhilis, þis

20   greuaunce comeþ of a corrupte wynde þat is inclosid in þe
herte, and þan it is clepid leping of þe herte. Oþirwhilis,
it comeþ of corrupt humours and kene þat ben in þe mouþ of
þe stomake and goiþ vp to þe herte by smale veynes and

[199v]   greueþ þe herte. Oþirwhilis, it comeþ from suche humours

---

5 ii° titles] *corr. from* oon chaptir. **6** *4-line initial in gold.* **12
maner]** *in r. h. margin.* **18-19 and brekiþ . . . withoutenforþ]** *in l. h.
margin.*

The Herte

þat comen from þe lyuer to þe herte. Oþirwhilis, it comeþ
of wormes þat ben in þe stomake eiþir in þe guttis, and

f. 185   prickeþ hem, and þe herte haþ / compassion of her
greuaunce and is y-greued also.   And þis greuaunce of þe

5   herte eiþir it comeþ of blode þat haþ moche colere, eiþir
of blode þat haþ moche malencoly.   The tokenes of þis
sekenes ben, trembling and leping of þe herte and of oþer
membris, hote swote withoutenforþe, and moche passing awei
of hete bi poores, feblenes of senewis, pale coloure, lene

10   and y-wastid awei as men þat han þe tisike eiþir etike,
with moche ache and greuaunce aboute þe herte.   And þei
mowe not slepe but litil, and oftesiþis þei ben costif, and
her pouse is swifte, and her vryn is reed, and þei tremblen

f. 185v   as men / doon for grete colde.   And whan it is of colere,

15   þe herte trembliþ, and þei han moche hete, moche þirste,
and depe breþing.   And when it comeþ of malencoly, þe
herte trembleþ, and þe man haþ moche sorowe, and sleuþe,
and is not þirstful.   And whan þis sekenes comeþ of ony
oþir sekenes of ony oþer membre, let 3yue þe pacient

20   suche þingis þat comfortiþ þe herte while þe oþer membre is
in heling.   But if þe greuaunce is principali of þe herte
and it be of coler, lete him blede at þe arme veyne þat is
clepid basilica if þou seest þat it is nede, as if þe man
be replet of blode and 3onge.   Ellis let garsen him in /

---

12 not] *ins. above.* slepe] *corr. from* sleple.   22 him] *prec. by* it
canc. in red.

places þat ben acording þerto and ny3e þe herte. And syþ
3eue him a sirip of borage, and siþ 3eue a cologoge to purge
him of coler. And siþ 3yue him þe iuse of borage, and of
scariole, and of pomgarnard. And in þe same maner do aftir
5 a feuer whan þer is mater y-lefte þat he is not y-purgid
of. Aftirwarde, anoynte al his body with þe muscilage of
sillie, and with þe white of an ey, and a litil popilion;
eiþir with þe watir þat draga[ga]gantum haþ be resoluid yn,
y-medlid with þe muscilage of sillie. Aftirward while þe
10 body is moist, let strowe þeron poudir of roses, of galles,

of bole, of acasie, of ypoquistidos, and of suche / oþir
strictories. And let him vse coolde electuaries, as

triasandri, rosata nouella, diarodon, diacameron, diantos
muscate, diamargariton, pocio muscata, diacitoniton muscata,
15 and medle with hem oþir hote electuaries. But let þe colde
haue þe maistrie. Also, sugir roset, and sugir of violet,

and diapapauer ben good for hem. A special sirip for þis
sekenes: Take borage, and maces, and spodie, and horshel,
and þe sede of citonies, and lignum aloes, galengale, canel,

20 þe rynde of pomgarnard, white coral, and make vp þi sirip
with sufficient sugir. Her dieting must be of suche metis
þat ben esi to defie. And let hem vsen oftsiþis þe for/-

seide anoynting of her body. And let hem also smelle
oftetymes colde þingis þat ben aromatike, as roses, and

---

5 he] *ins. above.* **6 al]** *corr. from* as. **7 of]** *ins. above.* **8
dragagantum]** dragantum. **14 muscata (2)]** *in l. h. margin.*

[200]

floures of violet, of borage, of basilicon, of baume. And
make poudir of þe same þingis, and do it in a bagge, and ley
it on þe stomake. And let þe house þer he lyueþ be strawen
with saleyn leues, or feren leues, and vyne leues, and roses,

5   and leues of violet, and watir-lilies, and of suche colde
herbes. And if it comeþ of colde, 3yue him poudir of canel,
of spike, of cardamomum, and zeduare, of eueriche, yliche

Hote
medicines

moche. And if it comeþ of malencoly, purge him with
mirabolanis indie, epitimi, sene, and with gotis mylke, and

10   suche oþer þingis. And if þe cardiacle comeþ of malencoly
and of coler togedir, let his purgacion and his oþir me/-

f. 187v

dicines be made of þo þingis þat purgen coler and malencoly:
iera fortissima Galieni, and þe grettir stoma[ti]con. And
siþ 3yue him comfortable electuaries and wel-smelling. And

15   medle with hem þe lymail of gold and þe poudir of þe boon þat
is in a hertes herte. And let his breest be anoyntid with
hote oynementis and aromatike, and oþer hote oylis þat ben
moche bettir. And let him vse good metis and good drinkis
þat engendren good blood. And let him vse oftetymes in his

20   metis lymail of golde and þe poudir of margerie peerles þat
ben good for þe cardiacle þat is with a feuer also. And in
þat cardiacle þat is with grete hete let þe soles of his fete

f. 188

and þe pavmes of his handes be wel rubbid with cold oy/les.
And wete a lynen clooþ in watir of roses and ley to his

13 stomaticon] stomacon.   **21 þat is**] *corr. from* is.

noseþirllis. And ley him in a colde place þat is ful of cold floures and cold leues and y-spreynt with cold watir. And anoynte him aboute þe templis with þe iuse of sorel, and of syngrene, and of suche colde herbes. And anoynte

5 his necke and his chyn with oile of mirtis and of saleyne. And siþ cast þervpon þe poudir of roses and of sandris.

Oyle of mirtis is y-made of þe leues of mirtis y-soden in comen oile and leide xxx daies in þe sunne.

Oile of mirtis

Comen oile is mete oile, þat is, oile de olif. And ri3t

10 as oile of mirtis is y-made, so is y-made al maner oiles þat ben made of leues eiþir of floures, as oile of roses or oile of violet, and suche oþir. Also anoynte his

f. 188v brest / with þe white of an ey and with þe iuse of citonies y-medlid togedir. Eiþir make a plastir of þe þre kyndes

15 of sandris, and roses, and þe shaving of yvery y-medlid togedir with oile of violet and with watir of roses; eiþir of þe poudir of hertis horne and sandris y-medlid with watir of roses. And if þe cardiacle comeþ of þe stomake, make him to caste, eiþir 3eue him a purgacion of mirabolani

20 citrini, of cassia fistula, of manna, and plumbes. And make him a plastir withouten of sandris, and barly mele, and smyþþes asses. And 3yue him cold electuaries as it is y-told tofore, and if it comeþ of þe lyuer, as it shal be told in his sekenes. And if it comeþ of moche waking

---

1 noseþirllis] *corr. from* noseþrillis. 6 þervpon] to *canc. in red after* þer. 19 a purgacion] *in l. h. margin.* 20 fistula] *corr. from* fistule. manna] *corr. from* manne. And] *corr. from* of.

f. 189

[200v]

f. 189v

A special
gargarisme

Special
medicines:
þis sekenis

eiþir of moche fasting, ȝyue him diaanisum, diacitoniton, /
eiþir diaspermat[ic]on.   And if þou may not gete þes, take
anese and seþe it in watir.   And in þat watir wete wolle
þat is y-shore of an vnwasshid shepe, and ley þat vppon
5 þe herte.   And ley oþir medicynes in diuerse places
þat ben dissolutiues and moun dissolue þe corrupt humours
þat ben boþe in þe stomake and in þe herte.   And if þis
sekenes come of fleumatike mater eiþir of colerike þat is
aboute þe liȝte, it is clepid a trembling cardiacle, for
10 whan a man lyeþ his honde on þe herte, he trembleþ.   And
she haþ not hir kyndli meving as it shuld haue.   And to
þis cardiacle is profitable to make a gargarisme of
louage, ysope, and sauery, and þe iuse of liquoris,
and radiche, / and yreos, and origanum, and calamynt,
15 and horehovne y-soden in meþe.   Let him vse þis gargarisme
on morewe and at even, and let him swolowe doune of þe
same decoccion into his stomake.   And siþen let purge
him with iera y-medlid with þe poudir of radiche and of
yreos.   And siþen let anoynte him with mel roset wel-
20 despumed. Symple medicines and nameliche for þe cardiacle
ben, coral, margaritis, golde, and þe boon þat is in an
hertes hert, carpobalsamum, clowes, and a precious stone
þat is callid iacinctus.   And to hem þat han þe cardiacle
of colde and of malencoly, it is a profitable medicyn to

1 **diaanisum**] *corr. from* dianisum.   2 **diaspermaticon**]
diaspermaton.   7 **if**] *prec. by* fo *canc. in red.* 11 **she**] *corr. from* it.   16
swolowe] solowe.   21 **coral**] *ins. above.*   23 **iacinctus**] *corr. from*
iacintus.

drinke wiyn. And to hem þat han a cardiacle of corrupt
humours of þe stomake and namely of grete hete, þou shalt

f. 190   not 3eue / hem hote metis þat wolen sone be defied, but
oþer metis þat wolen be longe in defieng.

Chapter XI, Part 2
Syncope

5   Sincopis is a greuaunce of þe herte and may be

· [201]   y-clepid a cardiacle, for-asmoche as it is a sekenes
of þe herte. But it comeþ not of humours as þe oþer
cardiacle doiþ, but of þe greuaunce of þe spiritis of
þe hert, and þat is in ii° maneris. Oon is when þei

10   ben gaderid togedir in þe herte and þe herte haþ mo þan he
sholde kyndly haue, as it hapneþ whan a man falliþ
from a sodeyn gladnes into a sodeyn sorewe, eiþir falliþ
from a grete hete into a grete colde. But þe toþir maner

f. 190v   is whan a mannes spiritis goon soden/ly oute of his herte

15   and ben y-sparplid abrode in al þe body, as it happneþ whan
a man falliþ into a soden ioy aftir his sorowe, eiþir into
a grete hete aftir a grete cold. And of boþe þes maneris

Peril of
deeþ   a man may li3tly dye but if he be þe raþir y-holpe. This
sekenes comeþ also of to grete plente of humours in a

20   mannes body þat þristiþ þe hert togedir; oþerwhilis of a-
nyntishing of a mannes body and of to grete feblenes, as

Long
stonding
in þe
sunne is
perilous   it happneþ bi suche men þat han had a long-during fluxe,
eiþir sum oþir maner lesing of blode, eiþir þoroughe moche
stonding in þe sunne þat haþ y-drawen oute a manis kyndli

---

5 *2-line initial in blue.* **6 sekenes]** *corr. from* senes. **15 happneþ]**
corr. from happeþ. **23 maner]** *in l. h. margin.* **moche]** *prec. by* longe
canc. in red.

f. 191

f. 191v
[201v]

hete and his spiritis.   Oþerwhiles it comeþ of plente of
hu/mours þat ben in þe stomake, and þan a man shal volate
moche, and casten oftensiþes, and þe hyndir parte of his
hede wole ake, and nameli bifore mete.   And whiles he haþ
5   his accesse, him semeþ þat he seeþ moche þinge bifore his
y3en þat is not þer.   And þis cardiacle þat comeþ of
stomake lestiþ not long.   Oþerwhiles it is of plente of
humours þat ben in þe guttis.   And if it be of malencoly,
þen is heuynes and greueunce in þe wombe and swelling.   Of
10   colere comeþ ache and pricking.   Of flevme comeþ heuynes and
swelling, and oþer suche tokenes aftir þe kynde of þe
humour.   Oþirwhiles it comeþ of an-oþer sikenes.   But how-
euer it be, þou shalt hi3e to hele þis sekenes, / 3ee wel
raþir þan þe sekenes þat it comeþ of.   And if it be of to
15   grete plente of spiritis þat be inclosid in þe herte and
ben y-runne from withouten into þe herte, eiþir if it be a
sekenes bi himselfen, eiþir com of an-oþer sekenes, let
bynde his fyngris with þongis and his toon also, þat þe
spiritis and þe blode movn drawe outeward from þe herte.
20   And close þe noseþirles, and open his mouþe þat þe fume
mowe cum oute at his mouþe.   And wring him wel by þe
nose, and pulle him by þe heris of his berde and also of his
hede.   And let sum frende of his kisse him þat tendirly
loueþ him.   And rubbe wel his hondes, and þis shal

---

2 shal] *in r. h. margin.* **5 his** (1)] *ins. above.* **13 be]** *prec. by* com
canc. in red. **15 plente]** *in l. h. margin.* **21 at]** *corr. from* of.

make him to arisen vp of his accesse.   And if it comeþ of

f. 192 anentising / and of feblenes of his body, ȝyue him in tyme

of his acces wiyn þat clowes and sage ben y-soden yn. And

if it be of moche plente of blode eiþir of oþir humours,

5   let þat be abatid bi blode-letting or bi sum oþir purgacion

aftir þe kynde of þe humours. And if it be of grete plente

of humours of þe stomake, make him to caste. And if it be

Remedi for
hote
humours and
cold see in
þe chaptir
of þe
stomake of hote humours, ȝyue him colde medicines. And if it be of

colde humours, ȝyue him hote medicines, as Y wole seie in

10   þe sekenes of þe stomake.   And if it be of fulnes of

þe guttis, purge him with a clistre or a suppository. And

if it be of þe ouer-guttis, purge him with an-oþir

purgacion, as Y shal sey in þe sekenes of þe guttis. And

f. 192v if it comeþ of / hete of þe sunne or of suche oþer hete,

15   let springe his face with watir of roses, and ley on his

visage and aboute him saleyn leues. And if it comeþ of

grete fleume þat is in a mannes guttis, and he haue þe

feueris, let heten a tiyl stoon and put it in vinegir.

A tild
stoon
leide
warme to
þe herte And þan wrappe him in a clene lynen cloþe and ley to his

20   herte.   And if he haþ not þe feueris, ȝyue him triacle

diatesseron with wiyn þat auence and rue ben y-soden yn.

Triacle diatessaron is þus y-made: Take of mirre, of

[356v] aristologie rotunda, of gencian, of baies of lorer y-

made clene, ana, oz. i & sc. ii; of ditandre, of pigami,

---

3 yn] *followed by* eiþir *canc. in red.* 10 it] *in l. h. margin.* 11 a (2)]
ins. above. 13 purgacion] *in r. h. margin.*

[357]

f. 193

of camedreos, ana, dr. i & sc. ii; and viii greynes of þe gumme of yuy; of calcant y-brent, sc. i; of hony, quantum sufficit. Oþir men don herto / femigreke, nigelle, and zedwarie, of eueriche on, oz. i & sc. ii; and of aspalte, 5 as moche. Al þes shullen be y-poudrid and y-medlid with þe forseide hony. This triacle is good for men þat ben y-poisened or biten of venemous bestis or wormes, or of a woode ho[u]nde. And it shal be drunken with þe iuse of myntes. And it is good to ley on venemous 10 postmes in þe maner of an oynement. And it is good for þe feuer quarteyn, and for þe cotidian feuer to drinke it with þe iuse of pigami or of gencian. And it is gode for hem þat ben greued in her stomake, or in her lyver, or in þe splene. And if sincopis com of bleding at þe nose, 15 if it be at þe lifte noseþirile, let him be cuppid aboute þe splene on þe lifte side, withouten garsyng to drawe þe blode doun/warde from þe nose. If þe nose blede on þe ri3te þirile, do so on þe ri3t side. And if it comeþ of anentising of þe body, eiþir of moche bleding, let him 20 drinke good wyne y-medlid with colde watir. If he haue no feuer, let him smel swete-smelling þingis, as roses, and violettis, and suche oþer. Also it is good to hete a pece of golde or of siluer in þe fier and qwenche it oftsiþis in þe wiyn þat he shal drinke. And suche men shulen not

[202]

f. 193v

A pece of
gold or
siluer
y-hete

---

5 þes] *in r. h. margin.* 7 wormes] *in r. h. margin.* 8 hounde]
honde. 20 wyne] *in l. h. margin*

baþen hem, ne be y-lefte to blede, for þat wolde drawen
þe spiritis of her herte outeward. And þerfore it behoueþ
to lye him in a colde place, and maken it cold with cold
leues, as it is y-tolde in þe cardiacle of þe herte. /

f. 194   5   And if þis greuaunce comeþ of moche beyng in þe sunne, or
of long abidyng in a baþ, caste no colde watir on his
visage but it be medlid with wiyn. But set him in þe
wynde, or by craft blowe wynde on him. And þe smel of
gourdes is good for hem. And if it comeþ of grete cold,

  10   let him vse hote electuaries, and let him drinke good wiyn
and smel to wel-sauerid þinges and good of smel. /

Chapter XII, The Stomach
Part 1, Difficulty in Swallowing

f. 221   Here beginneþ þe xii chaptir of þis boke whiche
[?]   conteineþ xii titles or practi[s]es.

A man-is stomake haþ many greuaunces. Þe firste
  15   is greuaunce in swolewing of mete and drinke. Anoþir
is vnresonable appetit to mete and drinke. Anoþir is
defaute of appetit to mete and drinke. Anoþir is þirste;
f. 221v   anoþir is defaute of þirste. / Oþir greuaunces þer ben,
as balking, zosking, abhominacion to mete and drinke, and
  20   wille forto caste, turnyng vpsodoun of a mannes stomake,
grete hete of þe stomake, and a postem of þe stomake.

Greuaunce of swolewing comeþ in þre maners and
Greuaunce
of swolwing   of þre enchesons. Of greet hete and of greet coold
[206v]   of þe wesaunde: but þan whan he swolewiþ, it is greuous,

---

12 *In the margins of f. 221 the scribe has written* Aftir trev stonding
þis chaptir shulde stonde nexte aftir þe title of sincopis, and nexte
þis: þe chaptir of þe guttis. And aftir þat, þe chaptir of þe lyuer, and
aftir þat þe chaptir of þe spleen, and þen þe chaptir of þe reines, and
soforþ as it is writen. *The text has been rearranged accordingly.* **xii]**
xiiii. **13 xii]** xi. **practises]** practies. **14** *4-line initial in gold.*

but so he may swollewen a litil and a litil. And he is
þirstful if it comeþ of hete, and haþ moche hete and
row3nes in his wesaunt. And to helen him of þis greuaunce,
3yue him cassia fistula, and plumbes, and innibes. And if

5 him nediþ, let him blede. And ellis purge him. And siþ
3yue him colde siripis to akelen him with, as violet, and

f. 222   of plumes with þe iu/se of gourdis. And let him ete
colde erbis, as purselane, gourdis, violet, arage,
letuse, and suche oþir. And anoynt him with oynementis

10 and ley colde plastris also þerto to abaten þe hete. And
if it comeþ of colde, let him vsen electuaries þat
is y-made of hony roset, and scariole, and þe iuse of
marche y-medlid togedir.

Hony roset is y-made of hony and of roses y-hackid

Hony roset
15 smale and y-soden in hony ouer þe fier. In-to a pounde

[?]   of roses þou shalt put ii° pounde of hony. Also let
him vse hoot electuaries þat weren tolde in þe coughe.

[206v]   In anoþir maner þis greuaunce comeþ, as of a postem
þat is in wesaunde. And þan he haþ grete greuaunce

20 þerin, and nameli while he swolewiþ. And if þe postem

f. 222v   is hoot, / þou may knowe bi þe foreseide tokenes. And if
it comeþ of colde, þer is heuynes in þe wesaunde withouten
þilke tokenes. And if it is an hoot postem, do as it was
seide raþir. Whan it comeþ of hete withouten postem, leye

11 electuaries] alectuaries. **16 put**] *corr. from* haue. **22 it**] *ins. above.*

colde plastris withoutenforþe and cold pillulis vndir þe
tunge, and norisshe him with almonde milke, and with gourdes,
and tisan, and suche oþir þingis. And if it be a coolde
postem, ȝyue him ysope y-soden in hony, and þe sirip of

5   horehone þat was y-spoke of in þe couȝ. And if it be
with a feuer, ȝyue him tysan wiþ almonde mylke and with
sugir. And if þe postem breke, clense him with tisan, and
almonde milke, and calamynte y-medlid togedir. And if he
be riȝt feble, ȝyue him gotis milke to drinken þat a reed

10   glowing stoon haþ be oftesiþes quenchid yn. And if it /
be an hoot postem, let þe plastir þat shal make him repe
be made of sillie and of lynsede y-temprid with milke. And
if it be of colde, let maken þe plastir of femigreke and þe
seed of coton y-meynd with bottir. In þe þridde maner, þis

15   greuaunce comeþ of a wounde of þe wesavnde. And þan he
feliþ þeryn boþe ache and pricking and nameli whan he etiþ
soure metis eiþir salte. And þes woundes shullen ben y-
helid with þe iuse of planteyn, bole, and turmentyne, and
hony y-medlid togedere. Þis medicyn is profitable þouȝ þe

20   wounde be oolde. And if þe wounde be withouten, þe
foreseide medicyn shal be leyde þerto in þe maner of an
oynement. And if it be within/forþe, let him swolewe his
medicyn. And if it be with a feuer, ȝyue him his medicyn
with a tisan. If he haþ no feuer, ȝyue it him wiþ

f. 223

f. 223v

---

11 postem] *prec. by a canc. in red.* **14 meynd]** *corr. from* mynde.
21 þe] *prec. by a canc. in red.* **24 he haþ]** *marked for reversal.* **no]**
corr. from noon.

mellicratum.

[?]

Mellicratum is made of wiyn and hony y-soden togedere, but þe two partis ben wiyn and þe þridde parte is hony. And oþir þingis ben profitable þat ben y-tolde in þe

5 woundes of þe li3t. And al medicines þat shullen be

[206v]

swolewid shullen not be sodenliche swolowid adoun, but al by eese. And þen þei shulen stond to profite.

Chapter XII, Part 2
Defective Appetite

Defaute and lesing of a mannes apetite is in two maneris, eiþir þorou3 colde humours þat ben in þe

10 stomake þat ben rawe and vndefied, and þan þe balking

f. 224

is soure, and he is not / þirstful, and þe stomake

[207v]

defieþ febely and swelliþ. It comeþ also of colerike humours þat ben in þe stomake. And þe tokenes of hem ben hoot balking, bitternes of þe mooþ, and grete þirste, and

15 swiftli he defieþ grete mete. And in þe secunde maner, it comeþ when a man haþ loste his desire and his wil to mete. And þis is in two maneris. Oon is þorou3 corrupcion of þe stomake. And þe token þerof is þat a man haþ abhominacion

[208]

to þat mete þat he louiþ bifore. And þis is a perilous

20 greuaunce in long sikenessis and nameliche in þe blodi fluxe. The toþir maner comeþ þorou3 corrupcion of a man-is witte, as in men þat ben frentike eiþir wode, and han

f. 224v

lost her witte, / and so þei lesen appetit to mete and to drinke. An vnresonable appetit is whan a man haþ wille

8 *2-line initial in blue.* **19 a]** *ins. above.* **23 to mete]** *in l. h. margin.*

[206v] to ete aftir þat he haþ eten ri3t ynow. And þer ben two
kyndes of þis appetit.   The toon is y-clepid an houndes
appetit.   And þat is whan a man etiþ moche more þen him
nediþ and sone aftir castiþ it vp as an hounde.   The
5 secunde maner is whan a man defieþ his mete þou3 he etiþ
moche more þen him nediþ; eiþir þou3 he defieþ it not, he
castiþ it not, but let it passe forþe þorou3 his guttis.
And þis vnresonable appetit comeþ of þe stomakes cooldenes
[207v] and of malencoli þat is in þe mooþ of þe stomake.   For
10 þou shalt vndirstonde þat þe stomake desiriþ mete and
f. 225 drinke boþe for sustenaunce of himsilf and for al þe bo/di.
And in þe ouer-parti of þe stomake þer is feling.   And
whan þat þe humour of malencoli droppiþ on þat ouer-parti
of þe stomake, þe stomake feliþ þe keneship of þis malencoli
15 and willeþ and desireþ more mete kyndli.   But whan þer is
to moche of þis malencoli in þe mooþ of þe stomake, it
makiþ þe appetit vnresonable, and wileþ more þen he mai
defie and makiþ him to casten it vp.   For men þat han þis
[208] greuaunce, it is profitable to drinken good reed wiyn, and
20 moche fasting, and nameliche suche wiyn þat is þicke in
þe mouþe and swete.   And let hem vsen hoot electuaries þat
ben sumwhat bitter, as diatrionpipirion, diacalamentum,
diapigamum, diacene, diaprassium, diacinimum, and suche
oþer.   And let her stomake be anoyntid with hoot /

f. 225v

oynementis, and ley hoot plastris þeron. And let hem not ete soure þingis. But if þei desiren vnctuous þingis, 3yue hem, boþe in þe beginning of her appetit, and in þe myddel, and in þe ende.

Diatrion-
pipirion

5   Diatrionpipirion is to dissoluen corrup wyndes and humours of þe stomake, and comfortiþ þe stomake and þe guttis boþe, and is þus y-made: Take of pipir boþe white and blacke and longe, of canel, of ginger, of fenel seed, of anyse, of mastike, of asarum, ana, oz. i; of zilobalsamum,

10 of cassie, of spike, of amomum, ana, oz. 1/2; of cardamomum, of marche, ameos, citre, clowes, coost, and of macis, ana, oz. iiii;   of hony, quantum sufficit.   Also   let   him   vsen diazinziber, dia[ga]lange, and suche oþer electuaries þat clensen þe stomake of corrupt humours. And if þe stomake

15 be feble þat he may not holden þe metis þat he resceyueþ,

f. 226

þan / vnctuous metis ben noiful. Vnctuous metis ben fat metis and alle maner fatnes and oiles.   But 3yue him smelling electuaries and bitter also, and saueri soure metis. And if it comeþ of hete þat anentishiþ þe stomake

20 and makiþ him feble, let him vsen reste, and slepe, and colde eire, and anoynte his stomake with oile of roses and of violet.   And 3yue him colde siripis to drinke, as of violet and roses.   And in suche vnresonable appetitis þat comen of corrupt humours of þe stomake, it is profitable to

13 diagalange] dialange. **19 anentishiþ]** *corr. from* entishiþ. **24 is]** *ins. above.*

make him caste, and þan purge him of þat humour. And þat
þou may doo by anet and hony. And þis shal make him caste
withoute greet traueil. But firste let him ete freisshe
fisshe and rotis of erbis with oximel. And siþ let him

5 drinke good wiyn, and þan he shal eseli caste. And

aftirwarde, let / him be dietid with deintes. And make a
plastir withoutenforþe on þe stomake of mastike, spike,
roses, wormod, and suche oþir þingis.

A sirip þat doiþ awei an vnresonable appetit, and

10 makiþ a good appetit, and lettiþ a man of casting: Take
of clowes, canel, notemig, maces, quibibis, calamynte,
origanum, mynte, seen, sandris white and reed, and
cardamomum. And put þerto a sponful of vynegir. And
make vp þi sirip wiþ sufficient sugir. But oþirwhilis þis

15 vnresonable appetit comeþ of humours þat ben rawe and
vndefied. And þan it is profitable to make him caste and to
purge him with sum purgacion bineþeforþe. And siþ 3yue him
good metis and good drinkis to make good humours. And 3yue
him comfortable electuaries, and siripis, and sweet-

20 smelling / emplastirs. And among al erbis, þe moost
profitable ben mynte, and wormod, and rue. And if þe
humours ben collerike, let him be purgid. And siþ 3eue him
soure metis and cold. And eueriche defavte of appetit þat
comeþ of yuel complexion of þe stomake, as of to greet

2 him] *ins. above.* **20 smelling**] *followed by* and *canc.*

160

hete eiþir of to greet colde, shal be helid bi þe contrari,
[208v]   as if it is of hete, bi colde medicines.

Chapter XII, Part 3
Lack of Thirst

Defaute of þirste comeþ in four maneris, eiþir
of yuel humours þat ben in þe stomake þat ben colde and
5   moist.   And þat is y-helid if þe stomake be y-purgid
of þo humours, and siþ is y-fed with good drie metis and
leviþ moist metis.   And let him vse hoot electuaries and
drie, as diatrionpipirion.   And let him vse hoot sauces
with his mete and no vynegre. Also it comeþ of greet colde
f. 227v 10   of þe stomake, and it is y-he/lid bi hote medicines.   And
þis defaute of þirste comeþ of feblenes of þe stomake, and
it is y-helid also bi hote medicines.   Also defaute of
þirste þat comeþ of feblenes of þe stomake and corrupcion
of þe feling of þe stomake is incurable and token of deeþ.
15   And if it comeþ of lesing of mannes wit, if þe man be brou3t
to his wit a3en, it may be holpe, ellis not.

Chapter XII, Part 4
Excessive Thirst

Miche þirste comeþ in meny maneris, eiþirwhilis of
grete hete of þe brest, eiþirwhilis of þe metis þat a
man etiþ, eiþirwhilis of hete of þe eire, eiþir of moche
20   traueil.   Thriste þat comeþ of þe stomake is in two
maneris: eiþir for to hoot metis, and token þat a man haþ
f. 228   y-ete; eiþir of corrupt humours þat ben in / þe stomake,
as coler, eiþir salt fleume.   And if þis þirste com of
coler, þe mooþ is hoot and bitter, and nameli aftir þat a

3 *2-line initial in blue.* **6 drie metis**] *marked for reversal.* **17** *2-line initial in blue.*

man haþ y-dronken colde watir. And he may feel hou þe smoke comeþ vp into his þrote. And if it is of salt flevme, he shal fele saltnes in his mooþ. And his þirst is y-kelid þorou3 drinking of warme watir. And if it comeþ of heet,

5 colde watir wole quenche it. Þirste þat comeþ of hete of þe brest is raþir y-staunchid þorou3 drawing breeþ of colde eire, þan þorou3 ony drinke. Neþeles, if suche greet þirst com of corrupt humours, eiþir in þe stomake, eiþir bineþe in þe guttis, eiþir in þe brest aboue, let him be purgid

10 with a medicin þat is acording to þe humour. And if it
f. 228v comeþ of moche blode, let him / bleed. And siþen 3yue him cold siripis, as of gourdes eiþir of violet with sugir. And norisshe him with tisan, and purselane, letuse, vinegir, and blitis. And let him be in reste, boþe of bodi and of

15 speking. And let make him a plastir of gourdes, of portulake, and of suche oþir cold þingis. And if þe þirst com of coler þat is in þe stomake, let him be purgid with sum cologoge, and make him to cast. And siþ 3yue him þe sirip of violet eiþir þe seed of citonies. A drinke forto

20 staunche moche þirst: Take of drie roses, dr. v; of
oxifistula, dr. v; of fenel seed, dr. i. Do al þis in two pounde of hoot scalding watir al any3t. And on þe
[209] morewe, 3yue him þerof to drinke fasting halfe a pounde. But if þe þirst com of salt flevme, 3yue him a purgacion

4 it] *in r. h. margin.*

f. 229 and siþ let him drinke þe watir þat fe/nel seed and marche seed ben soden yn. And ȝyve him to drinke mellicratum y-medlid with warme watir eiþir good white wiyn. Dieting of him shal be of gode metis þat ben not salt. And if

5 a man is a-þirste anyȝt, lete him sleep. And þat shal kele his þirste. Or ellis ȝyue him drinke.

Chapter XII, Part 5
Burping

Balking: Sum is smoky and hoot and sum is soure. Þe first comeþ of heet and of hote humours þat ben in þe stomak. Þe secunde is of coold humours eiþir of feble

10 heet of þe stomake. For balking þat comeþ of hete and of colerike humours in þe stomake, let him be purgid of þo

[209v] humours. And siþ let him vse colde þingis boþe in medicynes and also in his dieting. And let him vse colde electuaries, as þe colde diacitoniton, triasandri, diarodon

15 abbatis, sugir roset, sugir violet, and þe sirip of roses

f. 229v and þe / sirip of violet y-made vp with vinegre. And her dieting shal be of metis and drinkis þat ben not ful hoot, as shalid fisshe, and wiyn medlid with watir, and colde frutis, and cold anoyntinges aboute þe stomake, and cold

20 plastris y-leide þerto, and a temperat baþ neiþir to hoot ne to colde. But if þe balking comeþ of colde of þe stomake, it may be in two maneris: eiþir of cold humours þat ben in þe stomak and makiþ þe stomake to swelle, and heuy, and makiþ a man deliueren him of wiynd byneforþ,

---

7 *2-line initial in blue.* **19 anoyntinges**] *corr. from* anoyntis.

eiþir ellis it comeþ of coldenes of þe stomake withouten
suche humours.   And þat greuaunce is y-holpen bi hoot
medicines and with hoot oynementis and emplastirs.   And if
þer waxe miche wynde boþe abouen and bineþen, make him

f. 230   5   a poudir of mastik, comyn, louage, a/nise, ginger, carewei,
long pepir, and suche oþir þingis.

A good medicyn for balking and to destroie corrupt
wyndis of þe stomake: Take of mastik, comyn, louage, anise,
fenel seed, squinantum, gynger, carewei, ameos, amomum,

10   sileris montein, long pipir, zedeware, galengale, ozmi,
calamus aramaticus, cassia lignea, macis, maiorone, of eche,
yliche moche. Poudir hem and medle hem with hony roset.

A good electuari for coldenes of þe stomake, and
Electuari   for wyndis, and for soure balkingis, and for vnresonable
for
coldenes
of þe   15   appetit, and it makiþ a mannes mooþ wel-y-sauerid, and
stomake   is þus y-maad: Take of canel, and of long pipir and of
blacke, of clowes, of lignum aloes, cassie, citre, spike,
f. 230v   azarum, squinantum, / galengale, calamus aroma[ti]cus,
carpobalsamum, zilobalsamum, ameos, ginger, ana, dr. iii;

20   of sugir, dr. iiii; of mastik, oz. i; of aristologie þe
rounde, of macis, of polie, of liquoris, ana, dr. iiii &
1/2; of honi, quantum sufficit.

A good poudir for men þat ben discolerid and han feble
si3t and feble digestion: Take canel, gynger, cardamomum,

18 aromaticus] aromacus.

pepir, sauery, maioran, anise, fenel, carewai, netlis seed, galengale, eufrase, of eueriche, oz. 1/2; of notemig, squinantum, folie, ana, dr. ii; of citre, dr. i & 1/2; of iera yreos, oz. ii. Let him vse þe povdir þat is y-made of

5 al þes y-medlid togedir in his metis and in his drinkes.

A good sirip and an hoot, for coldenes of þe stomake, and for soure balkingis of þe stomake, and for wyndes of þe stomake: Take xx pounde of watir and put to hem /

f. 231   halfe pounde of reisenes, of calamynte, mynte, and nepte,

10 of eueriche of hem, oz. iii. And let al þes ben a day and a ny3t in þat watir. Aftirward, clense þat watir and do þerto v pounde of hony. And seeþ þat ouer an esi fier. Aftirward take mastik, cardamomum, black pipir and long, of eueriche, dr. ii. Poudir hem and put hem to

15 þis foreseide watir and hony.

Diaspermat[ic]on is good for heuynes of þe hede, and turning of þe brayn, and for aking and swelling

Diaspermat-
[ic]on for   of þe chechis, and for siking, and streitnes of breþing,
þe hede
and narewship of þe breste, and for men þat han loste

20 her speche, and for ache of þe stomake and hardenes, and soure balkingis, and for a feble stomake þat may not holden his mete but sone aftir hit is receyved, castiþ

f. 231v   it vp, eiþir lettiþ it passe doun / vndefied, and is good also for þe spleen, and is þus made: Take of longe

---

4 **iera]** *in l. h. margin.* **8 put to hem]** *corr. from* do him *in a.* **12-13 an esi fier]** *copied* þe fier an esi *with* þe *canc. and the words following marked for reversal.* **16 Diaspermaticon]** Diaspermaton. **18 of (2)]** *ins. above.*

pepir, dr. ix; of gynger, dr. viii; of carewei, of louage,
ana, dr. vi; of parsely, macedo, ameos, femigreke, dauke,
sileris montein, amomum, comyn, marche sede, fenel seed,
[210]   anise, ana, dr. ii; of hony, quantum sufficit.   Anoþir
5   diaspermat[ic]on þat is good for swelling of þe wombe
and for hem þat movn not wel defien her mete: Take
carewei, anise, cardamomum, canel, ameos, marche, ana,
dr. iii; of pepir, oz. iii; of hony, quantum sufficit.

Chapter XII, Part 6
Hiccups

Zosking comeþ in meny maneris, eiþirwhilis of excesse
10   of etyng eiþir of drinking þat makiþ þe stomake to
[210v]   ful.   And þat mai be in two maneris, for al þe stomake
mai be to ful of mete, eiþir þe mooþ of þe stomak may /
f. 232   be to ful, and suche zosking comeþ aftir mete.   And þis
mai be staunchid in making a man agaste, eiþir ashamid,
15   eiþir ri3t glad, eiþir if he puttiþ his fyngir deep in his
mooþ and holdiþ him þer awhile.   Eiþirwhilis zosking comeþ
of corrupt humours þat ben in þe stomake and makiþ þe
[?]   stomake feble.   And þis zosking comeþ raþir bifore mete þen
aftir.   And þis is y-holpen if þe stomake be purgid of þo
20   humours bi casting, eiþir anoþir purgacion þat is acording
to þe humour þat is encheson of þe zosking, and siþ in
norisshing þe man with good metis and with good drinkis and
leuing surfet.   Eiþirwhilis it comeþ of cooldnes þat is in
þe ouer-parte of þe stomake þat makiþ þat party han a

---

5 diaspermaticon] diaspermaton. **9** *2-line initial in blue.* **10
makiþ**] *in r. h. margin.* **14 be**] *in r. h. margin.* **21 encheson**] *corr. from*
enchesons.

f. 232v

crampe, and is vnmiȝti to deliuere him of þe corrupt humours þat / ben in þe stomake. Eiþirwhilis it comeþ of anentishing and of feblenes of þe stomake. And þat mai be in two maneris: eiþir of colerike humours þat han long y-

5 leien in þe stomake and y-made þe stomake feble, eiþir of sum oþir sikenes þat haþ y-feblid þe stomake, as of flux eiþir of a feuer. And whan it is of a feuer, it is perilous. But if þe stomake be y-feblid and zoskiþ of a long fluxe þat a man haþ y-had, þou shalt dieten þat man

10 with comfortable þingis. And ȝyue him electuaries þat wole maken him moiste withynforþe, as diapenidion and diadraga[ga]ntum. And ȝyue him tisan to drinke, and þe sirip of violet, and þe sede of citonies. And make a plastir to leye on his stomake of lynseed and of femigreke

15 y-soden in oile. And anoynte þe stomake with oile of

f. 233

violet / and of roses. And if zosking comeþ of kene metis, þe same þingis ben profitable. And let him þat haþ zosking of anentishing of þe stomake vse sugir roset and cold erbis

[210]

and moist, as purselane, and letuse, and cheries, and soure

20 plumbes, and suche oþir. And wete a clooþ in warme watir þat violet and hockis ben y-soden yn, and ley þat clooþ from þe mooþ of þe stomake doun to his membris and to his sidis. And if it comeþ of humours þat filliþ þe stomake

[210v]

and þe humours been hoot, make him þis sirip: Take þe

---

12 **diadragagantum**] diadragantum. **him**] *in l. h. margin.*

rotis of fenel, and of parseli, and of wormod, hertistonge, endiue, comyn, spiknard. Stampe hem togedir and þen seeþ hem in watir. And make vp þy sirip and ȝyue it him to drinke. Aftirwarde purge him with a laxatif. And

f. 233v 5 siþ ȝyue him cold þingis boþe in me/dicines and in metis. But if it be of colde humours, ȝyue him oximel componed. And siþ ȝyue him a purgacion. And ȝyue him þe iuse of wormod with hony, and siþ ȝyue him hoot electuaries. And make a stufe for þe stomake of wiyn þat þes þingis

10 ben soden yn: origanum, souþerenwode, sansuke, rue, mynte, and suche oþir. And of þe erbis make a plastir and ley on þe stomake. Anoynte also þe stomake with oile of lorer, oþir with siche oþir hoot oil. And if he be replet of blood, let him blede. And ȝyue him cassi[a] fistula with

15 warme watir. And if þe stomake be harde, take dates, and cast awey þe stones, and stampe hem with fresshe grees. And make a plastir þerof and ley vppon þe stomake. It is

f. 234 good also for zosking þat comeþ of heet eiþir of / colde, and siþ comforte þe stomake as Y tolde tofore. And if

20 zosking comeþ of colde of þe stomak withouten suche humours, it mai be y-holpe bi drinking of warme wiyn and anoynting of hoot oynementis withouteforþe. Let al her metis and her drinkes be warme. Snesing also staunchiþ þis zosking, and zosking also þat comeþ of to moche eting and drinking. And

14 cassia] cassi.

pillulis þat ben made of aloes, and mastike, and þe iuse of wormod ben good here also. Eiþir ȝyue him to drinke wiyn þat rwe is soden yn y-medlid with hony, eiþir þe sede of carewei, eiþir anees, eiþir calamente, eiþir reubarbe, eiþir

5 ginger, eiþir ony hoot electuari þat Y spake of bifore. And anoynt him with oil of lorer or suche oþir hoot oil.

f. 234v And if zosking come of keen metis þat a / man haþ y-ete, let him drinke colde watir, eiþir þe sirip of violet, eiþir of plumes. Also þou maist staunche eueri maner of zosking

10 bi making a man aferde, eiþir a-shamid, and by snesyng. And if a man holdiþ his breþe, his zosking wole cese. A good poudir for corrup windes of þe stomake: Take of fenel seed, a pounde; of ameos, anet, carewei, ana, half a pounde; of ysope, piliol, origane, calamynte, ana, oz. i; of

15 cardamomum, of canel, ana, oz. 1/2; of folie, of gynger, ana, dr. ii. Make poudir of al þis and ȝyue him þerof with his metis and bi itsilf also.

Chapter XII, Part 7
Vomiting

Casting and spuyng and wil forto caste comeþ of corrupt humours þat ben in þe stomake. And of suche corrupt

20 humours þat ben in þe stomake comeþ anoþir greuaunce þat

f. 235 is abhominacion and volating of mete and / drinke, for suche corrupt humours, if þei ben in þe mooþ of þe stomake, þei distroien a man-is appetit. And if þei ben withinforþ in þe stomake, þei maken þe stomake feble þat he may not

18 *2-line initial in blue.*

defien þe mete þat he resceiueþ. And þes two enchesons
maken a man to volaten his mete and haue wil forto caste.
And if þes humours ben in þe mooþ of þe stomak, þan
a man shal caste li3tli and deliueren him of þilke
5   humours. And if þei ben bineþeforþe, he shal caste
with more greuaunce. But if þei ben in þe poores of
þe stomake, a man whan he haþ grete wil to caste, shal
caste but litil, and þat shal be with grete greuaunce.
And if þei ben bitwene þe two skynnes of þe stomake,
10   a man shal haue grete wil to caste, but he shal cast

f. 235v   noþing. And þis is clepid nausea. Þes ben / þre greet
greuauncis of þe stomake þat comen of corrupt humours.
But if colerike men haue abhominacion to mete þorou3

[211v]   suche corrupt humours, vnneþe þei may be helid, but
15   fleumatike men moun li3tli. And þei han wil to cast and
moun cast wel, þat is a good token, for þan þe corrupt
humours þat ben in þe stomak moun li3tli be brou3t oute.
But if a man volatiþ his mete and haþ wil to cast and mai
not, þat is a feble token, for þan þe humours ben in þe
20   poores of þe stomake. And eiþirwhilis þes greuauncis comen
of distempering of þe stomake withoute suche corrup humours.

[211]   And eiþirwhilis þei comen of hoot humours and eiþirwhilis
of cold. If þe greuaunce comeþ of hoot humours þat ben in

f. 236   þe stomake, þe mooþ of þe stomak / is heui and hote, and

---

10 shal] *in r. h. margin.*

þer is pricking aboute þe mooþ of þe stomake, and þe mooþ is bitter, and þei han hoot balking. But if þe stomake is distemperid with heet and haþ noon suche corrupt humours, a man shal haue alle þe forsede signes and heuynes of þe

5 stomake. And if þes greuauncis ben of cold humours, þe stomake is heuy and colde, and þe mooþ is vnsaueri, and his balking is soure. But if þe stomake is not distemperid with cold ne haþ noon corrupt humours in him, þan he shal haue al þe forseide tokenis, saaf heuynes of þe stomake.

10 And of þis sikenes comeþ aking of þe heed, scotomie,

[211v] and turnyng of þe brayn, lesing of appetit, feblenes of al þe bodi; and whan þei han y-ete, þan þei ben ful

f. 236v feble. And eiþir þei han a flux, eiþir a grete / wil to cast. And if suche corrupt humours ben bitwixe þe two

15 skinnes of þe stomake, wheþir þei ben hoot eiþir colde, þei han þe forseid signes, saf if þe humours ben cold and ben aboute þe mooþ of þe stomak, þei maken a man to haue apetit to mete. But whan he haþ y-ete, it makiþ him to haue wil to cast. Casting eiþirwhilis comeþ of feblenes of þe stomac,

20 and þan comenli a man haþ more wil to casten aftir mete þan bifore. And þis feblenes may be in two maneris, eiþir of þe ouer-parti of þe stomak, eiþir of neþir-parti. And if þe feblenes be of þe ouer-parti of þe stomake, a man shal cast li3tli and þat mete þat he haþ last y-ete.

13 þei] *in r. h. margin.*

f. 237   But if it be of neþir-parti, he shal / caste with greet
         greuaunce þat mete þat he haþ first y-ete.   And in alle þes
         sekenessis þat comen of corrupt humours, it is profitable to
         caste and purge þe stomac of corrupt humours.   And if þe
5   humours ben colerike, make him cast bifore mete, and nameli
         if þe humours be not in þe pores ne bitwene þe two skynnes.
         And þou may maken him cast with esi medicines, as with
         tisan, mellicrate, eiþir with warme watir; eiþir stampe þe
         seed of arage, and radiche, and rapis togedir, and seeþ hem
10   in watir, and let him drinke þat; eiþir þe iuse of lilie
         rotis, and sal gemme, and mete oile, of eueriche, yliche
         moche.   And let him drinke þerof fasting.   But if þe
         humours ben in þe middle of þe stomake, eiþir in þe
f. 237v   grounde, eiþir in þe poores, eiþir if þe / humours ben
15   viscouse, it is bettir to caste aftir mete þan bifore.
         And if þes distemperancis comen of an hoot distempere of
         þe stomac withouten humours, it sufficeþ him cold watir.
         But er þan þou 3eue a man þes medicines forto caste, firste
[212]   defie þe humours þat ben in þe stomake, if þei ben colerike,
20   with þe sirip of violet eiþir with þe sirip of vinegir,
         and with erbis, as hockis, and blitis, and arache, and
         suche oþir.   And if þer be moche mater þat heueiþ þe stomac
         miche, make a plastir withouten of hockis, and of radiche,
         and of þe holihock, and of betis, and of lynseed, and leye

17 him] *corr. from* it.

þe plastir bifore on þe stomake, and bihinde on þe rigge, of hockis y-stampid and y-fried in grece. And anoynte his brest

f. 238 with deute and with bot/tir two daies eiþir þre or þou make him caste. And if þou make a man to cast aftir mete, let

5 him ete rotis and fruyt aftir his oþir mete. And siþ withyn two oures aftir mete, make him cast. But if þes greuauncis comen of cold humours, firste defie þo humours. And ȝyue him oximel squillitik eiþir oximel of radiche þre daies togidir. And siþ make him to cast with þe iuse of radiche,

10 eiþir of walwort, eiþir of serpentarie þat wole slee an addir in a mannes wombe, eiþir þe iuse of spurge. And him nediþ strengir medicines, ȝyue him þe iuse of gourdis, or of þe les centory. And if a man abhorreþ to resceive ony of þes, þen take þe galle of a bolle or of ony oþir beste,

15 and anonynte his bodi fro þe navel vpward, and he shal cast.

f. 238v And if þou anoynte him fro þe / nauel dounward, he shal haue deliuerance bineþe. And þe same werking iera rufa. And if þou anoynte þe ouer-lacertis of a man-is arme with drastis of oile, he shal caste. And if þou anoynte þe

20 neþir-lacertis, he shal go to priuy.

An oynement laxatif with whom, if þou anointist a mannes stomake, he shal caste, and if þou anoyntist his navel, he shal go to priuy. And if þou anoyntist þerwith his reines, it wole make him costif: Take þe rote of

---

13 to resceive] *in r. h. margin.* **14 of** (3)] *ins. above.* **17 And þe ...**
iera rufa.] *in l. h. margin.* **21 An oynement]** *corr. from* Anoyntement.

electarie, dr. vii; of coconidie, of scamonie, dr. ii; of
þe iuse of titimalle, dr. v; of turmentine, dr. iiii; of
siclamen, dr. iiii; of eleborus niger, dr. vi: of hony,
quantum sufficit.

5   Anoþir oynement with whom if þou anointist a mannes
hondes it wole make him casten. And if þou anointist
his feet, it wole make him haue sege. And if it deliuereþ

f. 239   to moche mater, / anoynte his feet and his hondis with
popilion: Take peletre of Spayne, and eleborus niger,

10   hermodactalis, henbane, accorun, þe iuse of synegreen, and
brionie, of eueriche of þes yliche moche. And medle hem
with swynes grece. If þou can-not make a man to caste by
þes, make him a purgacion to deliueren him bineþeforþe aftir
þe kinde of þe humour þat noieþ þe stomake, as if it be of

15   coler, ȝyue him colo[go]ge of mirabolani citri, eiþir
reubarbe with þe iuse of plantein. If it be of flevme,
ȝyue him a fleumagoge of mirabolani keber eiþir iera pigra
with þe iuse of calamynte. If it be of malencoli, ȝyue him

[212v]   a mala[go]ge of mirabolani indie eiþir diacene. And

20   aftir his purgacion, wheþir it be abouen eiþir bineþen, /
f. 239v   comforte þe stomake with comfortable metis and drinkis,
and electuaries, and siripis, and poudirs, and anoyntingis
withoutforþe, with hoot oynementis eiþir colde, aftir þe
kynde of þe humour þat greueþ þe stomake.

2 titimalle] *corr. from* titmalle. **14 noieþ]** moueþ. *Add 30338*
noieþ. **15 cologoge]** cologe. **19 malagoge]** malage. **20 aftir]** *in r. h.*
margin.

A sirip
for þis
greuaunce
of þe
stomake

A good sirip for þis greuaunce of þe stomake is y-made of þe iuse of myntis y-clarified.   And þen put þerto sugir aftir þe quantite of þe liquor.

A good emplastir for þe stomake is y-made of mastike,

5   and roses, and myntis, y-stampid togedir, eiþir þe iuse of myntis, and vynegir, and soure brede.

Chapter XII, Part 8
To Stop Vomiting

But eiþirwhilis it is nedeful to let a man cast, for so longe a man my3t vsen it, þat it shuld be harde to destroien it.   And þerfore it is nedeful to telle medicines

10   to staunche casting. Firste, purge þe stomak of þe humours þat maken him to cast.   And if he is costif, make him

f. 240   neisshe-/y-wombid.   And if he is on þe flux, stoppe him with strictories.   And diete him with metis þat wole make a

[213]   man costif, as with barliche brede and rostid metis.   And

15   let him vse vynegre for sauce.   Siþ 3yue him a sirip constrictif, and make him a plastir strictory of myntis, and comferie, and mastik, and vynegre, and citonies, and soure breed.   And reyn watir þat gold is oftensiþes qwenchid yn cesiþ casting.   And if þe stomake be feble and

20   þe sikenes olde, make a sirip of clowes, and notemiggis, and canel, and lignum aloes, and mastike, and myntis, and spodie, and acacie.   Eiþir if þe greuaunce be of hoot humours, take mastike and ley it on an hoot tiyl stoon, and siþ ley it on his stomake al warme.   And seeþ galles, rosis,

---

7 *2-line initial in blue.* **8 a man]** *corr. from* he.

f. 240v and myntis, and þe rynde of an oke in vy/negre. And þerin
wete a sponge of þe see and ley it al warme to his stomake.
Eiþir make a plastir of bole, and mastike, and sandragon
distemperid with þe white of an ey. Eiþir let him drinke
5 watir of roses þat poudir of mastike is soden yn. Eiþir
make a plastir of mele, and of þe iuse of myntis, and of
roses, and of planteyn, and vynegre. And if it be of cold,
make him a poudir of comyn, and of baies of lorer, and
mastike, and olibanum. And anoynte his stomake with oile
10 of lorer. And þe foreseide sirip of myntis is good for al
þes greuauncis. And if casting comeþ of feblenes of þe
stomac, let him vse comfortable þingis. And if it comeþ
of moche etyng, let him vse abstinence: Þat is moost
f. 241 souereyn medicyn. Calament y-soden in gotis / mylke and
15 oþir medicines þat weren y-tolde in spitting of blood
[213v] ben good here. If a man-is stomake be y-feblid bi long
abstinence and fasting, let him be dietid with comfortable
metis, and drinkis, and electuaries. And make him leue þe
occupacions of his soule, but it be mirþe and gladnes.
20 And let him vse a plastir on his stomake of myntis, aloes,
mastike, and wormod, of eueriche yliche moche. And
stampe hem and medle hem with oile of roses and ley to
þe stomake. And oftsiþes anoynte þe stomake with oile
of roses. And let him vse a poudir y-made of clowes, of

---

18 him] *in r. h. margin.* **24 him]** *ins. above.*

galengale, canel, gynger, maces, quibibes, and lignum alloes, amonie, calamus aromaticus, storace, carewei, and anet, of sugir, as moche as of al þe oþer. And let him vse of þis poudir at his mete, þe wiȝte of a dramme. /

Chapter XII, Part 9
The Mouth of the Stomach

f. 241v 5   The mouþ of þe stomake is eiþirwhilis y-turned vpsodoun and makiþ a man to haue a continuel wil to caste. And þis comeþ of a wood colerik humour þat is in þe stomake: Whan he meueþ vpward, he drawiþ oþir humouris with him. Eiþirwhilis it comeþ for þe mooþ of þe stomake

10   is feble, and þe botme is stronge to put oute þe humours þat ben in him. If it comeþ in þe firste maner, þou must ȝyue him colde þingis in medicines to destroy þilke hoot

[214]   colerike humours. And if it comeþ in þe secunde maner, it is profitable aftir his oþir medicines þat he vse fruitis

15   þat wole make him costif. And let him ete litil, and drinke litil, and trauel litil. And make a plastir to his stomake of mastike and of myntis. And let him ete þe

f. 242   lymaile of gold with an ey, eiþir let him drinke / watir with wiyn þat gold haþ ben oftsiþes y-qwenchid yn. Eiþir

20   make him þis plastir: Take galbanum, and opoponac, serapinum, amoniac, and lei hem in vynegre al anyȝt, and aftirward seeþ hem. And þen put þerto mastike, olibanum, coost, mirre, sandragon, notemig, and put þis in a clooþ and ley on his stomake. Also medicines þat were y-tolde

---

5 *2-line initial in blue.* **10 is feble]** *in l. h. margin.* **12 in]** *ins. above.* **17 him]** *ins. above.*

for casting ben good here for þis sekenes. Eiþirwhilis, þe neþir parte of þe stomake is febler þen þe ouer-parte and for feblenes is y-turnid vpsodoun. And þis may come of two enchesons, as of grete abstinence eiþir of grete surfet.

5 If it be of grete abstinence, he must be dietid with comfortable metis and drinkis and also medicines. If it
f. 242v be of surfet, he must caste / þat he be deliuered of þe corrupt humours þat ben in his stomake. Siþ, he must be rulid with abstinence and with reste. And siþ ȝyue him
10 electuaries and oþir medicines to comforte wel þe stomak, þat he moun wel defien his mete. And make a plastre of gallis and of planteyn. And let him vse metis and electuaries þat ben of kynde to make a man costif, as it shal be tolde when Y speke of þe fluxe.

Chapter XII, Part 10
Stomach Ache

15 Ache of þe stomake comeþ eiþirwhilis of heet, eiþirwhilis of colde. And þat is in two maneris: eiþir of corrupt humours þat ben in þe stomake, eiþir of distempering of hete eiþer of colde withouten suche humuris. Tokenis of heet is a smert ache, þirstfulnes,
20 hoot balking þat brenneþ þe roof of þe mooþ, and hoot metis
f. 243 and drinkis encresiþ þe ache. / His vryn [is] of an hiȝe colour. And if þer be hoot corrupt humours in þe stomake,
[214v] his mooþ is bitter and he haþ wil forto caste. And þat þat passiþ from him at his fundement is forbrent. And

---

4 **surfet**] *corr. from* suffet. 13 **ben**] *in r. h. margin.* **make a**] *ins. above.* 15 *2-line initial in blue.* 21 **is of**] of. 22 **be**] *prec. by* stomake *canc. in red.*

þes han oo maner cure: Saaf if þer be corrupt humours
in þe stomake, þe stomac must first ben y-purgid of hem,
and siþ haue oþir medicines to abaten þe heet. But
if þe ache comeþ of colde, he balkiþ ofte, and hoot

5 metis comforten him, and colde metis greuen him. And if
þer ben colde humours in þe stomake, his balking is soure,
and þat he castiþ is fleumatike and so his drit is also.
And eiþirwhilis, whan þe ache comeþ of colde withouten
suche corrupt humours, a man is costif. But þes humours

f. 243v 10 moun be eiþirwhilis bitwixe / þe two skynnes of þe stomake,
eiþirwhilis in þe poores of þe stomac. Eiþirwhilis ache of
þe stomac and also of þe guttis comen of corrupt wyndis
þat ben in hem, and is y-knowe bi noise and hurling in þe
wombe. And when þei ben deliuered of suche windes, þei

15 ben moche y-liȝtid. And þei balken moche, but þei ben
not deliuered of noon corrupt humours. And in þe same
maneris comeþ ache in a mannes guttis. And riȝte as þe
stomac may be y-greued with þre maner humours, þat is to
sey, with colere, and fleume, and malencoli, riȝt so þe

20 guttis moun. But whan þe stomac is y-greued bi ony
of þes humours, it may be y-knowe bi what humour, bi þat
þat Y haue tolde bifore. And if þe guttis ben y-greued bi

f. 244 ony of þes humours, it may be y-knowe / of what humour it
is bi a mannes drit; for of kindliche fleume comeþ white

16 same] *in l. h. margin.* 21 bi (1)] *followed by* þat *canc. in red.*
22 bifore] *in l. h. margin.*

drit and þynne; of glasi flevme comeþ white drit and þicke, with moche fleume y-medlid þerwith. And but if a man be þe raþir y-holpen, he shal falle into a flux eiþir into anoþir greuaunce of þe guttis þat is y-clepid collica

5 passio. Of salt fleume comeþ pale drit and þinne. Of swete fleume comeþ drit þat is neiþir ri3t þicke ne ri3t þynne, and þei felen heet in her guttis. Of soure flevme comeþ drit þat haþ moche fome and many bollis. And þei ben eiþirwhilis blac eiþirwhilis swart 3elew, and þei

10 felen cold in her guttis. Of colere þat is in þe guttis þe tokenes ben, þe drit is citrin eiþir green, and /

f. 244v þei felen hete, and smerting, and biting in þe guttis, and þei ben þirstful and her mooþ is drie. And but þei ben þe raþir y-helid, þei shulen falle into a blody flux.

15 Of malencoli, þe tokenes ben swarte 3elewe drit eiþir blac, moche noise and hurlyng of wyndis in þe guttis, and colde. Eiþirwhilis, þis ache comeþ of a postem of þe stomac þat is not wel y-helid. Eiþirwhilis it comeþ of etyng of sum sory metis. Eiþirwhilis þe stomac akiþ

20 and swelliþ, for þe drit is y-hardid in a mannis wombe. Eiþirwhilis ache and swelling comeþ of þe dropesi. If it comeþ of hoot corrup humours, purge þe stomake of þilke humours as it is y-tolde bifore with mirabolanis eiþir reubarbe. Aftirward, take þe iuse of syngreen and of

8 haþ] *prec. by* is *canc. in red.*

f. 245

penyworte, and anoynte / a clooþ þerwiþ, and ley to þe
stomak. Eiþir make a plastir of white sandris and of reed,
and of oile of roses, and vynegre y-medlid togedir; eiþir
of white sandris and of reed, and of spodie, and barliche

5   meel, and camphore, and þe iuse of syngreen. Eiþir
anoynte þe stomake with oile of roses and oile of violet.
And of electuaries, let him vse triasandri, and oximel
simple, and stomaticon þat is colde. And let him vse
cold siripis, as of violet and also watir þat þe seedis of

10   colde erbis ben y-soden yn. Also seeþ þe iuse of planteyn
til þe halfendel be y-soden awey. And make it vp in þe
maner of a sirip, and put þerto a litil reubarbe and let
him drinke þerof. And anoynte þe pavmes of his hondes and

f. 245v   þe soles of his feet with oile of / violet, eiþir of roses,

15   eiþir popilion, eiþir with vynegre y-sprent on hem. And

[215]   let him vse to ete purslane and oþir colde erbis.
But if þis comeþ of colde humours, let þe stomake
be anoyntid with hoot oynement. And let seeþ peritorie
in white wiyn and leye it al warme to þe stomake, and

20   oftesiþis renewe it. And if þer is ony wiyndi mater in his
stomac, it is profitable to setten an horne eiþir a cuppe
on þe stomake withouten garsing. And if he be a riche
man, let him drinke bavme, eiþir let him drinke of þe
gumme of an yuy tree þe quantite of þre peesen at ones.

12 a (1)] *ins. above.*

And make him a plastre of mastik, and of olibanum, and
of baies of lorer, and of oyl y-medlid togedir.   Calamynt

f. 246   is also ful profitable / for him, and a plastre y-made
þerof.   And of rue and of hony y-soden togedir is ful

5   good also.   And so is a plastre of rue and of origanum
y-soden in hony.   And let him vse diaspermat[ic]on, and
diacinimum, and diamargariton.   And let seþe auence with
his rotis and sauge in white wiyn and þerwith let stufen
his wombe. And let him drinke of þat wyn.   And þis is good

10   also if a man-is stomake akiþ for drinking of cold watir.
And let him vse a poudir y-made of comyn, and canel, and
coliandre seed.   And let him drinke wyn y-medlid with
watir.   And oft vse þe watir þat fenel seed, and parseli
seed, and mastike, and olibanum han be y-soden in.   And

15   þe same medicines þat distroien þes wyndes distroien soure
balkingis.   And for swelling of þe stomake, take þe sede of
rue, and þe baies of a lorer tree, and þe sede of parseli,

f. 246v   and of mar/che, and of carewei, of dauke, hemloc, and of
peritorie.   And stampe al þes and seþe hem in a litil

20   wiyn til þe wyn be consumed.   And siþ put þerto a litil
oile of lorer, eiþir of rue, eiþir of piliol.   And make
þerof a plastir and ley on his stomake.   And let him vse
þe electuaries þat ben y-told bifore.

A good drinke also for swelling of þe stomac and forto

---

6 diaspermaticon] diaspermaton.   **7-8 let seþe . . . his rotis]**
copied let auence with his rotis seþe *and marked for reversal.*   **9 is]**
prec. by a canc. in red.   **13 þe watir þat]** *in r. h. margin.*   **22 him]** *ins.*
above.

distroie suche corrupt wyndis: Take of fenel seed, comyn,

anise, ana, dr. vi; of long aristologie, squinante,

carpobalsame, dr. iii; of calamynt, spike, ameos, spodie,

ana, dr. ii; of macis, gynger, clowes, ana, dr. i.   Stampe

5   hem and siþ seeþ hem in iii pounde of þe iuse of fenel.

And siþ cast þerto a quantite of sugir.   And of þis drinke

let him drinke þe wi3te of iii drammes at oones.

Diacalamentum is gode also for cold of þe stomake,

f. 247   and for wyn/dis, and for eueri greuaunce of þe brest þat
Diacalamentum

10   comeþ of cold, and nameli for olde men, and for hem þat

han þe colde cou3 and it is þus made: Take of calamynt,

of piliol, of melanopipir, sileos, of parseli, ana   dr.

iii & sc. ii; of louage, dr. i & sc. i; of ameos, tyme,

anet, canel, gynger, ana, sc. i; of hony, quantum sufficit.

15   Diacitoniton þat is hoot is gode for casting, and
Diacitoniton
hote   for corrupt wyndis, and comfortiþ a man-is kindeli hete

of his bodi.   And it is good for men þat han to neisshe

wombe, et cetera.

Diacitoniton þat is cold is þus y-made: Take of
Diacitoniton
cold   20   citonies, and firste seþ hem and pille of þe rynde, and þen

make hem cleen withynforþ. Þen take of hem a pounde and an

halfe; of roses, of sandris, ana, dr. iii; of reubarbe, of

liquoris, of þe seed of purslane, of letuse, ana, dr. i; of

f. 247v   clowes, of canel, / dr. 1/2; of anise, of gynger, ana, dr.

---

4 **ana (1)**] *ins. above.* **10 cold**] *corr. from* gold. **17 neisshe**] *corr.*
from nesshe. **20 of**] *ins. above.* **21 hem**] *in r. h. margin.* **23 of (2)**] *in*
r. h. margin.

i; of þe sirip of roses, quantum sufficit. And put to þis a pounde of sugir. And let him vse herof aftir mete and aftir sopir.

Chapter XII, Part 11
Apostem of the Stomach

[216]   Apostem is eiþirwhilis in a mannes stomac. And
5   þat mai ben in diuerse wisis; for eiþirwhilis he is within þe stomac, eiþirwhilis withouten, eiþirwhilis bitwene þe two skinnes of þe stomac. If it be within þe stomac, or þan þe postem be rotid, sum of þe mater comeþ oute bi casting. And whan þe postem haþ y-cau3t his rote,
10   he is moche heuied aftir þat he haþ y-eten. If þe postem be withoute, þe swelling is a-seen withouten. And þou3 he cast, þer comeþ no-þing from þe stomac þat bitokeneþ þe postem. Whan he is bitwene þe two skinnes, he feliþ heuynes and greuaunce in þe stomac withouten þes oþir

f. 248   15   signes. And þes postemes co/men eiþirwhilis of hote corrupt humouris, eiþirwhilis of cold. If þe postem be of hote corrupt humours, eiþir it is of coler, eiþir it is of blood. If it is of coler, he feliþ greet heet and brening, and moche leping and heuynes in his stomac, and
20   his mooþ is drie and bitter, and his herte failiþ him oftsiþes, in-so-moche þat he falliþ adoun as þou3 he were y-sovned. And he haþ moche greuaunce boþe to swolewe and to drawe breeþ, and comenli he haþ a feuer tercian þerwith. If it is of blode, it haþ þe same tokenes, but þei ben not

---

1-3 And put . . . sopir] *copied* and let him vse þerof aftir mete and aftir sopir. And put to þis a pounde of sugir *and marked for reversal.* **4** *2-line initial in blue.* **5 wisis]** *prec. by* causes *canc. in red.*

so violent. But if þe postem com of cold humours, eiþir it is of flevme, eiþir of malencoli. If it be of flevme, þe postem swelliþ and is neisshe, and he feliþ moche heuynes in his stomac. But his ache is not ful greet, and he haþ no þirst. / And he spitteþ moche and al his bodi is heuy and slow, and al his wittis ben stonied and y-dullid as þou3 he had litargie, and he haþ an esy feuer. But if þe postem be of malencoli, he feliþ moche hardnes in his stomake. And þe mater of þe postem is y-gaderid togedir, and moche heuynes he feliþ also. And he haþ a soure balking and he feliþ moche greuaunce in his stomake. And he may sleep but a litil for a greet corrupt wynde þat smyteþ vp into his heed. And whan þe postem is in þe botme of þe stomake, he febliþ þe stomac moche, so þat þe stomac eiþirwhilis mai not holde þe mete þat he resceiueþ, and þan he haþ a continuel flux. Eiþirwhilis, þe stomac is so feble þat he mai not deliueren him of þat mete þat is in / him, and þan a man is continuel costif.

If þis postem come of heet, let him blede at his arme, if he haþ greet plente of blood. And aftir, let him be dietid with holsom good metis, as with letuse, purselane, and gourdis, endiue, bletis, and þe clensing of bran, and almond mylke. And let him ete walisshe-notis,

f. 248v 5

10

15

f. 249

20

---

5 he (1)] *ins. above.* 14 febliþ] *corr. from* feliþ. 22 holsom] *in r. h. margin.* 24 and] *ins. above.*

and also peres and apples y-soden, and chesteynes, not
harde but neisshe. And 3yue him þe sirip of roses, eiþir
of violet, eiþir of þe iuse of solatre and of scariole,
with cassia fistula and with manna. And whan þey ben wel
5 y-soden, cast þerto sum sugir. And lei cold repercussiues
withoutenforþ in þe vii dai. And anoynt him with oile of
roses, eiþir of violet, eiþir of mirtis. And with þe
watir of roses, and with þe iuse of planteyn, and of letuse,
and of purslane, and of pimpernel, and of turmentil, and

f. 249v violet, and solatre and / of saffren, of eueriche of þes,
take iliche moche. And medle hem wel togedir. And þerwith
anoynte þe stomac. And wete coton eiþir a lynen clooþ
þerin, and ley it on þe stomac. And twies renewe it in þe
wyntir daies, and þries in þe sommer daies. Also in þe
15 beginnyng of suche postem, make a plastre of sandris,
roses, vynegre, and of oile. And ley it on þe stomac. But
if þe mater mai not be remeuid from her place bi þes cold
plastris, þou muste make plastris to make þe postem ripe,
as it is y-told in þe chaptir of squinacye. Eiþir make a
20 plastre of barli mele and of 3olkis of eggis. But if þe
postem be of cold, let him be dietid with temperat hoot
metis. And make him potage of þe clensing of bran and of
almond mylke. Eiþir make him furmenti, eiþir riys y-made

f. 250 with almonde milke. And roste him good ap/ples and fulle

1 **also**] *in r. h. margin.*

hem with sugir. And make him þis sirip: Take a litil
spike and as moche of azarum, of anise, anet, ozimum,
yreos, femigreke, horshel, caparis, calamus aromaticus,
[216v] cassia lignea, mastike, mynte, wormod, and fenel seed, of
5 eueriche of þes, ix dr. Seþe al þes in watir and put þerto
a pounde of sugir. And let him vse þis sirip boþe in
fourme of medicyn and of drinke, and let him not blede.
Also take marche seed, dauke, comyn, anise, fenel sede,
spike, squinant, bavme, maioran, lynsede, femigreke,
10 mastike, cardamomum, quibibes, aloes, cassia lignea,
camomil, þe fleisshe of dates, of eueriche of þes, yliche
moche. Put þes in watir and let him seeþ a good while
þerin. Þen take þe erbis when þei ben y-soden, and put in
a lynen bagge, and leẏ to þe stomake. And with þis watir
f. 250v 15 wasshe þe wombe bifore þe stomake. / And wete wol þerin and
ley on þe stomake. Eiþir take lily rotis and betis and
medle hem with wiyn and with oile in a mortir. And siþ
warme it and plastir it on þe stomake. Eiþir seeþ oynons
and comyn in wiyn and in oile togedir and plastir þat on
20 þe stomake. And whan þe postem is broken, þou must vse
mundificatiues to clense þe stomac of quitere. Token of
þat breking is þat þe quitere brekiþ awei fro þe stomake.
And whan þe postem is within þe stomake, þe quitere passiþ
awei bineþe, eiþir aboue þorouȝ þe mooþ. And if it is

6 sirip] *prec. by* sugir *canc. in red.* 7 and let him not blede] *in r.
h. margin.*

withouten, it passiþ forþ bineþen also. And if he is within bitwene þe skynnes of þe stomake, þan þe quitere passiþ awei with þe vrin. And forto clense þe stomake of þis quitere, seeþ barliche in gotis mylke. And siþ clense
5 it and seeþ þerin dragagant, and gumme arabike, liquoris, penides, horshel, orobus, reisens, / yreos, zilobalsamum, and sugir. And clense it and drinke herof in þe mornyng and in þe euentid in a good quantite. And if þe quitere greueþ him soore whan it passiþ awei fro him, 3yue him
10 triacle with watir þat it is soden in, a-iii daies or iiii. Also to make him cleen, 3yue him meeþ bi himsilf, eiþir y-medlid with white wyn. And if he be purgid bi his vrin, 3yve him of þe medicines þat ben told in stranguria. And siþ, 3yue him consolidatiues to souden þat place þat is to-
15 broke, as reyn watir þat mirtillis and gallis ben y-soden in, y-medlid with sugir. And withouten, ley plastirs þat ben strictories, as it shal be told in þe flux.

Stomaticon þat is cold is good for al vnkinde hetis of a manne[s] stomake and quenchiþ a mannes þirste.

20 Stomaticon þat is hoot is comfor[ta]ble for þe stomake and helpiþ to defie a mannes mete. And it is go/de for þe greuaunce þat is in þe ouer-guttis of a mannes wombe, þer is stomaticon a laxatif.

f. 251

f. 251v

Chapter XII, Part 12
Colic of the Stomach

[217]   Colides is a greuaunce of þe stomake eiþir of þe

---

7 **herof**] *corr. from* herfore. 11 **him** (1)] *in r. h. margin.* **him** (2)] *ins. above.* 15 **þat**] with. 19 **mannes**] manne. 20 **comfortable**] comforble. 24 *2-line initial in blue.*

guttis þat makiþ a man haue so greet wil to shite þat him semeþ þat he shuld shite oute his guttis. And if it be in þe stomake, it makiþ a man boþe to cast and to shite. And þis greuaunce comeþ oþirwhilis of corrupte humours þat ben

5 in þe stomake eiþir in þe guttis, and þat may ben of coler eiþir of fleume. If it is of coler, it is ful violent and ful perilous and with grete hete. If it is of fleume, it is not so perilous. Eiþirwhilis, it comeþ of to moche eting and drinking; eiþirwhilis, for a man-is wombe haþ

10 leyn vnhelid, and þerof y-cau3te cold in his slepe. But wherof-euer þis sikenes com, þou shalt not encresen his flux ne his casting, for þat shulde make him þe more feble.

f. 252 But / þou shalt 3yue him comfortable medicines and medicines þat ben strictories. But þou shalt not be aboute

15 to staunche him sodeynli, ne no maner flux, but easli, for drede of more peril. And þerfor let him vsen sugir roset, and diarodon abbatis, and rosata nouella. And if colerike humours ben encheson of þis sikenes, let him be anoyntid with cold þingis. And let him baþen him in a baþþe

20 to ceesen his flux, as it shal be told in þe chaptir of þe flux. But if it comeþ of cold, let him vsen an electuarie þat is y-clepid dianthos, eiþir zinziber Alexandrium. And 3yue him þe sirip of mynt and make him a baþþe of myntis and of oþir erbis þat ben hoot and

strictories.   And if it comeþ of hete, let him drinke þe

f. 252v   si/rip of roses.   And if þe man is stronge of complexion

þat haþ þis sikenes, wheþir it be of hete eiþir of cold,

þou must ȝyue him esi medicines to make him cast, as meþ

5   y-medlid with a litil warme salt watir and a litil oile.

And let him be anoyntid with oile of rosis if it comeþ

of heet; if it comeþ of cold, with sum hoot oynement.

Mynte is ful profitable for þis sikenes if it comeþ of cold,

and for al cold greuauncis of þe stomake: Medle þe iuse

10   þerof with warme watir if it comeþ of hete, and with wyn

if it comeþ of cold.   And let hem þat han þis sikenes to

[217v]   drinke no cold watir but if þei han a greet lust and desire

þerto.   And ȝiue hem a litil cene.   But if þe flux be of an

hoot colerike humour, let hem drinke a good drauȝt of cold

15   watir if þei desire it.   And so þou mai do þerof if a

mannes liuer is distemperid with heet and in dissinterie

f. 253   also. / And if al þis helpiþ him not, ȝyue him gode

triacle, for þat staunchiþ eueri flux.

A good plastre if þat sikenes comeþ of hete: Take

20   spodie and barly meel, and tempere hem with þe white of

an ey and with þe iuse of planteyn and of meyntis.   And

ley þis plastir fro þe mooþ of þe stomak doun to þe priue

membres.   And in þe same wise ley it bihinde on his back.

But if it comeþ of cold, make a plastre of spodie and whete

---

12 **no**] *ins. above.* 13 **And . . . cene.**] *in l. h. margin.* 15 **do**] *ins.*
above. **þerof**] *in l. h. margin.* 17 **him not**] *marked for reversal.*

meel y-temperid with þe iuse of mynte. And plastre it fro
þe mooþ of þe stomake dounward, boþe bihinde and bifore.
And for þis sikenes is ful violent and drawiþ þe marie
oute of a mannes bones and wastiþ his kindeli moistnes, it
5 behoueþ to staunche þe flux as sone as it may be don, as it
shal be told in þe chaptir of þe flux. And it is nedful to
f. 253v 3yue him comfortable medicines to restore / him to his
kyndely moistnes as it is y-tolde in feuer etike, for moche
of his moistenes is y-wastid þorou3 violence of þe flux.

Chapter XIII, The Guts
Part 1, Dysentery

[?] 10   Here begynneþ þe xiii chaptir of þis boke þat
conteineþ viii titles or practi[se]s.
     In a mannes guttis þer ben meny sikenessis: þe flux,
and anoþir greuaunce þat is clepid collica passio, and
wormes ben y-gendrid also in a mannes guttis þat greueþ a
15 man ful moche. Anoþir greuaunce is whan a man may not
shite and 3it he haþ grete wille þerto. Anoþir greuance
is whan þe gut þat goiþ to a mannes fundement falliþ oute
at þe ers. Of fluxes, þer ben foure maner of kindes. Oon
is clepid dissinterie, and þat is whan a man shiteþ blood
f. 254 20 y-medlid with þe / shauing of his guttis. Anoþir flux is
[217v] whan blood passiþ from a man withouten suche medling,
and þat is clepid þe bloodi flux. Anoþir þer is þat is
clepid a simple flux, and þat is whan a man is deliuered
of þat þat is in his wombe soon aftir þat it is defied,

---

10 Here] *followed by* N a *canc. in red.* **xiii]** xv. **11 practises]**
practis. **12** *4-line initial in gold.*

but it passiþ awei from him al neisshe.   But þe iiii^e
maner of flux is whan a man is deliuered of his mete
as hool as he etiþ it, and þat is clepid lienterie.

[219]   Dissenterie comeþ of diuerse enchesons,   eiþirwhilis
5   from withouten, eiþirwhilis from within.   From withouten,

Dissenterie   it comeþ as of ful-kene medicines,   eiþir of metis and
drinkis þat ben ful laxatif; eiþir of falling a-doun from
an hi3e place;   eiþir of a stroke on a man-is rigge;

f. 254v   eiþir of a cold þat a / man haþ y-cau3t on his wombe eiþir
10   in   his   feet.   From withinforþe, þis sekenes comeþ of
corrupt humours þat ben in þe guttis, as of coler, eiþir
of sori blood,   eiþir of salt fleume,   eiþir malencolie.
Eiþir it is of a feble retentif, eiþir of a strong expulsif,
þat is to sei, eiþir þe guttis ben feble to holden þe
15   mete within, eiþir to put oute þat þat is within hem.

Thre   Of dissenterie þer ben þre maneris: Oon is in þe
maneris   ouermost guttis, anoþir is in þe middel guttis, and þe
of
dissenterie   þridde is in þe neþirmost gutis.   And in oon maner of
dissenterie, þat þat passiþ from a man is as þou3 it
20   were waisshing of flesshe,   and   þat flux mai be li3tli
y-helid.   In anoþir dissenterie, þer passiþ from a man
as þou3 it were þe shauyng of parchemyn.   But in þe þrid

f. 255   maner of dissenterie, þer / passiþ from a man hool gobetis
of his guttis, and þat is incurable.   Whan þis sekenes

---

1 neisshe] *corr. from* nesshe.   **15 oute]** *prec. by* it *canc. in red.*

comeþ of þe ouer-guttis, þei felen greuaunce aboute þe
navel. And þe mater þat passiþ fro hem is like þe wasshing
of flesshe without suche shauyng, for þei ben so þyn þat
þer comeþ no suche shauing fro hem. But when þis sikenes
5   comeþ from þe neþir-guttis, þan þe greuaunce is bineþe
þe nauel, and þei ben deliuerid of mater like þe shauing
of guttis and of blood togedir. And þe blode is not medlid
with þe drit, but lieþ gobet-mele bi himsilf. But whan þe
flux comeþ from þe ouer-guttis, þe blood is y-medlid with
10   þe drit, for it goiþ a long wey, and me shal not wel
perseyuen þe blood. But when it comeþ of þe middel-gut/-
f. 255v   tis, þen þe greuaunce is aboute þe nauel, sumwhat aboue and
sumwhat bineþe. And of what humour þis comeþ, þou maist
knowe bi þat þat was y-tolde in þe ache of þe stomake.
15   Neþeles, of colere, þe drit mai be in two maneris y-colorid,
eiþir 3elewe, eiþir grene and y-medlid with blode. Of
malencoli, it is black and y-medlid with blode. Of salt
fleume, it is a derke pale colour and medlid with blood.
Of corrupt blode, it is ni3e of black colour and y-medlid
20   with blood. Eiþirwhilis dissenterie comeþ in certeyn tymes
and in a certeyn cours, and a man is moche y-li3tid aftir
[219v]   his flux. And suche a maner flux shal not be y-staunchid
til he wol cese himsilf. But þer is anoþir dissenterie
f. 256   þas comeþ vncerteyn/liche, and greueþ a man and febliþ

13 **humour**] *corr. from* humours. 19 **is**] *ins. above.* 23 **is**] *ins.
above.*

him ful moche. And he must be staunchid with medicines.

For dissenterie þat comeþ of heet and of hoot kene humours þat ben in þe guttis, make him a purgacion of mirabolani: citri and indi.   And if it is of oþir humours,

5   purge him with medicines þat ben apropried to þe humours: Mirabolani citri purgeþ coler, and þat þat purgeþ colere purgeþ blode.   Kebulis, indi, purgeþ fleume.   Bellrici, emblici, purgeþ malencoli.   But whan þou shalt make þi purgacion, if it be a stronge boistous man of complexion,

10   poudre þi medicin, and let him ete þat poudre eiþir drinke it.   But if it be a feble man of complexion, eiþir a man þat haþ ben y-norisshid with deintis, take of þy medicin,

oz. i eiþir oz. 1/2, and do / þe poudir herof in rein watir, eiþir in watir of roses, eiþir in watir þat mastik

15   eiþir plantein haþ ben y-sode yn.   And clense þat watir and let him drinke þerof.   But whan þou ȝeuest a man suche clensing, do þerin þe more of mirabolani.   And when þou seest bi a man-is drit þat he is wel y-purgid of þat humour þat is cause of his sekenes, þan þou shalt staunche his

20   flux bi medicines þat ben strictories.   And þan ȝyue him an electuarie y-made of diacodion, and miclete, and athanasia y-medlid togedir.   And if he is a delicat man, do þerto a litil sugir, and a litil of sandragon, and of bole, and of mastike, and of a stoon y-clepid amachites.   And ȝiue him

---

6 purgeþ (1)] *corr. from* purgen. **15 ben**] *ins. above.* **17 of**] *ins. above.* **21 diacodion**] diaconidion. **24 him**] *in r. h. margin.*

þis wiþ þe iuse of plantein in þe morewetid or þan he ete

f. 257   or drinke. / And let him set his feet in warme salte watir

þat resta bouis is soden in: Þat is gode for eueriche flux.

Eiþir, aftir þe medicine, make him a baþ þat roses, and

5   plantein, and resta bouis, and sangrinari, and sheperdis

3erd, and gallis ben y-soden in, and suche oþir strictories.

And when he comeþ oute of þe baþ, let him haue rest.   And

3iue him diacodion, and athanasia, and miclete y-medlid

togedir.   Anoþir good baþ for þis sikenes to staunche þe

[221v]   10   flux: Take roses, plantein, comferi, daies-i3e, and þe

rinde of a blac þorne, and þe rinde of an oke, and

chesteines.   Seeþ al þes in watir, and when þei be wel y-

soden, put þerto þe fyueþe part of vynegre.   And let him

sitte a good while in þat baþ.   A good plastir for þis

f. 257v   15   sikenes: Take of acacie, and ypoquis/tidos, and of þe

iuse of plantein, of eueriche, yliche moche; of whete meel,

quantum sufficit.   Medle hem togedir and make a plastir

A plastir
for þis
sikenes

þerof from þe nauel to þe sheer. A good fumigacion: Take

colofonie and þe poudir of oþir þingis þat wole make a man

20   costif, and strewe hem on brenyng cooles. And let þe smoke

þerof smyte vp into his fundement. Eiþir take quicke eelis

and ley hem on brenyng colis. And let þe smoke of hem

smyte vp into his fundement. Þis fumigacion is good for

al maner flux.

2 warm salte watir] *copied as* salte watir warme; salte *ins. above and marked for reversal.*   **5 sheperdis**] shaperdis.   **8 diacodion**] diagodion.

A Flux of Dissenterie

Dieting of hem þat han þe flux shal be of rostid metis, and noon broþþes but if þei be made þick with spiceri, as with poudir of canel, clowes, bole, sandragon, dragagant,

f. 258   and of suche oþir þingis þat wolen make a man / costif.

5   And make him brede of milfoile and plantein. And let him make riys eiþir frumenti with almonde mylke. Her drinke shal be, if þei han feueris, watir of roses, eiþir reyn watir þat mastike is soden in. If þei han no feuer, 3yue hem good rede wiyn y-medlid with a litil watir.

10   Eiþir bren mastike and gum arabike on a til stoon and make poudir of hem. And seeþ þat in cleen watir and 3iue him to drinke. Eiþir make him gruel of femigreke eiþir of letuse, and let him vse it vii daies if his stomake is anentishid.

[223]   And olde chese y-soden in hony is good for hem.

15   A good sirip: Take of roses, oz. ii; of þe sede of

A gode sirip   plantein, oz. i; of louage or mirtillis, of sumac, oz. ii; sirip of plantein, manipulus i; of sugir, ii pounde. And if þou wilt, put in þe sede of planteyn, of mirtillis, of sumac. Seeþ þe spicis in reyn watir. And siþ clense it and put in

20   þi sugir.

A good plastir
f. 258v   A good plastir for þis sikenes: Take of roses, oz. i; plastir of sumac, oz. ii; of bdellie, of mastike, / of encense, ana, dr. ii; of spodie, of sandragon, of bole armoniac, ana, dr. ii; of gallis, of psidie, of balaustia, ana, oz. 1/2; of

---

2 as] corr. from and. **10-13 Eiþir bren . . . is anentishid.]** in r. h. margin. **17-18 And if . . . of sumac.]** in r. h. margin. **22 bdellie]** corr. from bdelle.

196

wormod, dr. ii; of þe iuse of mynte, oz. 1/2; of þe iuse of plantein, oz. ii; of whete mele and of þe white of eyren, quantum sufficit. Medle hem togedir. Vndirstonde þat for

[222v]   myrte, þou mai take louage; and for mirtillis, louage seed;

5   for balaustia, take þe blosmis of okes; for psidie, þe rinde of okis. Also oþir medicines þer ben for þis sikenes: Stampe þe seed of plantein and medle it with þe white of

[223]   eiren. And þen roste it on a tiyl stoon and let him ete þat. Eiþir take milke of a coughe and þe iuse of mynte. And

10   let him drinke þoroughe ii° pipis, iliche moche of eiþir.

f. 259   A good poudir for þis sikenes: / Take roses, plantein, camomille, encense, mummie, canel, mastike,

[222v]   turmentil, bole, balaustie, psidie, sandragon, gallis, maces, of eueriche of þes yliche moche, and put sugir

15   þerto. And vse in medicines and in metis and in drinkis.

[223]   Coughe milke also is good for þis sikenes, if stones of a renning watir þat ben gloyng hoot be oftesiþes y-quenchid þerin. Athanasia is good for þe flux y-dronke with þe iuse of myntis. Alle þes forseid medicines ben

20   for þe flux þat comeþ of greuaunce of þe ouer-guttis and also of þe myddil-guttis. But if þe neþir-guttis ben apperid, þe most profitable worching is with suppositories and with clistres to make þe guttis cleen. But when

[222v]   þou ȝiuest a clesterie in þis sikenes, þou shalt not

---

4 **myrte**] *corr. from* mynte. 8 **roste**] *corr. from* rostid. **it**] *ins. above.* 12 **camomille**] *corr. from* camille. 17 **watir**] *in r. h. margin.* 21 **myddil**] *corr. from* neþir. 24 **a**] *ins. above.*

put it ful depe in ne ful hastiliche, but eseli, for

f. 259v   hurting of þe guttis. / And anoynte þe pipe ende with

oile or with sum oþer suche soft þing þat it mov go in

eselyche. And when a man deliueriþ him of þe mater of his

5   clistere, loke wheþir he be deliuered of as moche as he

resceiued. And if he is deliuerid of euen so moche as he

resceiued, þan it is wel. And þan let him resceiue a-þre

clistres or fovre til þe mater com as cleer oute, as it was

y-þrowe into his wombe. And whan it is so, þe guttis

10   ben wel y-clensid. And but þei be wel y-clensid, þei mov

neuer be wel y-helid. And aftir þat þou hast ȝouen him a

clisterie mundificatif, þou must ȝiue him a clisterie

strictorie to make his flux cese. A clisterie strictorie:

[?]   Take whete and breke it and seþe it in coughe milke /

f. 260   15   in þe maner of þin gruel. And cast þerto mastike, and bole,

and sandragon, and gallis, of eueriche, iliche moche. And

A clisterie
strictorie   when þou ȝeuest a man a clisterie, þou maist ȝyue him þe

quantite of a pounde at onis.

Chapter XIII, Part 2
Bloody Flux

[223]   Blodi flux comeþ eiþirwhilis of greet plente of

20   blode þat a man haþ, and þan a man-is veines ben ful of

blood. Eiþirwhilis it comeþ of sum wounde, and þat a

man mai knowe bi his iȝe. Eiþirwhilis, it comeþ þorouȝ

keneship of þat blood, þat persiþ and brekiþ þe veines of

þe guttis. And þan a man shal feel smerting and grete heet

2 **guttis**] *followed by* and whan. **15 þin**] *ins. above.* **19** *2-line initial in blue.*

in his guttis. Eiþirwhilis, it comeþ for feblenes of þe
luyer, and þat is y-knowe whan þes forseide signes lackiþ.

f. 260v   If it comeþ of greet plente of blood, / let him blede
[223v]   at þe arme at þe lyuer veyne. And diete him with metis and

5   drinkis þat gendren but litil blode, as erbis and fruyt.
And let him absteine from baþing of fresshe watir and fro
moche sleep and moche reste.

           If it comeþ of keneship of blode, let him be y-purgid
as it is y-told in dissenterie. And siþ staunche þe flux,

10   as it is told þer.

           If it comeþ of þe feblenes of þe lyuer, þer comeþ
a grete quantite of blood y-gloderid togedir at ones,
withouten ony oþir þing y-meynd þerwith. And þei
ben y-greued in þe riȝt side. And þan þou must ȝeue

15   comfortable electuaries to hem, as sugir roset. And
let þe iiii parte þerof be of diacodion. And ȝyue him
þerof boþe in þe morewe-tide and at myddai and at euen.

f. 261   And ȝyue him tri[a]sandri, and siþ / þe sirip of roses.
Also make cold plastris of þe iuse of þe erbis þat ben

20   strictories, and of watir of roses and vinegre, and of þe
iii kyndes of sandris. And put þerto cow milke, as moche
as þou hast of al þe oþer. And anoynte him bifore þe
lyuer with oile of roses y-medlid with camphere. Ellis
make þis plastir: Haue a good quantite of þe iuse of

3 it] *followed by* is *canc. in red.* **4 him]** *in l. h. margin.* **13 oþir]**
ins. above. **15 sugir roset]** *ins. above.* **18 triasandri]** trisandri. **19 þe**
(2)] *ins. above.*

plantein, and of myntis, id est, ana. And with oon parte
þerof medle barli meel, eiþir whete meel, and plastir þat
on a clooþ. And with þe oþir parti of þe remenant of þe
iuse, anoynte þe place bifore þe liuer. And siþ strawe
5 þeron white sandris and of rede y-poudrid. And siþ ley þe
cloute with þi plastir al aboue. And let him absteine him
[?] from moiste metis. And if al þis helpiþ not, ȝyue him
strengir medicines. /

Chapter XIII, Part 3
Diarrhea

f. 261v Diarria is a flux of þe wombe withouten flowing of
10 blood and wiþoute shauing of his guttis, and his mete is
[223v] sumwhat defied or þan it passe fro him. And þis sekenes
comeþ of þe same enchesons þat dissenterie doiþ and þe
same tokenes haþ. And þe same medicines helen hem boþe,
saf þis sikenes nediþ not so stronge medicines as
15 dissenterie doiþ. But neþeles, if colerike humours ben
[224] þe encheson of þis sikenes, purge him with watir þat
cassia fistula is y-soden yn, and tamarindis and mirabolani
citri ben y-soden yn. If it be of fleume, purge him with
þe watir þat oz. i of polipodi, and oz. vii of agarike,
20 and oz. iii of kebulis ben y-soden yn. If it be of
malencolie, purge him with watir þat sene, and epithime,
f. 262 and mirabolani / indi ben y-soden yn. And aftir his
purgacion, ȝyue him medicines þat ben comfortable, and
strictories, as it is told in dissenterie. If it comeþ

7 þis] in r. h. margin. 9 2-line initial in blue. 17 cassia fistula]
corr. from cassifistula. 19 polipodi] polipidi. agarike] corr. from
agarilke. 22 indi] and indi.

200

[223v]

[224]

of a revme þat falliþ adoun from þe hede into þe guttis,
his drit is white and ful of spumes and of bollis.   Þan
þou shalt hele þe revme as it is y-told bifore.   And þen
purge þe guttis of fleume and hele him as it is seid in
5 dissinterie. Miclete is good for þe fluxis.

Chapter XIII, Part 4
Lienteria

[224v]

10

f. 262v

[225]

15

20

Lienterie is a flux whan a man is deliuered of his
mete al hool as he etiþ it.   And þis sikenes comeþ of
corrupt humours þat ben in þe stomac and in þe guttis,
eiþir of sum postem þat is in hem, eiþir of feblenes þat
is in hem, eiþir of to moche eting and drinking at oon
mele.   And / wheþir-of-euer it be, þou maist y-knowe bi
þe tokenes þat ben y-told bifore.   And þe medicines þat
ben good for dissen[te]rie wol heel þis flux.   Neþeles,
þer ben special purgacions for þis flux as, if it be of
cold humours, þan take þe þynne iuse within a gourde, and
polipodie, and fenel seed, and squinante.   And seþe hem
in watir, and do in þat oz. i of kebulis, and let it stonde
so al ny3t. And on þe morewe, let him drinke of þat watir.
Eiþir take of polipodie, dr. iiii, and seþe hem in watir.
And clense þat watir and resolue þerin agarike, turbit,
hermodactalis, ana, oz. ii.   And let it stonde so al ni3t.
And on þe morewe, clense it and let him drinke of þat watir.
Eiþir let him drinke watir þat fenel seed, and pollipodi,
and anise, and a litil mastike ben y-soden yn.   And

6 *2-line initial in blue.*   **13 dissenterie]** dissenrie.   **18 on þe
morewe]** *corr. from* a-morewe.

f. 263 put / þerto dr. ii of esula. Aftir his purgacion, 3yue him hoot electuaries and comfortable, as diacinimum, diatrionpipirion, and suche oþir. And let him ete kene metis, as onions, and leke, and garleke, and mustard, and

5 carses, and salt metis. And siþ 3yue him a litil to make him cast. And aftir his purgacion, let him baþe him in suche a baþe as it is y-told in dissenterie. And whan he comeþ oute of þe baþ, 3iue him miclete and athanasia with þe iuse of mynt. And anoynte him boþe bihinde and

10 bifore, from aboue þe stomake doun bineþe þe share, with dispumid hony. And springe þeron þe poudir of mastike, and of encense, and of syneuie, and of myntis. But if þis flux come of hoot humours, purge him with oz. 1/2 of /

f. 263v þe cold dia[dra]gagantum. And medle þerwith oz. ii of

15 mirabolani citri. Aftirwarde, make him a baþ of roses, planteyn, and of suche oþir colde strictories. And aftirward 3yue him miclete and let him be in reste. And anoynte his wombe and his rigge also with þe gleyr of eyren. And springe it al þicke with þe floure of benes

20 in þe maner of a plastir. And in boþe enchesons, triacle drunken with þe iuse of myntis is ri3t good.

Chapter XIII, Part 5
Colic

[225v] Collica passio is a greuaun[ce] of a gutte þat is clepid colon. And yllica passio is a greuaunce of anoþir smal gut þat is clepid ilion. And þes

---

14 diadragagantum] diagragantum. **22** *2-line initial in blue.*
greuaunce] greuaun.

f. 264

[226]

f. 264v

greuauncis acorden moche boþe in enchesons, and in tokenes
and in cures; and sumwhat þei discorden, / for colon
lieþ aboute þe nauel and is toward þe sher along:
eiþirwhilis in þe ri3t side, eiþirwhilis in þe lifte side.

5 Eiþirwhilis it goiþ a-þwert, ouer þe wombe in þe maner of
a girdil. Eiþirwhilis it is bifore, eiþirwhilis it is
bihinde. But þe greuaunce of ylion is lower: eiþirwhilis
bifore, eiþirwhilis bihinde vp to þe reynes, and eiþirwhilis
in þe ri3t side, and eiþirwhilis in þe lift side. And

10 it walkiþ from o place to anoþir, and it is a ful greuous
peyne as it were of a woman þat traueliþ with child. And
þe ache makiþ a man eiþirwhilis to lese his wit, and
oftsiþes makiþ a man fal into a feuer. And sum men clepen
þes greuancis stiches. And boþe þes greuauncis comen of

15 diuerse enchesons. Oon is / greet hete in þe guttis þat
drieþ þe drit, þat it may not passe fro þe guttis. Anoþir
is mete and drinke þat makiþ a man costif. Anoþir is
viscous fleume þat wiþholdiþ þe drit þat it may not passe
awei. Anoþir is a greet corrupt wynde þat is in þe gutte,

20 and lettiþ þe drit of his issu. Anoþir is a postem þat
is in þe guttis. Anoþir is greet plente of wormes þat ben
in þe guttis. Anoþir is feblenes of þe guttis þat moun not
deliueren hem of þe drit and of oþer corrupcions þat is in
hem.

10 a] *ins. above.* **13 fal]** *in r. h. margin.* **16-19 Anoþir is mete ...
Anoþir is viscous ... awei.]** *2 sentences copied in incorrect order and
marked for reversal.* **20 his]** *ins. above.*

If it comeþ of heet of colere þat is in þe guttis,
he is costif and he withholdiþ his vrin. And þe ache is
ful kene and ful sharp, and his face citrin, and he feliþ
greet hete in his guttis, and he is þirstfulle.

f. 265 5   If it comeþ of costif metis and drin/kis, þe pacient
mai knowe þat himsilf, bi þe metis and drinkis þat he haþ
y-ete. If it comeþ of salte fleume, þe greuaunce meueþ not
moche aboute, but abideþ stil in oo place, and þe ache is
ful kene and ful trauelous. His vrin is of feble coloure,

10   and his face pale, of þe coloure of leed; and he is not
þirstful, and his greuaunce is most any3t. And þe drit
þat passiþ from him, it is litil, and þat is ful of spume
and of bolles, and viscouse, like þe gleir of an ey whan
it is wel y-sterid. And greet wil he haþ to go to priuy,

15   and may no-þing deliuere. If it comeþ of corrupt wynd,
þe wynd makiþ moche hurlyng and miche noyse in his wombe,
f. 265v and / renneþ aboute from place to place to haue his issu
oute. And whan he is deliuered of þat wynde, eiþir aboue
eiþir bineþe, he is moche y-esid. And eiþirwhilis suche a

20   wynd wrestiþ a man-is gutte aboute, as who wold winde a
3erde. And if a man blowiþ þat tyme in his fundement, he
is moche y-esid and þe gutte is brou3t into his kynde. If
it comeþ of a postem þat is in þe guttis, it is y-knowe
[226v] bi þe grete greuaunce þat a man haþ euermore abiding

---

11 þirstful] *corr. from* þirful. **17 renneþ]** *corr. from* walkiþ. **haue]**
in l. h. margin. **24 man]** *corr. from* aman.

stille in oon place. And þerwiþ he haþ a feuer and grete
ache in his guttis, and grete hete, and miche þirst, and
litil slepe, and he volatiþ his mete, and is y-helid
as a postem of þe stomake is. If it comeþ of wormes,

[?] **5** þou maiste knowe it bi þe tokenes þat shal be tolde in

f. 266 þe nexte chaptir. If it comeþ / of feblenes of þe guttis
and of longe wiþholding of drit, þe pacient may knowe þat

[226v] himsilf if meny daies han y-passid siþen he was at sege.

For þis greuaunce if it comeþ of hete eiþir of hote

10 colerike humours: Seþe colde erbis in watir and to þat
watir put a litil oile of roses, eiþir of violet, eiþir
bottir. And wete in þat watir wol þat is y-shore vnwasshe
eiþir a lynen clooþ. And þerwith waisshe his wombe wel to
abaten þe ache. Eiþir waisshe him with watir þat violet,

15 and roses, and wormod, and louage ben soden yn. Eiþir
anoynte his wombe with oile of violettis eiþir of roses.
Eiþir seþe þe holi-hocke and make a plastir þerof and ley
to his wombe. Eiþir make him a suppositorie of larde whan
his greuaunce comeþ to him, and put it in his fundement.

f. 266v **20** Eiþir 3yue him a clisterie / in þis wise: Seeþ myntis,
wormod, and betis in watir, and þen clense it. And with
þat watir medle whete bran. And þen clense it and put
þerto dr. iii of oile, and dr. i of sal gemme, and dr. 1/2
of þe electuarie þat is y-made of þe iuse of roses. And of

4 is] *ins. above.* **6 feblenes**] *prec. by* wormes *canc. in red.* **12 is**]
ins. above. **18 him**] *ins. above.* **suppositorie**] *corr. from* supporie.

þis medicyn let him resseyue a pounde at oonis þorouȝh a
clisterie warme.   And forto make þe clisterie go esili in,

[?]   anoynt his fundement with þe oile of violettis, or comon
oile, or buttir.   And let him be baþid in a baþe of

5   mercurie, and of hockis, and of groundswili, and purselane.

[226v]   Þis is good if þe sekenes comeþ of hote humours.   And ȝyue
him a cold sirip and let him be purgid with a colog[og]e
as it is y-told bifore.   And reule him boþe bi medicines

[?]   and metis, as it is y-told in þe ache of þe stomac þat comeþ

f. 267 10   of hete. / But if it be of cold humours, purge him softli of
þo humours, as it is y-tolde in þe [ache] of þe stomac.   And
his dieting shal be as it is y-tolde þer, in al þingis and
medicines.   And anoynte þat place þat is y-greued with
deute, arrogon, marciaton.   And siþ ȝyue him a clisterie

15   mollificatif to make þe mater neisshe, and siþ a biting
clesterie to make him to be deliuerid of þat mater.

A mollificatif clistere is y-made of watir þat hockis,
eiþir lynsede, eiþir mercuri, eiþir oþir moist erbis ben y-
soden yn, and bran, eiþir barliche eiþir whete.   And siþ

20   caste þerto a litil hony, and oile, and salt, et cetera.
Let him neuer take a biting clisterie but if he had a

[227]   mollificatif bifore, for drede of peril.   Eiþir let him ete
triacle diatesseron.   Eiþir seþe in salte watir wormod,
comyn, anise, betis, marche, maiorone, watir-carsis, and

---

7 **cologoge**] cologe.   **11 ache of**] of.   **11-13 And his ... medicines**]
in r. h. margin.   **15 neisshe**] *corr. from* nesshe.   **16 to (1)**] *ins. above.*
18 eiþir lynsede] *in r. h. margin.*

f. 267v 3erde-carsis, myntis, origanum, souþer/enwode, baume, and
horehovne, of eueriche of þes, oz. 1/2. And as þe erbis
seþen, breke hem. And in þat watir, wete wolle þat is y-
shore vnwasshe, and ley to þe wombe, and renewe it

5 oftsiþes, and al warme ley it þerto. Eiþir take olde oile,
eiþir olde bottir, and hony, and stronge vynegre, and salt,
of eueriche, iliche moche. And medle it wel togedir ouer
þe fier til it be þicke. And þerin wete wolle þat is
vnwasshen, eiþir a felte, and ley to þe wombe, for þis wole

10 helpe a man þou3 þe sekenes haþ holde him longe. But renewe
it oftesiþes. 3yue him no laxatif til he haue wil to go
to sege.

And if þis sekenes comeþ of wynde, it is y-helid in
f. 268 þe / same maner as þou3 it com of colde humours. Neþeles

15 þer be special medicines þerfor. Oon is, make a plastir
of comyn y-soden in wiyn and ley to his wombe. But first
make him a suppositorie. Also make him a fumigacion of
[227v] peritorie y-soden in wiyn. And let him drinke of þat wiyn
and plastir þe erbe on his wombe. Peritorie is a special

20 medicin for suche wyndis, boþe withinforþe and withouten.
Eiþir take þe erþe þat liyþ bifore an oxe stalle eiþir an
horse mangir, þat is y-troden and bipissid, and hete it wel
a3enst þe fier, and al hote ley it to his wombe. And let
him vse diaspermat[ic]on and oþir electuaries þat distroien

---

2 horehovne] *corr. from* horehone. **as**] *ins. above.* **24
diaspermaticon**] diaspermaton.

f. 268v   corrupt / wyndis. And let him absteyne him fro metis þat
                 ben wyndi, as benen, and pesen, and erbis, and fruitis.
                 Neþeles, carsen ben good boþe within and withoute. And let
                 him vsen suppositories, and clisteries, and medicines þat
           5   ben laxatif, and let him leue al costif metis.   If þis
                 sikenes comeþ of a postem, heel it as þe postem of þe
                 stomac.   If it comeþ of wormes, hele it as it shal be
                 told in þe nexte chapitir.   If it comeþ of feblenes of þe
f. 269   guttis, let him vse comfortable / electuaries, as dianthos,
           10   diamargariton, with watir þat baume, and mynte, and
                 maiorone, and carses ben soden yn.

Chapter XIII, Part 6
Worms in the Guts

                 Worms ben y-gendrid in a man-is guttis of diuerse
                 shappe, boþe for diuersite of a man-is guttis, and for
                 diuersite of mater þat þei ben y-gendrid of.   Of salt
           15   fleume, þer comeþ longe wormes and smale, and þei ben in þe
                 smale guttis.   Six guttis a man haþ in his wombe: þre smal
                 and þre grete. And in þe smal guttis ben smal wormes y-
                 gendird, and grete wormes ben y-gendrid in þe grete guttis.
[228v]   Of swete fleume ben y-gendrid long wormes and brode.   Of
           20   soure flueme ben y-gendrid shorte wormes and rounde.   Of
                 kindeliche fleume ben y-gendird shorte wormes and brode, of
f. 269v   þe shap of a gourde. Of glasi / fleume ben noon wormes
                 engendrid, for coldenes of þe mater. And þe greuaunce of
                 þe wormes is ful kene, and makiþ men eiþirwhilis as þei

---

1 *The scribe has marked the first 7 lines of f. 268v* vacat. *They are
a duplication of the first 7 lines of f. 265.* **4 vsen]** *in l. h. margin.* **12** *2-
line initial in blue.* **21 brode]** *prec. by* and rounde *canc. in red.*

weren frentike. Eiþirwhilis, men han lost her myndes for sorew. Sum men þei maken to lese her speche, as þou3 þei hadden þe litarg[i]e. Sum men fallen doun to ground, as þou3 þei hadden þe epilencie. Sum men han ache in her

5 wombe, as þou3 þei hadden collica passio. Tokenes of þes wormis ben, yching of nose-þirllis and of þe lippis, stinking of þe mooþ, hurling of þe wombe, and meuing within þe guttis as þou3 it were a quicke þing. And þe wormes goon vp and doun in a mannes wombe, and eiþirwhilis crepen

10 oute at his nose and eiþirwhilis at his mooþ. And his teeþ grinnen and stinken.

f. 270 And þer falliþ a gre/te yching ouer al her bodies. Eiþirwhilis þei maken a man rise up of his slepe as þou3 he were wood. And þei maken a man to haue a feble coloure,

15 and haue ache in his stomake and in his guttis, and also pricking and aking in hem, and nameli bifore mete. And eiþirwhilis, þei volaten mete, and eiþirwhilis, þei han an houndis appetite. And eiþirwhilis þei han wil to cast. And eiþirwhilis, þer comeþ dropis of blood of a man-is

20 fundement as when þe wormes biten þe guttis. And þei maken a man-is bodi ful feble. Ther is a difference bitwixte men þat han wormes and hem þat ben frentike eiþir wode, for wode men pleinen hem of her heed, and þes of her wombe. Frentike

f. 270v men han þe feueris in her acces and lesen / her wit for

---

1 myndes] *prec. by* wittis *canc. in red.* **3 litargie]** litarge. **6 nose-þirllis]** *corr. from* nose-þrillis. **8 guttis]** *prec. by* as *canc. in red.* **16 and aking in hem]** *in r. h. margin.* **20 as]** *ins. above.*

þe tyme; þes men don not so. A man þat haþ þe litarg[i]e
haþ a feuer comenli þerwiþ; þes men han not so. And he
þat haþ þe epilencie vomeþ, and he þat haþ cathalempsie
castiþ, but þes men doon not so. And he þat haþ apoplexie

5   haþ ache in his hede, but þes men han it in her wombe.
Alle þes men þat ben vexid with wormes han more eese when

[229]   þei ben ful þan fasting. And þerfore þei must dine bitymes,
lest þe wormes for defaute of mete gnawen þe stomac and þe
guttis.   And generali bitter medicines, and wel-smelling,

10   and soure medicines sleen wormes.   And swete metis
engendren watri blode, and þat engendriþ wormes and

f. 271   norisshiþ hem, and also erbis and fruit and nameliche / þe
substance of þe erbis and þe parels of þe fruit.
And in þe sleyng of wormes, it is profitable a-þre daies

15   a man to ete swete milke, þat þe wormes mowon fillen hem
þerwith.   And aftirward 3yue him a bitter medicyn, and þat
shal slee hem soon. And whan þou 3euist a medicin, medle
bitter þingis and swete togedir, as wormode sede with worte;
or þe iuse of wormod with milke, eiþir with hony.   Special

Special
medicines   20   medicines þat sleen wormes ben alloes, þe iuse of wormod, of
for wormis   centori, of cokil, þe poudir of hertis horne y-brent, þe
poudir of bitter lupines, þe leues of a beche tre, þe leues
of capparis.   A plastre for children: Take centorie, cokil,
A plastir   and vinegre, and þe iuse of wormod, and a litil salt,
for children

1 litargie] litarge. **5 her]** *in l. h. margin.* **7 dine]** *corr. from* dien.
18 with] *prec. by* with sede *canc. in red.* **19 or]** *ins. above in red.* **20
of** (1)] *ins. above.*

f. 271v   and oile eiþir bottir.   And medle hem to/gedir.   Eiþir
           anoynte him aboute þe stomake and aboute þe nauel with
[229]   bollis galle,   and   with   þe   iuse   of   centorie,   and   þe
           iuse of walwort, and of ellern.   And anoynte al þe wombe
5   þerwith oueral, for þis sleeþ wormes and bringeþ hem oute.

                   A   strenger   plastir   for   men: Take   wormod,
           and   þe   iuse   of   plantein,   of   marche,   of   biche   tre
           leues,   of   þe   iuse   of   þe   lasse   centorie,   of   bollis
           gal,   of   eueriche   of   þes,   iliche   moche.   And   make
10   þerof a plastir.   Also 3iue   a   man   gencian   to   drinke
           and it wole sle þe wormes, and an addir, if it be in
           a   man-is   wombe;   and   so   wol   þe   rote   of   dragance
           y-drunke,   and   also   þe   rote   of   asshe   tree   y-drunken
[229v]   in wyn.   But   whan   þe   wormes   ben   slayn,   þou must
15   3yue a man medicin to bringe hem oute.   And þat is with
f. 272   suche   þingis   þat   purgen   /   fleume.   Also   þe   iuse   of
           stancrop eiþir of orpyn y-drunke, and þe erbis y-plastrid
           to þe wombe driueþ oute wormes þat ben y-slayen.   And
           if þe wormes ben in þe ouer-guttis, mak him a clisterie
20   of þe iuse of wormod, of lupines, of scamone, of nitre, of
           salt, and of hony; eiþir of bollis gal, and of þe iuse of
           centorie, and of souþerenwode.   But first anoynt his ers
           with oile or bottir, þat þe clisterie mow esili go yn.   Whan
           þe short wormes ben ny3e a man-is ers, 3iue him sharp

---

5 hem] *ins. above.* **7 iuse]** *ins. above.* **11 sle]** *ins. above.* **18 þe]**
ins. above.

clister and kene, as iera pigra y-medlid with gal.

Chapter XIII, Part 7
Tenesmus

Tenasmon is whan a man haþ grete wil to shite,
and is vnmi3ti þerto. And it semeþ a man as þou3 he
shulde euermore shite, and whan he comeþ to priuei,

f. 272v 5   he mai noþing / do. Þis greuaunce is of a man-is gut þat
is clepid longaon, and þat gut goiþ doun to a manis ers.
And þis greuaunce comeþ of a kene colerike humour
þat is in þat gut, eiþir of a glasi fleume. If it
comeþ of a colerike humour, þer is hete and pricking,

10   and eiþirwhiles yching, and eiþirwhilis smerting
within a man-is ers; for þe keneship of þe colere fleeþ
oþirwhilis þe gut withinforþ, and makiþ it smert. And
eiþirwhilis, dropes of blode fallen oute. Whan it comeþ
of salt fleume, þat þristiþ and perssiþ þe gut adoun, and

15   þei felen cold withinforþe. And þat mater þat passiþ fro
hem is white, eiþir pale with musculages. And eiþirwhilis
þer comeþ þerwith dropes of blood, of þe grete enforsing þat
a man enforsiþ him to shite. And whan þis sikenes comeþ

f. 273   of colere / eiþir of fleume, him bihoueþ suppositoires, and

20   clisteries, and purgacions, as collica passio doiþ.
If it comeþ of sum kene medicin þat he haþ y-take,
make him a clisterie of watir þat whete bran is soden yn.
And if it be of colere, purge him with þe same eiþir with
sum oþir purgacion as it is y-told bifore. And sone ordeine

2 *2-line initial in blue.* **12 it]** *ins. above.*

þat he be purgid lest he falle into dissinterie.   Aftirward,
let him be baþid in freisshe watir, and siþ let him reste.
And þe nexte dai, let him blede vndir þe ancle withoutforþe.
And siþ seþe hockis, and violet, and holihockis, and betis,
5 eiþir barli mele, eiþir femigreke and lynseed, in reyn
watir.   And þerwith wasshe his wombe and his fundement.
And make him a fumigacion of old yren y-het and vynegre

[230]   y-spreynt þeron.   Eiþir take þe leues of like and make þe
smoke þerof passe vp into his fundement.   Eiþir take coton

f. 273v 10 and wete it in oile of / violet eiþir in shepis talowe, and
put it in his fundement.   And let seþe a bag with bran in
watir or in wyn, and let him oftesiþes sitten on þat bag
while it is hote.   But if it be of glasi fleume, let him be
purgid with þe purgacion þat is y-told in lienterie.   And
15 siþ make him a fumigacion of mirre, and of leues of
leke, and a litil castor y-soden in wyn.   And make him
also a fumigacion and a wasshing of ysope, puliol,
origanum, and betis, y-soden in watir.   Also make poudir
of ysope, calamynt, and origanum, eiþir her flouris and
20 do þat poudir in his fundement.   If þe gut falliþ oute whan
he goiþ to sege, springe þe poudir þeron.   Also hete wel a
til stoon and ley þeron peritorie eiþir wormod, and let him
sitte þeron.   Also hete a til ston and ley a bag ful of þe
poudir of baies of a lorer, of carse sede, of piliol, of

---

8 **y-spreynt**] *corr. from* y-sreynt. **12 or in wyn**] *in l. h. margin.* **14
is**] *ins. above.* **17 a (2)**] *ins. above.* **21-23 Also hete . . . sitte þeron.**]
in bottom margin.

f. 274   mastike, and of incense þerin.   And let þe / pacient sit

þeron.   And kepe him from colde.   A suppositorie for þis

sikenes: Take of mirre, dr. iii; of olibanum, dr. i; of

ameos, dr. i; of opium, dr. 1/2; of saffren, x greines.

5   Medle hem with hony eiþir stampe hem with an hote pestel.

Chapter XIII, Part 8
Prolapsed Rectum

Falling oute of a man-is ers is falling oute of

þat gut þat is clepid longaon.   And þis greuaunce comeþ

of diuerse enchesons, as of grete aforsing þat a man

enforsiþ him   to shite, as   it is in   dissinterie   and

10   in tenasmon.   Eiþirwhilis, it comeþ of   an hote heui

humour þat puttiþ and þristiþ oute þe gut at þe ers.

Eiþirwhilis it comeþ   of a grete cold þat makiþ [þ]e

gut feble and falliþ oute for feblenes.   And þat is y-

[230v]   clepid palesi of þe ers.   If it comeþ in þe firste maner,

15   it is y-knowe bi dissinterie or tenasmon þat a man haþ y-

f. 274v   had.   If it be in þe secunde / maner, it is y-knowen bi

heuynes and cold þat a man feliþ bineþeforþe, and he haþ

y-seten on a marbil stoon eiþir on sum oþir cold stones

in cold tyme þat haþ made him haue þis greuaunce.   If

20   it be in þe þrid maner, he feliþ cold bineþeforþ, and

þe gut is neisshe and slidiri;   and þat þat passiþ from

him goiþ aȝenst his wil, eiþir þat he woot not þerof; and

his colour is pale.   Forto helpe men herof, þou must ȝyue

a man an esi purgacion to purge him of fleume, and an esi

---

6 *2-line initial in blue.* **12 þe]** e. **16 þe]** *in r. h. margin.* **21 neis-**
she] *corr. from* nesshe.

clisterie also, as it is y-told in collica passio. Eiþir make him an esi clisterie of hony and of woman-is milke y-warmid. And þat purgiþ boþe fleume and coler and malencoli.

5 A souerigne medicin for þis greuaunce: Stampe garlike in cleen watir, and take þat watir, eiþir

f. 275 þe watir þat garlike is y-sode in, and let his / ers soke wel þerin. And aftirward, take þe poudir of hertis horne y-brent, and of a pine appil y-brent, and

10 of encense, and of mastike, and springe þeron. And make him a fumigacion of piche and encense y-cast on coles. And seþe otis eiþir barliche in a bag, eiþir in many baggis, and ley hem al warme in þe maner of a plastir boþe on þe sher and bineþe vndir his ers. And þat is gode boþe in tenasmon

15 and for hem þat han wormes. And ȝiue no strictorie medicin til þe gut be wel y-clensid of sori humours þat ben in him. And aftir þe cleensing with clisteries, ordeyne him þe foreseide baggis in þe maner of a plastir. A special medicin and oynement for þis sikenes: Take gotis talowe and

20 melte it, and cast þerin þe poudir of litarge, of ceruse, of

f. 275v amide, of gallis, / of balaustia, of accarnes, of emachites, of bole, of sandragon, of eueriche of þes iliche moche. And wete a cloute in þis oynement and ley on his ers. Also take piche and melt it and anoynt þe gut þerwiþ. And springe

---

14 þat] *in r. h. margin.* **18 plastir]** plastris.

þeron þe foreseide poudir and put yn þe gut. And let him vse souþing metis and laxatif metis, þat he haue no nede to a-forsen him to shyte. And let him vse þe souereigne medicin of garlike and oþir biforeseid til he be hole. /

Chapter XIV, The Liver
Part 1, Distemper of the Liver

f. 194
   5   Here beginneþ þe xiv chaptir of þis boke and conteineþ
[?]   iii practi[s]es or titlis.

[235]   The lyuer of a man haþ iii sekenes: Oon is distempering of þe lyuer in hete eiþir in colde, in moistnes eiþir in drynes; anoþir is stopping of þe lyuer;
  10 and þe þird is a postem of þe lyuer. Distempering of þe
f. 194v lyuer þat com/eþ of hete haþ þes tokenes: brenyng and pricking vndir þe riȝt side, drienes of þe tunge and of þe roof of þe mouþe, continuel þrist, þe vryn is of an hie colour, þe face is citryn and oþirwhiles grene. Colde
  15 þingis comforten him and hote þingis noien him. He is ofte costif, and whan he shetiþ, it is but litil. He volateþ his mete, and slepiþ but litil. And whan he slepiþ, he holdeþ his mouþ open. And oþirwhiles his visage and his yȝen ben infecte with a ȝelewe colour. And þen he haþ a
  20 grete ycching ouer al þe bodi and a scabbe. And if þis distempering be of sum corrupt humour, þei felen heuynes vndir þe riȝt side. And if it be of coler, þe vryn is of a
f. 195 ful hiȝe colour, / with moche spume. And he feliþ a smert pricking ache in þe lyuer. And al þe body is discolourid,

4 medicin] *ins. above.* **5** *See above p. 153, note to line 12.* **xiv**] xiii. **6 practises**] practies. **7** *4-line initial in gold.* **12 drienes**] *corr. from* drines.

and aboute þe veynes þer is moche hete and redenes, more
þan in oþer placis of þe body.   And if it be of blode, þe
veines ben to-swolle ouer al þe bodi.   And oþer tokenes ben
a-seen þat weren y-tolde in þe ache of þe heed.   And of
5   suche hote distempering of þe lyuer comeþ a dropesi.   But
if þe distempering be of cold, he feliþ colde vndir his
ri3t side, and his face [is] febleche y-colourid.   And if
þat colde come of a corrupte humour, he feliþ heuynes in his
lyuer, and namely aftir mete; and his face swelliþ sumwhat;
10   and his vryn is discolourid; and he defieþ febly his /

f. 195v   mete; and al his body wexiþ heuy, and namely aftir mete.
His wittis ben a-stonyed, and his hede is heuy of a greet
corrupte smoke þat smyteþ vp into his heed.   His mouþ is
vnsaueri and he is sluggi, but his slepe is trauelous.   And
15   oftsiþis he haþ ringing in his eeris and scotomie, and he
is disposid to a colde dropesi but if he be þe raþir y-
holpe.   Tokenes of drienes ben heuynes in þe lyver; þe
colour of his face is y-chavngid and apperid; þe lippis and
þe tunge wexen drie; and þe crampe goiþ al aboute þe
20   lyuer; þe tunge is drie; his vrin is þinne; his dritte is
of litil quantite and drie; and his body is leen.   Tokenes

f. 196   of moistnes ben swelling of þe visage; li/til þirste; þe
vryn is white and cleer, and oþirwhilis ri3t þicke,
oþirwhilis meneliche þicke; and his skyn is neisshe and his

7 is febleche] febleche. **16 he**] *in l. h. margin.* **17 drienes**] *prec. by*
deeþ *canc. in red.*

dritte also. And if distempering be of flevme, þou maist y-
knowe by þe tokenis of colde and of moistnes. And if it be
of malencoly, þou maist y-knowe by þe tokenis of cold and

[235v]   drienes. Neþeles þer ben special tokenes of malencoli: Þe
5   vrin is white and þinne, and he feliþ heuynes and ache
vndir þe ri3t side, and grettist aftir mete, and namely whan
he haþ y-ete malencolies mete. And he feliþ gnawing and
hurling aboute þe lyuer, and al his bodi is discolourid and

f. 196v   heuy. And oþer tokenes þer ben also þat / weren y-tolde in
10   þe ache of þe hede. Distempering of þe lyuer þat comeþ of
hete is helid by medicines þat ben cold. And if he haue
plente of humours þat ben þe encheson of his distempering,
purge him of þo humours. And firste defie þe mater with þe
sirip of violet. And let him vse þes electuaries,
15   oþirwhilis oon, oþirwhilis an-oþer: diacitoniton, to
restore his moistnes þat is wastid awei with hete; diaprunis,
sugir violet, triasandri, diarodon abbatis, rosata nouella.
And if his vryn wexiþ þicke and more þen it was, 3yue him
colagoge. But in distempering of þe lyuer þorou3 hete,
20   3yue him no medicin þat scamonia is yn, þou3 þe liuer be

f. 197   stoppid. But if þe sekenes / be olde, þou maist 3eue him
þe electuarie of þe iuse of roses, or oximel, or trifera
sarasenica with scamonia. A special sirip for hem: Take

Sirip   þe rotis of colde duretike erbis and þe erbis also; and

---

1 þou] *prec. by* þan *underd.* 2 tokenis] *corr. from* tokens. 9
tokenes] *in r. h. margin.* 11 he] *ins. above.* 24 duretike] *corr. from*
dureke.

cold duretike sedis, as of melon, of cucumer, of gourdis,
of purslane, of letuse, of violet, of watir-lilies. And
seþe hem and þen cast sugir to þe watir, and make vp þi
sirip. And cast þerto þe poudir of spodie, and of

5 mirabolani citri, and of reubarbe. And eueriche morevtid,
ȝyue him þerof, and on euentid also. And let him take it
with gotis whei, or with watir þat duretike erbis ben soden
yn, and lyuer-worte, and hertistonge. And whan þat watir
is soden, cast þerto a litil vinegre þat is made of white

f. 197v 10 wiyn. Duretike erbis ben þo þat / han kynde to open pores
in a mannes bodi þat ben y-stoppid. And sum ben hote
duretike erbis, as fenel, and parsely, radiche, marche,
and þe rotis of þes ben more duretike þan þe erbe. Cold
duretikes ben hertis horne, and meidenhere, and cicori, and

15 ceterake. Hoot sedes þat ben duretike ben fenel seed, and
parseli seed, and þe sede of marche, and of louage, and of
anyse, and of ameos, and of anet. Anoynte him withouten
with popilion, and oile of roses and of violet y-medlid
togedir. And cast a litil vynegre þerto or þe gleir of

20 eggis. And make him a plastre of roses and of watir-lilies,
or of þe poudir of þre sandris, and barli mele, and a litil

f. 198 spodie y-medlid with þe iuse of / solatre, and a litil
vinegre y-warmed and oile of roses. Eiþir make him a
plastre of spodie and of roses y-medlid with þe iuse of

---

2 purslane] *corr. from* puslane.

[236]

A plastre

[236v]

f. 198v

f. 199

endiue, of morel, and of scariole. Anoþir plastre: Take of white sandris and of rede roses, ana, oz. 1/2; of gum arabike, of dragagant, of purselane seed, of spodie, ana, dr. ii. Stampe hem with watir of roses and wete a

5 lynen clooþ þerin, and oftsiþes ley to þe lyuer. And ʒeue him a-morevtid þe iuse of scariole, of endiue, of purslane, and of planteyn with þe foreseid sirip. Oþer medicines also þat ben good for vnkynde hetis and feueris, ben good for þis sekenes. And if he be costif, make him a clister of

10 bran, and of hockis, and of lynseed y-soden in watir. Ei/þir make him a suppositori of scamonie and of sugir. And diete him as men þat han þe feueris. And if he haþ no feueris, diete him with gentil and sotil mete, and ʒyue him wiyn y-medlid wiþ watir. But þis shal not

15 be doon but if þe distempering be colde, or ellis þat þe hete be not ful grete. But if þis distempering be of cold, be war of al maner metis þat ben yuel to defien, and from grete metis, and from viscouse metis, and from wyndi metis, and rostid metis. But diete him as it seide in coldenes of

20 þe stomake. And if he be a riche man, let him vse þes electuaries a-morevtid fasting: diantos, diacinimum, diacalamentum, þe hote diacitoniton. And if he be a simple man, ʒyue him / diatrionpipirion and mel roset. Also, if he be a riche man, ʒyue him diamargariton, diacameron, diarodon

---

14 him] *ins. above.* **shal]** *corr. from* shalt. **19 coldenes]** *corr. from* colde.

of Galiens making or of Iuliens making. And if he haþ
plente of fleume, let him vse oximel duretike. And if his
sekenes be of malencoly, 3yue him oximel squillitike.
And whan þe mater is defied, purge him with a fleumagoge

5 eiþir a malagoge. And aftirward make him a stue of
souþerenwode, and wormod, and mugwort, and marche, and
origanum, and calamynte, and sauge, and mynte, and rwe,
and horehoune, and lorer leues, and fenel. Take of eche
of þes iliche moche and seeþ hem in lie. And let him

10 baþe him wel þerin. And let þat place þat is before
þe lyuer soke wel yn þat watir. And take an handful

f. 199v or ii° of þe erbis and ley / hem on þe lyuer in þe maner
of a plastir. Aftirward, anoynte him with hote oynementis
and with hote oiles. And in þe same maner þou shalt

15 worche in simple distempering of þe lyuer, þer-as þer
is noon corrupt humour encheson of þat distempering,
saf þat þou shalt 3eue him no purgacion. But þou shalt
vse þe same electuaries, and stufes, and plastres, and
in dieting, and in oile, and in oynementis. Eiþir make

20 a plastir of þe seed of fenel, of parseli, of marche, of
dauke, of carewei, y-poudird and y-temperid with þe iuse
of myntis, of wormod, and of mugwort. Eiþir make a plastir
of ysope y-soden. And make him a sirip of wormod, of
carses, and of calamynte. Aloes y-wasshen is gode /

---

1 he] *in r. h. margin.* 19 in (1)] *ins. above.* in (2)] *ins. above.*

f. 200 also. And eueriche morevtid let him vse to drinke oximel
with watir þat duretike erbis and sedes ben y-soden yn,
eiþir with piment þat is made with duretike sedis and
oþir good spicis, as gynger, clowes, canel.

5 Pyment is þus y-maad: Take viii partis of wiyn
Pyment and þe ix of hony þat is wel despumed, and medle hem
togedir, and þen medle þerwiþ þes spices y-poudrid:
galengal, ginger, clowes, canel. And medle hem wel with
a sklice. And siþ let it renne þoroughe a bagge and kepe
10 it. And if þis distempering be of moistnes eiþir of
drienes, it is not comonli withoute distempering of hete
or of cold. And þerfore þat may be y-holpen bi þat þat
is seide bifore, boþe here and in þe / chaptir of hosnes,
f. 200v and of þe coughe, and of streitnes of þe breste.

15 Dianthos is medicyn þat is good for þe tisike, and
for þe cardiacle, and for þe greuaunce of þe lyuer, and
[237] for al maner feblenes of þe bodi, and nameliche for
feblenes þat comeþ of long sekenes. And it is þus y-
maad: Take þe floures of anthos, ii° pound; and of
20 þe croppes also, ii° pounde; of white sandris, and reed,
oz. i; of clowis, spike, galingal, ana, oz. 1/2; of
cardamomum, canel, zedeware, and of notemiges, ana, dr.
iiii; of long pipir, ginger, maces, lignum aloes, ana, dr.
iii; of liquoris, half a pounde; and of his iuse, oz. i;

7 þerwiþ] *in r. h. margin.* **9 sklice**] *corr. from* slice.

of sugir, oz. 1/2; of roses, oz. iii; of honi, quantum sufficit.

f. 201   Anoþir diantos þat is more y-vsid, and it is go/de for al maner feblenes of a man-is bodi: Take of clowes,

5   galingal, ginger, spike, and of notemig, ana, dr. iiii; of canel, cardamomum, and anise, ana, dr. iii; of liquoris, of roses, of violetis, ana, dr. iiii; of þe floures of rosmarin, oz. vi; of hony, quantum sufficit.   And let him ete herof dr. iii at ones.

10   Iera pigra of Galienis making is good for greuance of þe lyuer, and of þe heed, of þe y3en, of þe eris, and also þei purgen þe stomake.   And if þe splene be y-hardid, it wole mak it neisshe.   And it is good for þe reynes and for þe bladdir.   And it is þus y-maad: Take of spike,

15   of   canel,   saffron,   squinantum,   asarum,   zilocassia, zilobalsamum,   carpobalsamum,   violet,   wormod,   epithime, agaricum,   roses,   gourdes,   wield   gourde,   and   of   mastike, ana, sc. ii; of alloes, take þe wi3t of al þe oþer spicis.

f. 201v   And let him vse / herof dr. iii.   And if þou wilt, 3eue

20   it him with pillulis. 3yue it with sufficient diagredii.

Iera pigra of Constantines making is good to make þe si3t cleer, and to recouer þe si3t, and to holden it in state.   And it is good for þe stomake, and for þe lyuer, and for þe splene, and for hem þat han dissinterii.

---

9 ete] *corr. from* vse.   **10 Galienis]** *corr. from* Galiens.   **13 mak]** *in r. h. margin.*

And it purgeþ þe humours and it is þus y-made: Take
of mirabolanis: of kebulis, indi, citri; of violet,
of wormod, ana, dr. iiii; of bellerici, emblici, cassia
fistula, epitimi, sene, agarici, cuscute, squinanti,
5   reubarbe, ana, sc. ii; zilocassie, spike, and anise,
and mastike, and ziloaloes, sal iem, nitre, ana, dr.
i; of honi, quantum sufficit.   Þis iera pigra is bettir
for þe heed þen þe toþir, but þe toþir is bettir for þo
parties þat ben byneþe þe mydrif. /

Chapter XIV, Part 2
Stopping of the Liver

f. 202   10   S[t]opping of þe lyuer is stopping of oon of þe
poris of þe lyuer.   Ther ben iiii pores of þe lyuer þat
movn be stoppid.   Oon is toward þe veynes þat comeþ from
þe guttis.   Anoþir is in þe ouer-parte of þe lyuer in
þe gibbe.   Anoþir is toward þe galle.   And þe fourþe is
15   in þe weie toward þe splene.   And þis stopping comeþ of
grete plente of blood, eiþir for þickenes of blode, eiþir
viscouse of þe blode.   And þis comeþ eiþir of blode,
eiþir of coler, eiþir of flevme, eiþir of malencoly.   Whan
þat wei is y-stoppid þat goiþ to þe veynes of þe guttis,
20   þan þilke moistnes þe veynes of þe guttis souken, þat
f. 203   it may not come to þe lyuer. / Wherfore þat þat passeþ
from hem is moche and nesshe as it is in lientery.   And
grete greuaunce þei han in þe ri3t side byneforþe.   And
þat is a comon token of al maner stoppingis of þe lyuer.

5 reubarbe] reubarberi. **sc.**] *prec. by* dr. *canc. in red.* **10** *2-line
initial in blue.* **Stopping**] Sopping. **21** *The scribe has written at the
bottom of f. 202v* Verte ad aliam partem folii subsequentis. *The
proper order of the text has been restored by reversing f. 202v and f.
203.*

The vrin is litil and of feble coloure, and þei slepen litil. And þerfore þe guttis defien febliche. And þey felen gnawing and heuynes bytwene þe stomake and þe lyuer, and þei ben þirstful.

5   Of þe stopping of þe pore in þe gibbe, þes ben þe tokenes: Þe vrin is sotil and watri, and þei felen heuynes and greuaunce from þe ri3t side, evene to þe ribbis and to þe rigge. And whan þei goon to þe priuei,

f. 202v   þei ben deliuered of litil mater. / And þe ache þat þei

10 han is more sharp þan þe pricking of nedles for stri3t passing of þe vrin þorou3he þe smale veines, and nameli if þei eten inflatif metis, as benes, eiþir peses, eiþir lentes, eiþir suche brede, eiþir þerf, and suche þingis.

    Of stopping of þe pore þat goiþ to þe galle, þes

15 ben þe tokenes: Coler is wiþholden in þe lyuer, wherfore þe vryn is of an hi3e coloure with moche spume, and vndir þe spume is a 3elewe coloure eiþir a grene, for þe galle þat is withholden in þe lyuer; and þei felen pricking as of netles or of nedles vndir her ri3t side. And

20 her face and her y3en ben y-colourid as of men þat han

f. 203v   þe 3elewe yuel of reed colere. And þei felen / ycching in her bodi, and ben þristful, and slepen litil, and han a feble appetite. And oþirwhiles, þoroughe casting, þei ben deliuered of colerike humours, and her mooþe

is bitter. And þis is oo kynde of þe ȝelewe yuel.   Of
þe stopping of þat pore þat goiþ to þe splene, þes ben
þe tokenes: Þe vrin is of swarte coloure, and oþirwhilis
þicke.   And þei felen moche heuynes vndir her riȝt side.

5   And her face is of þe coloure of leed or of a swarte
ȝelewe coloure, and al her bodi is ful heuy.   And þei
han dredeful dremes and a grete scab as þouȝhe it were þe
mormale.   And her dritte is black.   And þei han tenasmon

f. 204   of heuynes of ma/lencoly þat is in þe guttis.   And þis

10   is also oon of the spices of þe ȝelewe yuel.   And if þe
lyuer be distemperid with ony of þe foure humours eiþir

[237v]   of ony of þe foure humours bi encheson of his stopping,
þou maist knowe it bi þat þat was y-seide in þe last
chapitir.

15   Forto hele a man of þes sikenessis, þou must vse
suche medicines þat han kynde to open þe pores þat ben
y-stoppid, and oþer medicines þat han kynde to voide
þe mater awei þat stoppiþ þe pores.   And for-as-moche
as þe lyuer is a noble membre and a worþi, it behoueþ

20   þat his medicines ben comfortable as wel as openyng,

f. 204v   as purgynge. / And sum medicines þer ben þat comforten
þe lyuer.   Þe lyuer, if he be distemperid with hete,
openeþ þe pores þat ben stoppid and voideþ awei þe mater
stoppeþ hem.   Þes comforten þe lyuer: roses, and

10 if] *ins. above.* **14 chapitir**] *corr. from* chaptir.

spodie, and sandris. Endiue, and scariole, and
hertistonge, and meidenhere, þes comforten, openen, and
purgen. Oþer medicines þer ben þat comforten, and openen,
and purgen, if þe distempering and þe stopping be of

5 colde humours, as puleol, and letuse, and coste, and
gencian, and spike, and asarum, and cuscute, and marche,
[208] and epityme, and yue, boþe þo þat growen on trees and
þo þat growen on walles. But if a man wol heel on membre
of his sekenes, he muste beholde wheþir ony membre þat

10 is ny3e be distemperid also. And þer-aftir he muste
f. 205 worche; / for if þe liuer be distemperid eiþir y-stoppid,
þe stomake eiþir þe spleen mai be distemperid also in
þe same tyme. And þan þou shalt 3eue þi medicines
for þe lyuer to worche withinforþe, and for þe spleen

15 withoutenforþe. And if þe stomake be distemperid, ordeine
þi medicines for þe stomak withinforþe, and for þe liuer
withouteforþe. And þis is to vndirstonde if þe
distemperinges of suche ii⁰ membris discorden, as if þe
[239] oon by hete and þe toþir bi of colde, or ellis þus: As

20 if þe oon be hote and þe toþir be colde.

A good reule is a gret helpe for þis sekenes, and
þis reule stondeþ in many þingis: Oon is þat he baþe
him not aftir mete, ne walke he not aftir mete moche, /
f. 205v ne drinke not, vntil þe mete þat he haþ y-eten be defied.

18 ii⁰] *ins. above*; two *in margin*. **if**] *ins. above*. **19 of**] *ins. above*.

And ne vse he not swete mete ne swete drinke. And let
him vse þe medicines þat ben y-tolde in þe last chapitir,
if þe stopping be with distempering of hete eiþir of colde.
But speciali vse he þat sirip þat is specified þer if
5 his distempering be of hete, for þat openeþ þe stopping,
and it is profitable for him boþe in mete and in medicines;
and in metis, to vse parseli, and fenel, and sauge, and
gourdes, and melones, and þe iuse of citernes, and gotis
whei bi himsilf, eiþir with þe iuse of cuscute, eiþir of
10 scariole, eiþir of cicori, eiþir of þe lasse centori. And
[239v] oftesiþes, let him blede at þe veine y-clepid basilica
f. 206 for þe firs/te maner stopping, and of þe herte veine for
þe seconde, and of þe veine of þe splene for þe þridde
and þe fourþe. But if þe stopping comeþ of colde, do as
15 it is seide in þe last chaptir. And diete him with sotel
þingis, as with carses, skirewhites, and þe leues of
cineuei, and netlis, with þe branchis of radiche, and suche
oþir. And ȝyue him kene electuaries, as diacalamentum,
and diatrionpipirion, and suche oþir þat ben hote and
20 keen. And ones or ii in þe woke, ȝyue him foure chesteynes
eiþir fiue y-rostid. And let him ete hote brede in þe
morewtid. And if þou haue noon hote brede, ȝyue him tostid
f. 206v brede y-wette / in wiyn. And þat shal kepe him wel from
corruption of þe eire. Meidenhere is good for sikenes of

---

1 **mete**] *ins. above.* 2 **vse**] *ins. above.* 4 **specified**] *corr. from*
specied.

þe lyuer.

Chapter XIV, Part 3
Apostem of the Liver

Apostem of þe lyuer comeþ eiþirwhilis of coler, eiþirwhilis of fleume, and eiþirwhilis of malencoli. If it comeþ of blode, þe ache and þe greuaunce is vndir
5 þe ri3t side. And he haþ comenli a feuer, and his mooþ is swete. And þe white of his yen is reed, his veines
[240] ben ful, and his vrin is rede. If it is of coler, þer is brenyng and a sharpe kene ache vndir þe ri3t side. And his mooþ is drye and bitter, and he is þirstful.
10 If it is of fleume, þer is ache and greuaunce vndir þe ri3t side with a maner softenes. And þe face and al þe
f. 207 body is of feble coloure. And eiþirwhilis, he haþ / an heuy feuer. And in euery postem of þe lyuer, þe vrin is trouble. If it be of malencoli, þer is heuynes and
15 hardnes vndir þe ri3t side, and drienes withoutforþe, and his visage is of þe coloure of erþe, and al þe bodi drawiþ to þat coloure also. And eiþirwhilis, þei han an esi feuer, and eiþirwhilis noon. And eiþirwhilis, þe postem is in þe gibbe of þe lyuer, and eiþirwhilis in þe holewenes
20 þerof. If it be in þe gibbe, he feliþ his greuance ni3e þe rigge boon, and þer is swelling aseen. And he haþ greuance to drawe breeþ, and he haþ eiþirwhilis a coughe. And vnneþe he mai felen þe touching of a mannnes
f. 207v hande for greuaunce. But if it be / in þe holewenes

2 *2-line initial in blue.*

of þe lyuer, he feleþ heuynes and ache in þe depnes of þe
lyuer and adouvne to þe navel; and he haþ grete wil to
caste, and eiþirwhilis castiþ siþ and balkiþ. And if a
man putteþ his hande þerto, þe ache waxiþ more. If þis
5   postem comeþ of hote humours, lete him blede at þe veine of
þe arme. And in þe beginning of þe postem, þou shalt vse
colde repercussiues to smyte aȝen þe mater of þe postem.
And make a plastir of þe inner pilyng of henipe and of þe
iuse of solatre, and lei þat warme on þe lyuer. And
10 change it þries eiþir foure siþes a day. And anoynte
þat place with oile of roses eiþir of violet. And /

f. 208
let him vsen withinforþe colde erbis in medicines, as
endiue, purslane, and suche oþer. In waxing of þe postem,
vse dissolutiues, as barliche meel y-soden with þe iuse
15 of wormod, and þerof make a plastir and ley þeron. But
whan þe postem is ful y-wax and þe mater turneþ to quitour,
þan þe ache is most greuous. Þan þou shalt with
maturatiues make þe postem ripe. Seþe þan whete mele
with oile of violet eiþir with fresshe bottir, and make
20 þerof a plastir; eiþir of whete mele, and lynseed, and
femigreke y-soden in lye þat is not ful strong. Eiþir
in suche lye, seþe barly meel and make a plastre þerof.

f. 208v
And within/forþe let him vse duretikis. Eiþir make
a plastir of þe iuse of solatre, and of sandris, and a

---

3 siþ] and siþ; *prec. by* ȝocke *canc. in red.* **23 duretikis]** *corr. from*
durekis.

litil vinegre, and of þe iuse of wormod. And when
þe postem is to-broke, þe quiter wole passe forþe
with his vryn eiþir with his digestion. And þan
mundificatiues ben good to clense þe lyuer of þat
5 corrupcion, as diaprunis, sugir of violet, triafera
saracenica, reubarbe. Eiþir make a sirip of spikenarde,
and of hertis-tonge, and of endiue, and of þe iiii colde

[240v] sedis, and of sugir. But if þe postem be of colde humours,
let him blede as Y seid tofore. But neþeles, it is bettir
10 to ȝyue him hoot duretikis boþe in siripis and in

f. 209 electuaries, as fenel sede, parseli / seed, marche,
dauke. And withoutforþe, ley plastres of dissolutiues
þat moun opene þe pores and turne þe mater into smokes
and fumes, as ysope, origanum, centory, rwe, celidon, and
15 suche oþir. And make him suche plastres þat ben y-tolde
in þe postem of þe stomake. In þe waxing of þe postem, vse
plastres þat ben dissolutiues, as a plastre of wolle
vnwasshe y-soden in þe iuse of wormod. And when þe postem
is ful y-waxen þat þe mater drawiþ to quiter, vse plastres
20 maturatiues, as of whete mele, and of oile, and of violet,
and of hony y-medlid togedir. Eiþir make a plastir of

f. 209v snailes y-soden with hony, and whete meel, and lyn/seed,
eiþir of soure dowe y-soden in oile, eiþir of rwe y-soden
with wiyn and oile, eiþir of fenel seed, of marche, and of

1 **And**] Ande. **7-8 and of þe iiii colde sedis**] *in l. h. margin.* **24
with**] *corr. from* in.

rwe y-soden with wiyn and oile. And anoynte him with deute
and popilion y-medlid togedir. And whan þe postem is y-
broke, ӡyue him dia[a]nisum, and diacalamentum, and þe
sirip of wormod, and of spikenard, and of suche oþer. And

5 ӡyue him mirabolani, for þei ben good for boþe enchesons.
And make him a clistere mollificatif and an-oþer
mundificatif. And if þe mater be y-purgid by þe vrin, ӡyue
him watir to drinke þat duretike sedis ben y-soden yn.
And if he be purgid þoroughe þe wombe, helpe him with

10 þe decoccion of tyme, epitime, pollipodie, agarike,
and seen. / And vndirstonde þat in þe beginning of þes
postemes, þe wombe is nesshe as þough he had þe fluxe, for
þe lyuer is vnmiӡti to drawe to him moistnes from þe veines
of þe guttis. But in þe ende of þe postem, a man waxiþ

15 costif, for þen þe lyuer drawiþ to him miӡtili moistnes
from þilke veines. And vndirstonde þat in al sikenes of
þe liuer, þou shalt medle þingis þat comforten þe lyuer
with oþir þingis þat ben medicines.

f. 210

Chapter XV
The Spleen

[?] Here beginneþ þe xv chapitir of þis boke þat
20 conteneþ but oon chaptir.

[261] In a mannes spleen þer ben diuerse sekenessis, as
stopping, and swelling, and hardnes, and nesship, and
postem, and wyndnes. And eiþirwhilis, he is more replete

f. 210v of hu[mours] / þan he shuld be. And he may be replete

---

3 diaanisum] dianisum. **6 an-oþer**] *corr. from* oþer. **13 is**] *ins.*
above. **19 xv**] xiii. **20 chaptir**] *corr. from* captir. **21** *4-line initial in*
gold. **24 humours**] hu.

and ful of þre humours, principali of malencoli, for he is
ordeined to resceyue malencoli þat comeþ from þe lyuer,
ri3t as þe bladdir vndirfongiþ þe vrin; and þe bladdir þat
cleuiþ to þe lyuer vndirfongiþ coler and galle þat comeþ

5 from þe lyuer; and þe spleen also of fleume and of coler.
If it be ful of malencoli, þes ben þe tokenes: Þe vrin is

[261v]   white, and þyn, and cleer, eiþir-ellis swarte 3elewe, eiþir
blacke, of malencoly þat is y-medlid þerwith, þe whiche
also makeþ þe vrin þicke. And he feliþ ache and swelling

10 vndir þe lifte side, and moche hardnes þeras þe spleen lieþ.
And al his bodi is heuy and discolourid, and leen and

f. 211   feble. And he bal/keþ soure, and his spitting is soure
and keen. And his face is derke white eiþir pale. And
þe white of his y3en ben swarte 3elewe and þei ben turned

15 from her kyndli coloure. And þei feelen moche heuynes aftir
mete, and defien febeli her mete.

Of replecion of f[l]eume þe tokenes ben white vrin
and þicke, eiþir þyn, but not cleer; ache and hardnes
vndir þe lifte side, but not so grete as of malencoly.

20 His balking is withoute sauour and his spetting also.
And þe pawmes of his hondis ben hoot and þe soulis of his
fete also. And he haþ feble digestion, and þat þat passiþ
from him is white and rennyng, ful of spume, eiþir þicke

f. 211v   with muscilages. And þe bodi is discolourid and a / pale

---

17 fleume] feume. **24 discolourid]** *corr. from* discourid.

coloure and feble. And he wole be sone wery in goyng and
is slowe in goyng, and more aftir mete þan bifore.

Of replecion of coler, þes ben þe tokenes: Þe vrin
is of an hi3he colour and þynne; and swelling, and heuynes,

5 and hardnes þer-abouten as þe spleen liyþ, with hete þat
is y-felid in þe deepnes of þe spleen. And his mouþe is
drye and bitter, and he is þirstful. And he haþ grete
wille to caste. And his face and al his bodi is of a
citryn colour. And his dritte is citrin and rennyng,

10 and oþirwhilis is it þicke. And his bodi is leen and feble.
And þis is ful harde to ben y-helid. Nesship of þe spleen

comeþ of flevme þat renneþ into his poores, þat makiþ hem
nesshe. And þe token herof is þat / whan a man touchiþ þe
place with his hond, he shal fele al neisshe vndir his

15 fingris, as þou3he þe spleen were y-turned into humours þat
ben fleting and nesshe. And þei felen also ache vndir þe
lifte side. And oþir tokenes it haþ also of replecion of
þe spleen þat comeþ of fleume. Hardenes of þe spleen comeþ
of malencoli þat is y-dried and y-hardid in þe spleen. And

20 tokenes þerof is heuynes in þat place þat þe spleen lyeþ.

And þe vryn is discolourid and þynne, and eiþirwhilis blac
and þicke, of malencoly þat is y-medlid þerwiþ. And þat
makiþ a man defien yuel his mete. And eiþirwhilis, þei
fallen into a flux, and eiþirwhilis þei ben costif. Also

5 as] corr. from and. **6 is(1)]** ins. above. **12 hem]** corr. from him.
14 al] prec. by it canc. in red. **19 is]** ins. above.

f. 212v

[262v]

5

10

f. 213

15

20

[262]

þis hardnes of þe spleen comeþ of viscouse fleume /
þat is in þe spleen. And whan þe watrines þerof passiþ
awei, þe remenant abideþ stille and makiþ þe spleen hard.
And þis hardnes haþ þe same tokenes þat þe oþir hardnes haþ
þat comeþ of malencoly. And hardnes of þe spleen comeþ
also of coler, whan þe sutil moistnes vanisseþ awei þorou3he
hete, and þe gretenes abideþ stille and waxiþ hard. And
þe tokenes ben pricking and brenning vndir þe lifte side,
and contynuel þirste and bitternes of þe mooþ, and citrin
colour of þe face, and þe vrin is of an hi3he colour and
þynne. And he haþ þe flux, and al his bodi is 3elewe.

Stopping of þe spleen comeþ oþirwhilis of colde
humours, as of flevme and of malencoli, eiþirwhilis
of colere. Eiþirwhilis þe stop/ping is toward þe stomake,
and þan a man leueþ his appetite to mete. Eiþirwhilis
it is stoppid toward þe lyuer, and þan malencoli is
withholden in þe lyuer and is y-sente forþe ouer al
þe bodi. Eiþirwhilis it passiþ forþe þe wei þat þe vrin
goiþ and makiþ þe vrin þicke. Eiþirwhilis it abideþ in
þilke wey, so strei3te þat þe vrin may not passen þat wei
but it be clensid and y-made as cleere and as þinne as ony
watir. Eiþirwhilis þe spleen is stoppid toward þe guttis.
And þen þe guttis ben y-feblid þat þei moun not wel
withholden þat þat is wiþin hem, and so a man falliþ into

---

5 malencoly] *prec. by* fleume *canc. in red.*

a flux. Eiþirwhilis þe spleen is al-rounde and eiþirwhilis
euen-long. Eiþirwhilis þe spleen is þicke on þe toon side
and þinne in þe toþir side, eiþirwhilis abouen, eiþirwhilis
bineþen. Eiþirwhilis he is stoppid ouer eiþir side, /

f. 213v 5 eiþirwhilis in sum side. Eiþirwhilis it is y-stoppid of
colere þat persiþ into þe pores.

Swellling of þe spleen comeþ of humours þat fillen þe
spleen. And þat may be y-knowe bi þat þat was seid in
replecion of þe spleen.

10 Wyndines of þe spleen comeþ of grete humours þat ben y-
gendrid of a feble hete. And þilke humours letten þe wynde
þat is in þe spleen of his yssu. Eiþir it comeþ of humours
þat þorou3he violence dryueþ wynde into þe spleen. And
þat wynde makiþ þe spleen greet and moche. And þe token

15 herof is of walking aboute of þat wynde and horsing
from place to place. And now it comeþ, and now it goiþ.

A postem of þe spleen comeþ eiþirwhilis of hoot
humours and eiþirwhilis of colde. And þis same haþ þe

f. 214 same tokenes þat replecion / haþ. And also, if it be of
20 colde humours, þei felen colde and ache vndir þe lifte side.
And if it be of hete, þei felen brenyng and pricking in
þe lifte side. And þei han a contynuel feuer.

[262v] For nesship of þe spleen if it be of colde humours:
3yue him oximel to defie þe humours. Aftirward 3yue

---

7 fillen] *corr. from* fellen. **16 from place to place]** *copied* to place
from place *and marked for reversal.*

him iera pigra Galieni to purge þe humours. Aftir þe
iii^e day make him a stufe of hoot erbis, as of origanum,
calamynt, horehovne, tyme, rosemaryn, and suche oþir. And
þe nexte dai þeraftir, let him blede vndir þe ancle in
5 þe hyndrer side of þe lifte fote. And siþ make him hote
plastres þat ben during and consumeng þe humours, and
ley to þe spleen, as of rwe, celidon, netlis, and of
comyn y-soden. And let anoynte him bifore þe spleen
[263] with warme hony, and springe þeron þe poudir of syneuei,
f. 214v 10 and of / carse seed, and of comyn.

Hardnes of þe spleen and stopping of þe spleen
acorden moche in medicines, saf þat medicines þat ben
openyng acorden to þe stopping of þe spleen, and
purgacions and medicines þat ben mollificatif acorden
15 to þe hardenes of þe spleen to make þe mater neisshe.
And siþ þou shalt vse medicines þat ben dissolutif to
dissolue þe mater and to drawen it awei þat was encheson
of þe hardnes. And vndirstond þat hardnes of þe spleen is
incurable, eiþir ful hard to ben y-helid, wheþir it be
20 of heet eiþir of colde, and a man haþ it a hool ȝere
continueli. Neþeles, sum men seyen þat it wole raþir
be y-helid aftir ten ȝeer þen aftir þe firste ȝeer. And
whan þe mater is meving, and seen, and not y-hid, it
is bettir to be y-helid þan þoughe it were y-hid.

4 dai] *in r. h. margin.* **5 hyndrer**] *corr. from* hynderer. **15 neisshe**]
corr. from nesshe. **22 aftir** (1)] *in r. h. margin.*

f. 215   If þou touche þe / place þat is bifore þe spleen, if it
be so hard þat it synke not vndir þi fingris, it is
incurable. And þou shalt ȝyue him no laxatif medicyn
þorouȝhe his mouþ, ne duretike medicyn, ne no medicin

5   þat is ful dissolutif, ne within, ne withoute,
til þou haue y-ȝoue him mollificatiues to make þe
spleen neisshe; for ellis þe mater þat is sotel
wolde vanisshe awei and þe spleen waxe harder þen
it was. Ne suffre him to lete blode til þe mater be

10   y-made neisshe bi mollificatiues, and þat he be purgid,
lest þe spleen waxe harder þan he was. And
vndirstond þat þe spleen is purgid þorouȝ þe bladdir
with þe vrin. And if his hardnes com of hote humours,
ȝyue him oximel to defie þe humours, and a-morewtid

f. 215v 15 and on even and bifore mete. And anoynte þe / spleen
with bottir and oile of violet and rubbe it
sooftli. And let him stire wel his lift arme
as a renging bel or blowing beluwes. And let him
vse suche traueil from þe tyme þat it dawiþ til it

20   be liȝt day. And let him vse to walke in hilli
places on morewtides til he swete. And ȝyue him
oximel with watir to drinke þat þe flores of borage
and of violet ben soden yn. But let him vse bifore
diadraga[ga]ntum and diapenidion for his breest. And whan

---

4 **ne no medicin**] *in r. h. margin.* 10 **neisshe**] *corr. from* nesshe.
14 **him**] *in r. h. margin.* 17 **And let him**] *in l. h. margin.* 18 **a**] *ins.
above.* **beluwes**] *corr. from* belies. 20 **vse**] *in l. h. margin.* 24
diadragagantum] diadragantum.

238

þe spleen waxiþ nesshe, purge him with þe electuary of þe iuse of roses, eiþir with trifera saracenica, or with reubarbis.

[314v]

Electuary of þe iuse of roses is þus y-made: Take

5   of sugur, a pounde and oz. iiii; and of þe iuse of roses, as moche; of eueriche of þe þre kyndes of sandris, dr.

f. 216   vi; of spo/dye, dr. iii; of diagredium oz. i & dr. iiii; of camphore, sc. i. Make a sirip of þe sugir and of þe iuse. And herwiþ tempere þe poudre of þes oþir þingis.

10   And þe þrid dai make him a baþ of þe leues of a vine,

[263]   and of turmentil, and of lyuerworte, of hockis, violet, fenel, wormod, and of saleyn leues in a grete quantite. And siþ let him rest. And þe nexte dai aftir, let him blede on þe lifte arme in saluitica of þe lifte honde,

15   eiþir at þe veine vndir þe lifte eere, and at þe veine also þat is vndir þe ancle of þe lifte foot. And eueriche woke 3iue him a cologoge. And let him drinke warme wyne þat steel or gold is y-quenchid yn, for cold þingis noien þe spleen. Eiþir make a sirip of smyþþes watir and let

f. 216v 20   him / drinke þerof oftesiþes with warme watir. And 3yue him of þat watir þat þe iiii colde sedis ben y-soden yn, and lyuerwort, and meidenhere with hem. And 3yue him diaceraseos and sugur of violet y-medlid togedir eueriche morevtid.

6 þre] *in l. h. margin.*

[263v]   Dieting of hem shal be of temperat metis and
drinkes.   And be war of grete metis and of malencolies
metis.   And bifore mete, þei shulen traueil a litil,
and aftir mete reste hem.   And let hem vsen in her potage
5 planteyn, and hockis, and acori, and morel, and mercury.
And ȝyue hem also medicines þat ben good for þe ȝelewe
yuel and for stopping of þe lyuer þat comeþ of hete.
Oile þat is made of þe leues of mirte is good for hem.
And so is a plastre made of femigreke, of hockis; and
10 þe rote of holihocke and þe leues and þe stalkis of
f. 217   capparis y-ete in electuaries is good for þis / greuaunce
whan it is of hete.

[265]   Diacaparis is good for eueriche greuaunce of þe
spleen and of þe lyuer, boþe newe and olde.   And if þe
15 spleen is y-hardid, it makiþ him neisshe aȝen.   And if
it be y-dronke with wiyn, it sleeþ wormes in a mannes
wombe.   And if it be y-medlid with vynegre and y-put
in a mannes eere, it sleeþ þe wormes þat ben þerin.   And
if it be y-medlid with wiyn and y-holden in a man-is mouþ,
20 it doiþ awei ache of teþe.   And if it be y-medlid with
watir þat rue is soden yn and y-drunke, it is good for
ache of þe sides and for þe stomake.   And it is þus
y-made: Take of capparis, oz. iiii; of squille, asarum,
centorie,   piretre,   pepir,   tyme,   marche,   seen,   gith,

---

5 acori] *corr. from* cicori. **6 hem]** *ins. above.* **11 is]** *ins. above.* **15
neisshe]** *corr. from* nesshe.

f. 217v agrimonie, radiche, ana, oz. i; of honi, quantum / sufficit.
3iue him þat haþ þe greuaunce of þe spleen iii daies
herof, but if þe greuaunce and hardnes comeþ of cold.

[263v] Eiþirwhilis it comeþ when þe lyuer is distemperid with
5 hete.   And þan it behoueþ to doon rediliche boþe in
dieting and in electuaries, for þe lyuer wolde haue colde
þingis and þe spleen hoot. And temperat medicines wolen
helen euer eiþir.   And þerfor oon medicyn wole not serue
for hem boþe. But þou shalt vse medicines for þe lyuer
10 wiþinforþe in electuaries and in siripis.   And for þe
spleen, þou shalt vse medicines withoutforþe, as plastris
and oynementis.   And if þe lyuer be distemperid with
heet for þe same tyme, leie cold plastris to þe lyuer
and hoot plastirs to þe spleen.   And anoynte þe lyuer
f. 218 15 with colde oyne/mentis and oiles, and þe spleen wiþ
hoot.   And firste be aboute to make þe spleen neisshe
with deute and with botir, eiþir oile of asshes and
birches y-medlid togedir, eiþir lynseed y-stampid and y-
soden in bottir, and þerof make a plastir.   Eiþir make
20 an oynement of hockis, and of holihocke, betis, lilie
rotis, and of oynons y-leid in wiyn and in oile a-foure
daies eiþir fyue, and siþþen y-soden til þe wiyn be
consumed.   And defie þe mater wiþ oximel squillitik eiþir
oximel of radiche.   But bifore, let him vse diacene,

3 but] *corr. from* But. 7 medicines] *corr. from* þingis. 9 vse] *ins. above.* 16 neisshe] *corr. from* nesshe.

[263v]

f. 218v

eiþir diacapparis, eiþir diaspermat[ic]on, and sum oþir
electuaries with oon of hem, as diarodon eiþir triasandri.
And siþ purge him with diacene, eiþir iera pigra Galieni,
eiþir with þe fyue kyndes / of mirabolani, eiþir with
5 þis special medicyn: Seþe erbis þat ben duretike
in watir, and in þe same watir seþe time, and epitime,
seen, cuscute, and þe rynde of tamarindi, and of asshe,
and of capparis.   And siþ clense þat watir and put þerin
þe poudir of mirabolani indi, oz. ii; and of lapis lazuli
10 and [sal] armoniac, ana, sc. ii.   But waisshe wel þe stones
bifore, and let him   drinke   of þis   watir.   And aftir
þat he haþ vsid þis þre daies, make him a stufe of hoot
erbis   and   duretike.   And   þe   nexte   dai aftir,   let him
blede   at   þe   saluatelle of   þe   lifte   honde   eiþir vndir
15 þe lifte eere.   And ones a wike, 3yue   him a   clister
to   purge   flevme   eiþir   malencoly.   And   make   plastris
þat ben mollificatiues to   make   þe spleen   neisshe,   as
of amoniake,   and   mirre,   and   deute,   and   a   litil vinegre

f. 219

y-medlid / togedir   and y-leid   vppon a   clooþ vpon
20 þe spleen.   Eiþir make a plastir of amoniac and of salt
a[r]moniac.   And þis [is] good for swelling of þe spleen.
Eiþir   make a plastir of squillie y-soden and of amoniac,
eiþir of rue,   and marche,   and   vyne   assis, and   wiyn,
and   vynegre   y-stampid   togedir.   And   make   a   plastir

1 diaspermaticon] diaspermaton. 9 indi] and indi. oz.] ana oz.
20-21 salt amoniac] salt and amoniac. 21 is good] good.

[264]   and ley þerto.   And tempere þe wiyn þat he drinkeþ with
watir þat þe root of fenel is y-soden yn, and of marche,
and of parsely, and lyuerworte, and hertistonge, and
meidenhere, and filipendula, and ceterac, and   pollitricum
5   adiantos.   And if it be to him abhominable to drinke,
put sugir þerto and make þerof a sirip.   Also let him
vse watir þat capparis, and filipendula, and pentafilon
ben soden in.   Also a plastre y-made of turmentine, and a
f. 219v   litil oile, and barli mele y-medlid to/gedir on an esi
10   fiere doiþ awey þe hardnes of þe spleen.   Also make him
drinke camedreos and camapiteos and make of hem a plastre
also, and vse in electuari also.   Oile of ellerne doiþ
awei þe hardnes of þe spleen and so doiþ amoniac also.

[264v]   A postem of þe spleen is y-helid as þe postem of þe
15   lyuer, but þe medicines must be strenger þan þo þat ben
doon to þe liuer.

Windnes of þe spleen is y-helid bi plastirs,
oynementis, and oiles, and electuaries, and siripis, and
waisshingis þat ben hoot and extenuatif, þat is to sey,
20   þat han kynde to make þicke boisteis wynde more sotil
þan he was.   And let him vsen also medicines þat ben
duretike.   But þou shalt vndirstonde þat wyndenes of þe
f. 220   spleen comeþ oþirwhilis / of wyndi metis. And þen when a man
etiþ suche metis, his spleen is greued.   And whan he leueþ

5 **adiantos**] and adiantos. 19 **waisshingis**] *corr. from* wasshingis.
extenuatif] *corr. from* extuatif.

suche metis, his greuaunce passiþ awei. But when þe wyndnes
comeþ of þe spleen-silf, þan a man feliþ himsilf wheþir
he etiþ suche metis or do not. Alle oþir greuaunces of
þe spleen mowon be helid bi þat þat is seide bifore.

5 Diacene is good for alle sikenessis of þe hede þat comeþ

[265] of malencoly. And it shal be take þe morevtid fasting in
Diacene

wiyn. And it is good for hem þat han a feble brayn, and for
hem þat ben for3eteful, and for al greuaunce of þe spleen þat
comeþ of malencoly, and a special medicyn to purge þe blood

10 of malencoly. And þe best sirip þat is for woodnes þat comeþ

f. 220v of malencoly ys y-made of þe iuse of bo/rage, and seen, and
sugir. And diacene is þus y-made: Take of sene, oz. iii; of
canel, of clowes, of cardamomum, of galengal, of macis, of
lignum aloes, of long pipir, of ginger, of zedeware, of

15 spike, of notemyg, of eueriche of þes, dr. iii. And sum
putten þerto borage, and calament, and tyme, and suche oþir
þat purgen malencoli, and also nottes fifty; and of brent
silke, dr. ii; and of lapis lazuli, dr. iii; and of lapis
armenicus, dr. ii; and of sugir, dr. vi. Sum men doon as

20 moche seen to þis confeccion as of alle þe oþir þingis. 3eue
þis to þe pacient with watir þat sene haþ leyen yn al ny3te.

Diaceraceos
is good for Diaceraseos is good for greuaunce of þe stomake, and of
þe stomake

þe liuer, and of þe spleen, and is þus y-made: Take of

f. 221 þe iuse of chiries, iiii pounde; of dispumid / hony, iii

7 is] *ins. above.*

pounde. And seeþ hem togedir ouer an esy fier til it be
þicke. And þan put þerto oz. iii & dr. iiii of diagredium
y-poudrid; of canel y-poudrid, oz. i; of mastike, as moche;
and of þe pouderis of þe colde sedis, dr. iii. Of þis ȝyue
5 a man dr. iii at morwe. And let him faste aftirward til
mydday. Agrippa is a good oynement for swelling of þe
spleen and for al oþir swellingis and for greuaunce of þe
senewis.

Chapter XVI, The Kidneys
Part 1, Ache of the Kidneys

f. 275v / Here beginneþ þe xviþe chapitir of þis boke þat
[?] 10 conteniþ iii titlis or practi[s]es.

In a man-is reynes eiþir in his kidneiren ben þre
greuauncis: ache, postem, and stones. Ache comeþ
eiþirwhilis of cold, eiþirwhilis of hete: of hete, as of
blode eiþir of coler; of cold, as of fleume eiþir of
15 malencoli. Þe reines ben y-fillid, principali with oon of
f. 276 þes humours: / with blood, eiþir coler, eiþir fleume; with
malencoli but rit sildene.

Tokenes of blood ben, hete in þe depnes of þe reines,
and heuines, and greuaunce, and þe veine þat is in þe inner
20 side of þe leg vndir þe ancle is ful of blood. And þe vrin
is fat and wel y-colourid.

Tokenes of coler ben brenning and pricking in þe depnes
of þe reines, and a kene ache aboute þe reines, and heuines
also, and drines of þe skyn withouteforþe. And þe vrin is

---

4 and] *corr. from* as. 9 xviþe] xvþe. 10 practises] practies. 11 *5-
line initial in gold.*

of an hie coloure and þinne, and eiþirwhilis þicke, of coler þat is medlid þerwith. And meny smale þredis ben in þe vrin, eiþirwhilis bineþe, eiþirwhilis aboue.

[265v]

5 Of fleume, tokenis ben colde and heuines aboute þe reines, and þe vrin is white and fat, and if þe reume is y-gloderid togedir aboute þe reines, þer ben muscilagis in f. 276v þe vrin and smale white þredis. Tokenes of / malencoli ben, þyn vrin and ȝelew, eiþir swarte ȝelewe, and ful of bollis. And eiþirwhilis þe vrin is þicke, of malencoli þat is y-
10 medlid þerwith. And þei felen miche heuines aboute þe reines. And hem semeþ þat þe places aboute þe reines slepiþ. And þes humours þat þus greuen þe reines eiþirwhilis flowen from al þe bodi to þe reines. And þe token herof is, al þe bodi is y-greued as wel as þe reines.
15 And þan þe beginning of þe cure shal be to purge al þe bodi of þat humour þat greueþ þe reines. Eiþirwhiles, þe humour þat flowiþ to þe reines flowiþ from þe hede, eiþirwhilis from þe lyuer, eiþirwhilis from þe spleen. And þan þe cure shal be doon to þat membre with confortatiues and f. 277 20 strictories þat mown staunche þe flowing. / And if þis greuaunce of þe reines be of blood, if þe man haue miche blood, let him blede in þe riȝt arme at þe veine þat serueþ to þe lyver. And siþ hele him with þe same medicines þat seruen for coler. First ȝyue him diaprunis to defie þe

1 **coler**] colour.

mater, eiþir make him wortis of hockis and of oþir cold
erbis.   And anoynt þe reines with oile of violet and
with freisshe bottir.   And seþe otis and solatre in
watir, and wringe oute þat watir, and wete a cloute

5   þerin, and ley vppon þe reines.   But if þilke humours
flowe not to þe reines from noon oþir place, 3yue him
oximel to defie þo humours.   And siþ 3iue him þe electuarie
of rosis to purgen him of þe humours.   And if he haþ
not grete plente of blode, purge him with a clisterie

f. 277v 10   cologoge.   And siþ ma/ke him a stufe eiþir a baþ of cold
erbis.   And 3yue him a drau3t of wyne y-medlid with watir

[266]   þat incense is y-soden yn.   And on þe morewe, let him
blede on þe veine þat is vndir þe ancle in þe vttir side
of þe leg.   And eueriche moneþe ones, let him blede at þat

15   veine, oonis in þe oon leg, and anoþir tymes in þe oþir
leg; for þe veine undir þe ancle on þe inner side of þe
leg serueþ for þe lyuer and þe spleen, and to þe bladdir
and to þe guttis.   But þe veine of þe vttir side of þe leg
seruiþ to þe reines, and to þe ioynt þat þe leggis ben

20   tied to þe bodi bi, and for þe iunctis of þe chyn.   And
medicines þat Y told for distempering of þe liuer þat
comeþ of hete ben good here.   And if þe reines ben

f. 278   distemperid with hete and han not to moche blode / ne
colere, þei shulen ben y-helid with cold electuaries and

---

14 þat] *corr. from* þe. **15 in** (1)] *ins. above.* **18 veine]** *in l. h.*
margin. **22-23 ben distemperid with hete]** *copied* with hete ben distemperid *and marked for reversal.*

siripis, and oynementis and plastres, withouten purgacions, as distempering of þe liuer is. But if þe greuaunce be of cold, anoynt þe reines with sum hote oyl or with deute. And if þe humours flowen from oþir placis þidir, make him wortis

5 of betis and of carsis. And if þe humours flowen not to þe reines from noon oþir place, 3iue him oximel, and þen purge him, and make him a stufe of origanum, and calamynt, and suche oþir hote erbis. And whan he comeþ oute, let him drinke wyne þat incense is y-soden yn, if þe humours flowen

10 þidir. Ellis 3iue him wyne þat fenel rotis ben soden yn. And þe nexte dai aftir, let him blede vndir þe ancle in þe

f. 278v vttir side of þe leg. And let him / ben y-cuppid and y-garsid on þe reynes. And aftirward, anoynt him with hony þat is dispumid and hote. And strawe þeron þe poudir of

15 fenel, and of parseli, marche, dauke, carewei, ginger, spikenard, encense, mastike, and of wormod. And þen tose coton as smal as þou mai and strawe it aboue þe poudir. And let it lye so til it fal awei. And for-as moche as medicines passen meny weies or þei com to þe reines, it

20 behoueþ þerfore þat þei han sum-þing to bringe hem to þe reines þat wol not be consumid ne wastid awei anoon, as opium. But vndirstonde þat ri3t as opium quenchiþ a man-is kindeli hete, ri3t so mirre and baume tendiþ a mannes kyndeliche hete, as oile tendiþ and norisshiþ fier. And

---

3 sum] *in r. h. margin.* **oyl]** *followed by* as *canc. in red.*

þerfore medle hem togedir. /

Chapter XVI, Part 2
Apostem of the Kidneys

f. 279

[266v]

Apostem of þe reines: Eiþirwhilis he is in oon of hem, eiþirwhilis boþe þei han postemes. And hou-euer he come, eiþir he is of blode, eiþir of colere, eiþir of fleume,
5 eiþir of malencoli. If he is of blode, he feliþ hete, and ache, and heuines in þe depnes of his reines, and his hede akiþ, and he haþ wil forto caste. And his vrin is y-let of his cours. And eiþirwhilis it is rede, eiþirwhilis blodi, eiþirwhilis it is like þe drastis of quiter of þe postem
10 þat is y-medlid þerwith. And he haþ ache in his chyne, and þe veine is swol þat is vndir þe ancle. Of colere ben þe same, but þei ben more violent þan of blood. And he feliþ brening and pricking in þe depnes of þe reines and in þe

f. 279v place aȝenist þe reines. If it is of fleu/me, þer is ache
15 with cold, and with heuines, and oþir tokenes of fleume. Of malencoli, þe tokenes ben ache with grete heuines, and cold, and drines. And þer is a grete difference bitwixte þis and collica passio, for in þe collica passio, þe ache is vnstable, and aftir þat a man haþ y-go to priuy, his ache
20 is abatid. And comenli he is costife. But þis ache is stable and duriþ stille til þe postem be ripe to breke.

[267] And if þe postem be of hote humours, duretike medicines sufficen to hele him. But medle hote duretikis with cold, þat þe cold haue þe maistri. And if it be a cold

2 *2-line initial in blue.* **7 of**] *prec.by* fro *canc. in red.*

postem, let hote duretikis haue þe maistre, boþe in
siripis, and in electuaries, and in plastris. And þat þat

f. 280 is seid / in þe postem of þe liuer is good here. A good
plastir to make þe postem of þe reines ripe: Take hockis

5 and holi-hockes, and betis, and violettis, and seþe hem in

A plastir watir. And siþ grinde hem with gose grece, and hennis grece,
for postem
of þe reynes and shepis talowe. Whan þe postum is of colde, anoynt þe
reines with deute and make a plastir of fenel seed, and
comyn, and sileris mountein, and of datis, and of drie figis

10 y-stampid togedir with þe iuse of marche and a litil oile,
eiþir þe marie of a calf, eiþir bottir, eiþir gose grece.
And whan þe postem is y-broke, þou maist see þe quiter come
oute in his vrin. Þen 3yue him þe ballis þat souden woundis
þat ben withynforþe, þe whiche shulen be tolde in þe

15 pissing of blode. 3iue him þilke ballis with gotis milke,

f. 280v and make him a plastir / of barliche and of sape. And let
him sitte in watir þat barliche and hockis ben y-soden yn.
And if þe quiter be þicke, 3yue him þe iuse of solatre,
wormod, and marche wel-y-soden and y-clensid. And

20 aftirward, 3iue him goute milk or coughe milke, for þat
clensiþ, wheþir þe wounde be without or withyn. And ri3t
as þis postem is y-helid, so is þe postem of þe bladdir
y-helid. And þe same tokenis þat þis postem haþ aboute
þe rigge, þe postem of þe bladdir haþ aboute þe share.

---

13 oute] *prec. by* at *canc. in red.* **17 him]** *ins. above.* **sitte]** *corr.*
from sette. **20 3iue him]** *in l. h. margin.* **milk]** *ins. above.*

Chapter XVI, Part 3
Stones in the Kidneys and Bladder

Stones ben y-gendrid in a man-is reines and also in þe
bladdir. And þre enchesons þer ben of gendring of suche

[267v] stones. Oon is a viscous mater of whom þe stonis ben y-
gendrid. Þe seconde encheson is hete þat wastiþ awei þe

f. 281 5 watrines of þat viscous mater and turniþ þe / remenant into
stones. Þe þrid encheson is þe streitnes of þe pores and of
þe wei þat suche viscous mater shuld passe forþ bi. And
eiþirwhilis stones ben y-gendrid of hote viscous humours,
and eiþirwhilis of cold.   And eiþirwhilis þe stoon is newe

10 and eiþirwhilis elde.   Of hete, tokenis ben a kene pricking
ache, and greuaunce in pissing, and þe vrin is of an hiȝe

[270] coloure, and eiþirwhilis haþ dropes of blode eiþirwhilis
grauel, and þat is reed, eiþir grene, eiþir blac.   If þe
stone comeþ of cold viscouse humours, þer is grete cold

15 aboute þat place þat þe stoon lieþ in, and heuines, and
greuaunce, and þe vrin is white eiþir swart ȝelewe, and þe
grauel is white eiþir swart ȝelewe, eiþir of þe colour of
assis.   Eiþirwhilis grauel is in men-is watris þat han /

f. 281v not þe stoon, as in suche men-is watris þat han an hote

20 brening feuer eiþir þat han go[u]tis.   But þat grauel wole

[269] falle to smale poudir if it be rubbid bitwene a man-is fingris,
but grauel of men þat han not þe stone is not so.   Stones
also ben y-gendrid in oþir place as wel as in þe reines or in

[268] þe bladdir, for men han stones in her stomake and þei ben

1 *2-line initial in blue.* **5 into]** *corr. from* to. **11 of an]** *in r. h.
margin.* **12 coloure]** *prec. by* in *canc. in red.* **13 blac]** balac. **20
goutis]** gotis. **22 stone]** *corr. from* stones. **24 han]** *prec. by* þat *canc.
in red.*

deliuerid of hem þorou3 casting. Sum men han stones in her
guttis, and þei ben deliuerid of hem in shiting. Sum men
han stones in oþer placis, as þilke þat han goutis aboute
her ioyntis, wheþir it be in þe rigge, in þe leg, or in þe
5 armis. Tokenes of þe stoon: Þe foot on ilke side þat þe
[270]   stoon is, is a-stonied, and þe rigge-boon on þat side is
f. 282   y-greued. And þei han greua/unce in pissing, and grauel in
þe vrin. And if þe stoon be waxing, þe vrin waxiþ from dai
to dai ful of grauel. And whan þe stoon is ful y-waxe,
10 eiþir wexiþ lesse, þen þe grauel waxiþ lasse in þe vrin.
And þan þe vrin waxiþ white as milke. And þei ben y-greuid
as oftesiþes as þei pissen. And þe same tokenes ben of þe
stones in þe reynes and in þe bladdir, saf in þe reynes, þe
greuaunce is bihinde in þe rigge; and in þe bladdir, it is
15 bifore, in þe shere, and toward a man-is ers. A stoon þat
haþ be longe in a man wole not be wel y-helid but if he be
[270v]   kut awey. A newe stoon may ben y-helid with medicines.
And if it be of hete, 3yue him diaprunis on þe morewetid.
f. 282v   And þe euentid, 3iue him gin/ger with oximel. And let him
20 take it with watir þat hertistonge, and meiden-here, and
parseli sede, and þe iiii cold sedis ben soden in.
[271]   Aftirward, 3iue him þe electuarie of þe iuse of roses. And
þe þrid dai aftir, make him a baþ of mercurie, wormod,
saleyn leuyes, and vyne leues, and turmentil, sour-doc, and

---

1 casting] *prec. by* cou3hing *canc. in red.* **5 ilke**] *prec. by* þe *canc.*
in red. **9 stoon**] *prec. by* vrin *canc. in red.* **15 ers**] *in r. h. margin.* **18
on**] *ins. above.* **22 him**] *ins. above.*

burnet. And whan he comeþ oute of þe baþ, 3yue him þe
watir þat soure-doc, hertistonge, endiue, ben y-soden yn.
And þe next dai aftirward, let him blede at þe veyne vndir
þe ancle in þe vttir side if þe stoon be in þe reines,
5   and in þe inner side [if] it be in þe bladdir. And anoynt

f. 283   þe place with popilion and vinegre and ley / þis plastir
þeron: Take soure-docke, and purslane, and þe iiii cold
sedis, and arage, and sandris, and fenel sede, and parseli
sede. Poudir hem and tempere hem with vinegre and with
10   wyne, eiþir with vinegre and þe iuse of mercurie. And
medle diaprunis with þe electuarie of þe iuse of roses.
And let him eueriche wike ete þerof þe quantite of a
chesteyn whan he goiþ to bed. And þan he shal not drede hou
he diete himsilf. And 3iue him þe sirip of hertistonge, of
15   meyden-here, pollitricum adiantos, y-medlid togedir. And
let him vse it from þre daies to þre daies. But if it comeþ
of cold, let him vse oximel duretik eiþir oximel

[271v]   squillitike. And aftirward, make him a baþ of þe rotis of
fenel, of parseli, of marche, of carewei, of dauke, of /

f. 283v 20   saxifrage, and milium solis y-soden in watir. And let him
sit in þat baþ vp to þe nauel. And siþ 3iue him triacle
with wyn þat saxifrage and milum solis ben y-soden yn.
And amorewe, open þe veyne þat is vndir þe ancle. And if
þe stone be in his reines, let him vse þis baþ oftesiþes

    5 if it] it. **14 him]** *in r. h. margin.* **15 meyden-here]** meynden-
here.

in þe þrid eiþir in þe fourþe age of þe moneþe. And let
him vse þis sirip: Take of þe iuse of radiche and of
saxifrage yliche moche, and seþe hem ouer an esi fyer.   And
þen clense it and put þerto sugir.   Eiþir take þe rotis of
5   parseli,   marche,   dauke,   carawei,   radiche,   pentafilon,
and of saxifrage, and of breris þat growen in þe fildis,
burnet, and langdebef. And seþe hem in watir and put þerto
f. 284   sugir.   And ma/ke vp þi sirup.   An oynement for þe stoon:
Take þe iuse of saxifrage, radiche, burnet, watir-lilies,
10   langdebef, and medle þe iuse with oile of lorer.   And seþe
hem so long til þe iuse be consumed awei.   And siþ medle
swynes grees þerwith and make þerof an oynement.   And make
a plastir of ysope and of saxifrage y-soden togedir and
y-leide vppon þe share.   Eiþir stampe þe sede of fenel, of
15   parseli,   of   marche,   of   dauke,   of   saxifrage,   carewei,
radiche, and medle hem with her avne iuse.   And make a
plastir and ley vppon þe reines if þe stoon be in þe
bladdir.   And if þe stoon be fal doun into þe bladdir, and
[272]   siþ y-fal doun into þe 3erde and lettiþ a man forto pisse,
20   make him a baþ of hockis and of betis and let him sit þerin
f. 284v   vp to þe na[uel]. / And whan he comeþ oute þerof, anoynte
þe share bifore þe bladdir wiþ bottir.   And let him vse þis
baþing fyue daies.   And if he mai suffre wel, while he
sittiþ in þe baþ, let him rubbe from his ers to his 3erde

9 iuse] *in l. h. margin.* **21 nauel**] na. **22 vse**] *in l. h. margin.*

and so he mai with ofte-rubbing make þe ston com oute at his ȝerde. And let anoynt him with hote oynementis eiþir oilis. Forto breke þe stoon, meny oþir þingis ben good, as þe kirnels of chiry stones and of plumb stones, and þe seed of aisshis, and of gromel, and of cicori, and yue, and hertistonge, and meydenher, and þe seed of Oure Lady þistil þat is spekelid and beriþ blac seed. Eueriche of þes han vertu to breke þe stoon, and if þei be medlid togederis, þe medicin is of þe more vertu.

[?]

5

Chapter XVII, The Bladder
Part 1, Strangury

10

f. 285

In a mannes bladdir and longing to a mannes bladdir, þer ben diuerse greuaun/cis. Oon is y-clepid stranguria, and þat is whan a man haþ grete wil to pisse, and pissiþ but a litil, and þat is dropmele, as an eues of an house dropiþ. Anoþir greuaunce þer is, þat is an vnmesurable pissing of vrin fro a man. And þat mai com of greuaunce of þe reines, and þat is y-clepid diabetes. Eiþirwhilis, it comeþ of feblenes of þe bladdir, and þan it is clepid diampnes.

15

[274]

20

Stranguria is eiþirwhilis a sikenes bi himsilf, and he mai come of two enchesons. Oon is kene coler and hoot þat is in þe bladdir, and makiþ þat þe vrin dropiþ oute of þe bladdir into þe ȝerde, riȝt as it comeþ droping into þe bladdir from þe reines. And þe tokenes herof ben brenyng, and pricking, and swelling in þe ȝerde, and hiȝe coloure /

9 þe (2)] *ins. above.* **10** *The scribe neglected to introduce a new chapter here. 2-line initial in blue.*

f. 285v of þe vrin. Eiþirwhilis, it comeþ of a colde fleumatike humour þat makiþ þe senewis laxe þat ben aboute þe necke of þe bladdir. And þan þe vrin is discolourid and þicke, and litil in quantite. And þe wei of þe

5 vrin into þe bladdir is y-stoppid, eiþirwhilis with a stoon eiþirwhilis with a postem, and eiþirwhilis with blood þat is gloderid togedir. And þan it is y-helid bi þe same medicines þat þe stoon is, and as þe postem of þe reines. Eiþirwhilis þat wei

10 is al-togedir y-stoppid and eiþirwhilis but sumdel. Whan þis sekenes comeþ of a postem, it is y-knowe bi þe tokenes of þe postem of þe reines, saf þat þis greuaunce is aboute þe shar, as þe oþir of þe reynes is bihindeforþe. And þe same medicines þat

f. 286 15 helen þe oon postem, he/liþ þe toþir. If it comeþ
[274v] of þe stoon eiþir of grauel, þou mai knowe it bi þe tokenes þat ben y-told herbifore. And þat is y-holpe bi þe same medicines þat þe stoon is. And if it comeþ of humours þat stoppen þe wei of þe vrin, it is y-knowe bi

20 þicke gobetis þat is among þe vrin. And it is y-helid in þe same wise þat þe stoon is. If stranguri comeþ of hete, let him blede vndir þe ancle. And ȝyue him þe electuari of þe iuse of roses. And siþ baþe him in a baþ of cold erbis. And ȝiue him eueri day in þe morevtid and at euen

---

1 fleumatike] *corr. from* fleumeatike. **2 senewis**] sekenes; *Add 30338* sekenes; *L:* nervos. **3 discolourid**] *corr. from* discolorid. **5 y-stoppid**] *corr. from* stoppid. **10 is**] *ins. above.* **20 þicke**] þilke.

sugir violet, eiþir diapenidion, eiþir dia[dra]gagantum þat
is cold.   And let him drinke watir þat hertistong eiþir
endiue is soden yn.   And let him vse þe sirip þat is y-

f. 286v   tolde in þe hete of þe liuer.   And anoynt / him with oile

5   of roses eiþir of violet y-medlid with vinegre.   And make
him a cold plastir as is y-told in þe hete of þe lyuer and
of þe reines.   But if þe greuaunce come of cold, 3iue him
oximel duretike.   And siþ make him a stufe of hoot erbis.
And whan he comeþ oute of þe baþ, 3iue him triacle with þe

10   iuse of myntis, eiþir wyne þat castor is soden in.   And þe
nexte dai aftir, let him blede vndir þe ancle.   Contra

[?]   stranguriam: Take iii grana vel quatuor de palma Christi et
potatur cum aqua tepida, et statim minget, et est verum.   A

[275]   gode sirip for þis sikenes: Take þe rote of berdane, mynt,
A sirip for
þis   **15**   piony.   And stampe hem a litil, and seþe hem in watir.   Þen
sikenes   clense it and put þerto as moche honi as nediþ.   And let
him vse þis sirip.   And vndirstonde þat þou shalt not do in

f. 287   her / medicines neiþir euforbe ne scamony, but if þou be
aboute to make him pisse.   And if her greuaunce com of

20   feblenes, and þei ben vnmi3ti to pisse, make hem a baþ.   And
3iue hem triacle, and anoynte þe necke of þe bladdir with
hote oynementis and oilis.   But if þer ben cold viscouse
humours in þe bladdir, 3iue hem þe medicines þat ben y-told
for þe stoon.

---

1 diadragagantum] diagragantum.   **6 is]** it.   **7 reines]** veines.

An oynement for þis sikenes: Take encense, mastike, euforbie, and þe rote of berdane.   And stampe hem with grece of a cat eiþir of a gandir.   And roste þe cat and þe gandir and kepe þe fatnes þat dropiþ fro hem.   And medle it
5 with rede wexe and þerwith anoynt þe shere.   Þe grece of a foxe y-vsid in þe fourme of an oynement is good for þis

f. 287v   sikenes and for colde goutis. / Eiþirwhilis þer falliþ into þe bladdir grete plente of vrin þat streineþ þe bladdir and
[275]   strangeliþ hir þat þer mai noon vrin passen oute of þe
10 bladdir.   And þis is a grete greuance, and it falliþ eiþirwhilis in men þat semen al hool, eiþirwhilis in men þat han þe feueris.   If it fal in a feuer, let him be baþid vp to þe nauel in watir þat peritori is soden yn, and he shal pisse swyþe; eiþir in watir þat wormod is soden yn, and
15 plastre þe erbe on his shere. And þe same vertu haþ louage, for she makiþ to pisse anoon.   Also for hem þat han þis greuaunce and semen hool, make a plastre of louage and peritorie and y-soden in watir.   And with þat watir, medle

f. 288   whete bran and make þerof a plastir, and ley / to his shere.
20 Eiþir seeþ marche and louage in watir.   And wiþ þat watir medle whete bran and make þerof a plastir, and ley to þe share. And þat is good for þe stoon also.

Chapter XVII, Part 2
Pissing of Blood

Pissing of blode comeþ from withoutenforþ, as of
[276]   leping, of falling, of strokis, of trauel, eiþir of cold

---

9 þat] *ins. above.* **18 and]** *ins. above.* **23 2-line initial in blue.*

eyr. Eiþirwhilis, it comeþ fro withynforþ, as of þe lyuer, of þe spleen, of þe reines, of þe lendis, eiþir of þe bladdir.   Eiþirwhilis, it comeþ of grete plente of blood, and þat is y-knowe bi þe fulnes of a man-is veines.

5   Eiþirwhilis, it comeþ of keneship of þe blood.   And þe token þerof is pricking and hete in þe 3erde and aboute þe 3erde whan a man pissiþ.   Eiþirwhilis, it is for þinship of

f. 288v   þe blode þat makiþ it to swete oute of / þe veines. And þan þe blode is ful þin þat is y-medlid with þe vrin.   And þe

10   helping of þes þre maneris is by medicines, as it is y-told in þe nose-bleding, and in spetting of blode, and in þe blodi fluxe.   Whan it comeþ from þe lyuer, it comeþ in grete quantite, and is clene blode.   And þei han greuaunce vndir þe ri3t side.   And first þe vrin comeþ oute and siþ

15   þe blode.   Whan it comeþ from þe spleen, þei felen heuynes and greuaunce vndir þe lifte side.   And þe blode is litil in quantite, and trobelid and malencolious.   From þe reines comeþ blode withouten grete greuaunce.   And it is litil in

[276v]   quantite but is clere and y-medlid with þe vrin.   And þei

20   felen pricking aboute her reines.   Whan it comeþ oute of þe

f. 289   bladdir, / þei han greuaunce in þe shere and byneþe.   And þe blode comeþ first oute and siþ þe vrin, and þe blode is blac.   And if þei pissen blode and quiter togedir, it is a token þat þe bladdir is scabbid and haþ pymplis in hir, and nameli if it stinkiþ. But if þe blode comeþ from ony oþir veines, it is y-gloderid togedir alonge of þe shap of a watir leche, and so it comeþ oute with þe urin. And eiþirwhilis, it is so grete þat it stoppiþ þe wey of þe

5 vrin, and makiþ a man to haue strangury, and bringiþ a man to deþe. Eiþirwhilis, þer ben woundis aboute þe reines. And þan a man feliþ ache þer whan he pissiþ. And þe vrin is eiþirwhilis blodi, eiþirwhilis y-medlid with quitere.

f. 289v Eiþir/whilis, þer ben smale bodies in þe vrin yliche þredis.

10 And eiþirwhilis þei han ycching aboute her ers. If þis comeþ of grete blode, let him absteine him from metis þat gendren moche blode, and vse metis þat maken litil blode, as fruites and erbis. And if þe blood comeþ from þe liuer, let him blede in þe ri3t arme, and from þe spleen in þe lift

15 arme, and from þe reines vndir þe ancle in þe vttir side; and if it comeþ of þe bladdir, in þe neer side undir þe ancle. If it comeþ of keneship of þe blode, purge him of

[277] coler with þe electuarie of þe iuse of roses. And 3iue him siþ colde electuaries and siripis, as it is y-told in þe

f. 290 20 spetting of blode and in dissinterie. But in purga/cions, 3iue him neiþir aloes, neiþir scamone, ne euforbe. Aftir hir purgacion, 3iue him suche þingis þat wolen staunche þe bleding, as diacodion and sugir of roses, as moche as a chesteyn at oon tyme. And siþ 3iue him þis sirip: Take

16 þe neer] *corr. from* eiþir. **23 diacodion**] *corr. from* diaconidion.

roses, bole, and louage seed, encense, mastike, planteyn, mynt. And seþe hem in reyne watir and caste sugir þerto. And þeras he feliþ ache, anoynte it wiþ oile of roses and with þe white of eiren. And ley a plastir þeron of encense,

5 mastike, mummie, sandragon, and bole, and of planteyn. Stampe hem togedir with þe gleir of eiren. And if it be nede, make him a stufe of pentafilon, and planteyn, and of suche oþer erbis. And let him sitte þerin vp to þe nauel.

f. 290v And let him frote wel from þe / nauel to his ȝerde. And let

10 him vse þat oftesiþes. A baþ for þe same: Take louage leues, and bedegar, ribwort, comferi, daiesi, and planteyn

[277v] boþe þe more and þe lasse, and ypericon, and auence, and fenel, parseli, verueyn, columbine, and camomil. Take of eueriche of þes iliche moche, and seþe hem in

15 cleen watir. A good plastir to ley on a mannes reines and

[278] on his shere in þis sikenes: Take of roses, oz. i; of mastik, dr. iii; of bole, of white sandris, oz. 1/2; þe ȝolkis of fyue eiren; of oile of roses, dr. ii. Medle al þes with þe iuse of planteyn, comferi,

20 daiesi, fenel, parsili, columbine, verueyn, ribwort, camomil, and auence, of eueriche of þes, take yliche moche iuse; and of barliche mele, halfe a pounde, and medle al togedir. /

Chapter XVII, Part 3
Diabetes

f. 291 Diabites is an vnmesurable pissing of vrin þat comeþ of

---

14 hem] *ins. above.* **24** *2-line initial in blue.*

grete drienes of þe reynes, for whan þe reines ben ful drie,
þei soken moche moistnes of þe veynes þat comen from þe
lyuer, and þe lyuer moche of þe guttis, and þe guttis moche
of þe stomake and of þat þat is in him-silfen. And þat
5 moistnes whan it comeþ to þe reines and fyndeþ þe wei large,

[278v] passiþ swiftli to þe bladdir, and so passiþ forþe as it
comeþ. Enchesons of þis sikenes ben greet trauel, to moche
medling with wymen, chaccing of grete hete in a man-is bodi,
eiþir anoynting aboute þe reines with to hote oynementis,
10 eiþir of a long feuer, it mai come. And eiþirwhilis þis is
a simple distempring, and eiþirwhilis it is a distempering

f. 291v þat comeþ / of sum humour þat greueþ þe reines. And if it
is so, þer is ache, and heuynes, and pricking, and gnawing
aboute þe reines. And he haþ a continuel þirste and a grete
15 appetit to pisse aftir þat he haþ y-dronke. But suche
appetit comeþ eiþirwhilis of miche drinking of sotil wyne
þat persiþ þoroughe þe veines and comeþ sone into þe
bladdir. Eiþirwhilis it comeþ of drinking of stronge wyne
þat þe lyuer may not wel defie for feblenes. Eiþirwhilis
20 moche pissing comeþ of coldenes of þe lyuer þat mai not
defie þe moistnes þat is in him, and so it falliþ doun to
þe bladdir. But þes maners of vnmesurable pissing ben not
diabites ne diampnes, for þei ben neiþir of þe feblenes of

f. 292 þe reines / ne of þe bladdir; for whan þei ben distemprid,

22 **bladdir**] *corr. from* bladir.

a man shal pisse oftsiþes and litil at o tyme. Forto helpe
a man of þis greuaunce, first abate þe grete hete of þe
reyens. And if þe distempering be of hete of sum humour,

[279]   3iue him oximel to defie þe humours. And siþ 3iue him þe

5   electuari of þe iuse of rosis to purge him of þe humour,
eiþir diaprunis and sugir roset y-medlid togeder of þe
quantite of a chestein. Eiþirellis purge him with sum
colog[og]e, and þe þrid day aftir make him a baþ vp to þe
nauel of watir þat rosis, and plantein, letuse, purslane,

10   syngrene, pimpernel, violettis, ribbewort, ben y-soden yn,
eiþir suche oþir cold erbis. And let þe pacient rub wel
þat place þat greueþ him, þat þe vertu of þe erbis moun þe

f. 292v   raþir / perse þorou3 þe pores of þe skyn. And þe nexte dai
aftir, let him blede vndir þe ancle withoutforþe. And

15   aftirward 3iue him medicines as diaprunis and sugir roset,

Hou hony   as Y seide erwhil. Whan þou makist an electuari with hony,
shal be
purid   pure þe hony with watir þat plumbis or violettis ben y-soden
yn, if it be for an hoot cause. If it be for a colde cause,
take hote erbis in werking. And aftir þe foreseide

20   electuaries, 3iue þe siripis þat ben y-told in dissinterie.
And anoynt þe reines with oil of roses, eiþir of violet,
eiþir of mandrake, or watir-lilies. And take þe iii kindis
of sandris, and spodie, and poudre hem; and take as moche
of barli mele, and medle al þicke with þe iuse of solatre

---

6 togeder] *corr. from* togederis. **8 cologoge]** cologe. **15
3iue him]** *in l. h. margin.* **18 hoot]** *corr. from* cold. **22 iii]** iiii.

eiþir syngreen, and purslane, and plastre it vppon þe
reines. But þou shalt vndirstonde þou shalt not legge
euermore moist medicines to þe reines, for þei wold make þe
f. 293   rey/nes ful neisshe and feble, ne þou shalt not euermore vse
5   dry medicines, but eiþirwhilis oon and eiþirwhilis anoþir.
And let him vse þis poudir in his metis: Take þe sede of
hockis, and letuse, and purslane, and of plantein, of
eueriche, iliche moche. And poudir hem and medle þerwith as
moche of gum arabike and of dragagant as of al þes oþer.
10   And cast þerto sugir, quantum sufficit. Let him vse at oon
tyme of þis poudir as miche as he may take with his two
fingris and his þombe at ones. And let him be war of al
kene metis þat wolen make him þurstful. And his dieting
shal be of cold sotil metis. And let him drinke white wyne
15   y-medlid with watir, and let him be war of moche drinking.
And eueri monþe let him be purgid as Y haue seid bifore. If
[279v]   so is þat þe blode wole stop þe wey of þe vrin and make him
to haue a stranguri, þan make a plastir of rewe and comyn y-
soden in wyne and in oile and ley on þe shere. But if þis
f. 293v 20   sikenis / comeþ of cold aboute þe reines, ȝiue him pocions
of hote medicines þat ben confortatif and strictorie, as is
mynte and oþer þat ben y-tolde in dissinteri. And make a
plastir of þe same and ley vppon his reines. But first
purge him of þe humour þat is cause of þe sikenes, and

16-19 **If so . . . þe shere.**] *in bottom margin.* **22 mynte**] *ins. above.*

diete him wiþ temperat hote metis.   And eueri monþe, let him be purgid as it is seide bifore.   And let him be war of polipody, for þat openeþ þe veines and makiþ þe blode ren oute.

Chapter XVII, Part 4
Urinary Incontinence

5   Diampnes is an vnskilful passing of vrin þat comeþ of defaute of þe bladdir.   And þat may be in two maneris: eiþir of coler þat is in þe bladdir, and prickiþ þe bladdir, and makiþ þe vrin dropen oute ri3t as it comeþ to þe bladdir.   And þis coler is y-medlid with þe vrin and makiþ

10   þe vrin kene and biting.   Eiþirwhilis, þis sikenes comeþ of cold þat febleþ þe senewis of þe bladdir and makiþ þe

f. 294   bladdir fallen into a palasie.   And þis / falliþ comenli to hem þat goon barfote and goon a-cold on her bodies in colde wedir.   3it when þei pissen, þei perseiuen it, and han

15   grete greuaunce in pissing.   Eiþirwhilis, þe senewis and þe lacertis ben so laxe þat ben in þe necke of þe bladdir, þat þei moun not withholde þe vrin, and þan passiþ þe vrin awei fro hem þat þei felen it not, as it hapneþ in children and in drunken men þat bipissen her bed.   And þis comeþ

20   eiþirwhilis of humours þat ben in þe senewis of þe necke of þe bladdir, for þre humours þer ben wonte to be in þe bladdir þat greueþ hir: fleume, malencoli, and coler. Tokenes of fleume ben, þe vrin is of a feble colour and ful of musculagis and of smale þinne scales, and þei han

---

1-4 And eueri ... ren oute.] *in bottom margin.*   **5** *2-line initial in* *blue.*   **14 þei perseiuen it]** *in r. h. margin.*   **19 þis]** *ins. above.*

f. 294v greuaunce in pissing, and pis/sen dropmel. And þat is if
þe fleume be viscous and þicke. But if it be þin, þe
senewis drinken it vp, and þat makiþ hem laxe and slideri.
And þan þe vrin passiþ oute without greuaunce. Tokenes

5 of malencoli ben, þe vrin is swart 3elew and ful of þin
scalis. And þei han grete greuaunce whan þei pissen, and
aboute her ers-hole þei han no feling. Tokenes of coler
ben, þe vrin is of an hi3 coloure and þinne, eiþir þick of
coler þat is medlid þerwith. And þei han pricking and a

10 kene ache in þe bladdir, and pricking in þe 3erde whan þei
pissen. And þei han a grete hete aboute her ers-hole.

[280] Diampnes þat comeþ of hote colerik pisse is y-helid as
diabites þat comeþ of hete. And make him þis confeccion
þat is good for hem þat pissen hote kene pisse: Take of

f. 295 15 dragagant, of gum / arabike, of purslane, sede of gourdis,
of letuse, dr. iii. Make poudir herof and let him drinke
it with þe sirip of rosis. But if þis sikenes comeþ of
cold and of moistnes, 3iue him þe medicines þat ben y-told
in dissinterie, boþe in siripis, and in electuaries, and

20 plastirs, and oynementis, and baþes, for þe medicines þat
staunchiþ þe flux of þe wombe, staunchiþ also fluxes of þe
bladdir and of þe emeroidis. But if þis comeþ of humours
þat ben in þe bladdir, if þe humours ben hote, 3iue him
oximel to defie þe humours. And siþ purge him with a

cologoge, eiþir with þe electuari of þe iuse of roses.   But
if þe humours ben colde, purge him with a fleumag[og]e
eiþir with a malag[og]e.   And þe þrid dai aftir, make him a
baþ eiþir a stufe of hoot erbis.   And whan he comeþ out

f. 295v   5   þerof, 3iue him triacle with þe iuse of mynt eiþir / with
wyne y-soden in rewe or castore.   And let him   vse þis xv
daies.   Be war þat þou 3eue not yong men triacle.   Also
ackernes y-soden and y-eten ben gode, and þe watir þerof y-
drunke.   A gode plastir þerfor is y-made of triacle,   and of

10   oile, and of piliol y-medlid togedir.   And þes medicines
ben gode for hem þat bipissen her bed and for þe palesi of
þe bladdir.   And let him þat haþ þis sikenes of cold kepe
al his limes and his body from taking of colde. And anoynt
þe shar and þe places þat ben ny3 aboute with hote

15   oynementis as marciaton, and arrogon, and wiþ hote oilis.
And in eueri cold palesi of þe bladdir, make him a baþ þat
is ordeined for men þat han þe palesie.   And 3yue triacle.
And make a plastir of calamynt, and betein, and of comyn,
and of baies of lorer y-beten to poudir, and of oile of

f. 296   lorer y-medelid togedir, and al warme ley þe / plastre on
his share, and anoþir bitwene his ers-hole and his 3erde.
But old men ben incurable of þis sikenes.

Chapter XVII, Part 5
The Siphac

[280v]   Siphac is a skyn þat is bitwene þe guttis of a man and
his vttir skyn.   And þis skyn is eiþirwhilis y-made slacke

---

2 **fleumagoge**] fleumage.   **3 malagoge**] malage.   **9 plastir**] *in l. h.
margin.*   **12 haþ þis**] *ins. above.*   **16-17 And in . . . 3yue triacle**] *in bottom margin.*   **19 of lorer**] and of lorer.   **23** *This section should perhaps
begin a new chapter. 2-line initial in blue.*

þorou3 humours and moistenes, ri3t as leþir wole reche þat
is y-wet in watir.   And whan þe siphac is so slac þorou3
þirsting of the guttis, þer is swelling in þe side of þe
sher bisidis þe þi3, eiþir in sum oþir place of þe wombe of
þe shap of an ey.   And þe same maner swelling comeþ of
wynde.   But þe slacnes is y-know bi þe moistnes of al þe
bodi and of þe neisship of þe wombe.   Wyndnes is y-knowe bi
moche hurling and noise of wynd in þe guttis.   And in þe
tyme þat it be deliuered of suche wynd, þe swelling is
moche seen.   Eiþirwhi/lis, þat skyn is broken, so þat þe
guttis fallen doun into a man-is cod and makiþ him seme
broke-ballokid.   And þis breche is eiþirwhilis more and
eiþirwhilis lesse.   And þis breke comeþ eiþirwhilis of
falling, and eiþirwhilis of leping eiþir of bering of grete
birþens, eiþir of grete crieng of a man, eiþir of moche
weping on children, eiþir of a grete forsing þat a man
forsiþ him to shite.   And þer is a grete difference bitwene
þis and him þat is broke-ballokid, for he þat is broke-
ballokid haþ ache and greuaunce in his cod and in his
stones, but þes han swelling in þe neþir parti of þe shar
and greuaunce also.   And þe swelling is in þe cod and not
in þe stones.   This sekenes is y-helid bi putting yn of þe
gut þat is y-fallen into þe cod, and siþ bi souding of þe
ciphac bi medicines þat ben consolidatif.   Þis / is to

f. 296v 10

f. 297

5

15

20

---

8 in (2)] *corr. from* til. **22 y-helid**] *corr. from* helid.

vndirstonde if þe breche be new, for þat þat is olde may
not be holpe without kutting.   For in slacnes of þe ciphac,
behold of what humour it is bi þe tokenes þat ben y-told
bifore, and purge him of þat humour.   And if it comeþ of

5   wyndnes, 3iue him suche medicines as consumen wyndis, as it
is y-told in collica passio.   But if þe ciphac be to-broke
and þe guttis fallen doun into þe cod, let him lye vp-ri3t
and lift vp his þies, and putte in a3en þe guttis into his
wombe.   And siþ make þis plastir and ley þerto: Take

10   comferi, and sandragon, and mummie, and ypoquistodos, and
an hare-is skyn y-soden wiþ þe heris and man-is blood.   And
medle þes togedir and ley hem þeras þe breche is.   Eiþir
make a plastir of bole, and sandragon, and mummie, and
sumac, and of gum arabike, and of galles, and a litil

f. 297v 15   mastike.   Poudir al þes / and medle hem with þe gleir of
eiren.   And lei it on a pece of leþer and ley to þe sore,
and þeron ley a pece of lede and bynde it vp.   And let it
lye þer fourti dayes, for bi þat tyme it wole ben y-soudid.
And let him be war of al maner meuing, and fro trauel, and

20   fro snesyng, and wraþ, and cou3ing, and fro enforsing to
shiting.   And wheþir þe breche be vndir þe nauel eiþir in
þe side eiþir vndir þe share, ley þer þe plastir.   And whan
he goiþ to priuy, let him hold þat place fast with his hond,
lest þe gut fal oute þerat.   And diete him with suche metis

---

4 **him**] *ins. above.* 5 **him**] *in r. h. margin.* 6 **ciphac**] *prec. by* is fal
canc. in red. **be**] *followed by* s *canc. in red.* 8 **in**] *ins. above.* 11 **þe**]
ins. above. 19 **al**] *ins. above.*

þat wolen make him neisshe-wombid. And if his wombe be
harde, make him a ·clisterie mollificatif. And let him ete
aftir mete þe seed of fenel, of parseli, anise, and of

f. 298   marche to consume þe wyndis þat / wolen let þe souding.

5   Eiþirwhilis let him vse moist medicines, but noon erbis but
it be parseli eiþir auence. And bren columbine and þe
floure of calamynt and let him vse þe poudir þerof in his
metis. And eueri dai, anoynt þe place with þis oynement

[281]   þat is þus y-made: Take gotis talowe and melt it. And

10   medle þerwiþ þe iuse of þes erbis: comferi, daiesi,
plantein, oxi3e, pentafilon, ribwort, of eueriche of þes,
yliche moche iuse and of rede vinegre. And medle hem wel
togedir. And siþ cast þerto þe poudir of gallis, and þe
blosme of hockis, and of rindis of ackernes, and of

15   chesteines, and of bole, and of sangdragon, of mastik, of
nitre, mummie, of eueriche of þes iliche moche. And cast
oil of roses þerto, and medle hem togedir. And herwiþ
anoynt þe sore place. But waisshe it first with watir
þat strictorie erbis ben soden yn, but let þe watir be

20   ny3 cold. And aftirward lei þis plastir þeron: Take of

f. 298v   ypoquistidos, / acacia, mummie, bole, gallis, psidie,
comferi, daies-i3e, colofonie, picch, mastik, encense,
carseed, and cardamomum, ana, oz. 1/2. Medle hem with
gotis talowe and vinegre on þe fier. And do of þis plastir

6-8 And bren . . . his metis.] *in r. h. margin.* **8 eueri]** *prec. by* if
canc. *in red.* **12 rede vinegre]** *marked for reversal.* **18 waisshe]** *corr.*
from wasshe.

in a pece of leed y-made sumwhat holowe, and ley to þe
sore.   The best plastir is, to þis breche, to take of
amoniac, of galbanum, turmentil, mastik, gallis, litarge,
gipsum, bdellium, turmentine, mirre, olibanum, emachites,
aloes, serapinum, aristologie þe long and þe rounde,
colofonie, picch, bole, sandragon, comferi, daisi3e,
balaustie, spodie, acacie, mummie, of þe rinde of þorne and
of a sloo tre, ana, oz. iii; of gotis talowe and mannis
blode, ana, a pounde.   And make it on þis wise: Take a
newe weþires skyn, and / shaue of þe wol, and kit þe skyn to
smale pecis, and seþe hem in watir til þei ben tendir þat
þou mow esili put þi fingir þorou3 hem.   Þan wringe oute
clene þe watir and þerwith medle þi blode and þi talowe.
And cast þerto a quarte of vinegre, and as moche of þe
iuse of planteyn, and a pounde of wex.   And medle hem wel
togider, and siþ poudre al þin oþir þingis and cast hem
þerto, and medle hem wel togederis.   Of þis plastir ley to
þe sore aftir þat a man is purgid and haþ baþid him.   And
make him an electuari of honi, sandragon, mummie, acacie,
comferi, daiesi3e.   And let him vse þis electuari daili vii
wokes.   And xl daies, let him lye stil and vse þis plastir.
And if he be costif, help him with a clisterie mollificatif.
And eueri day, let him drinke in ale or wiyn þe poudir of
aristologie boþe þe longe and þe rounde, and of galles, and
of planteyn, of eueriche iliche moche.   Also for breche þat

f. 299

5

10

15

20

[281v]

Electuari
for þis
sekenes

[?]

23-25 **And eueri . . . iliche moche**] *in bottom margin.*

f. 299v

falliþ in a man-is brest eiþir in þe stomake, make / him
cakes of barli meel and of 3olkis of eyren. And make

A poudir
for þis
sikenes

[281v]

poudir of sauge, of mummie, of comferi, of canel, of þe
rinde of an aisshe, of aristologie boþe þe long and þe

5 rounde, of gallis, of planteyn, of eueriche, yliche moche.
And 3iue him to drinke in warme ale, in þe moretid and at

[?]

euentide a sponeful or half a sponful at ones. Anoþir good
poudir for him þat is broke: Take an vnce of þe shalis of
baies and an vnce of þe rote of turmentil, and of licoris,

Anoþir
povdir for
þis sikenes

10 iii vncis. And bet al into poudir, and 3iue to þe sike of
þis poudir half a sponeful at ones with warme ale þries
a day, nyne daies continueli. And see þat he be wel
trussid. And if þe breche or þe pacient be olde, let him
vse it þe lengir, and he shal be hole by þe grace of God.

Chapter XVIII, The Penis
Part 1, Satyriasis

[?]   15

Here beginneþ þe xviii chaptir þat conteineþ
iiii° titlis or practi[s]es. /

f. 300

In a mannes 3erde þer ben diuerse greuaunces:
to moche stonding þat is clepid satiriasis, and flowing of

[286v]

a man-is seed a3enst his wille, and pymples, and swelling,

20 and cancre. Satiriasis comeþ of a greet boistrois hoot
wynde þat falliþ doune into a man-is stones and into his
3erde and makiþ þe 3erde to arise. And þis comeþ of no
fleissheli desire, ne of no leking þat a man haþ þerto, but
wiþ ache, greuaunce, and swelling. And first þou shalt

4 aisshe] *corr. from* asshe. **9 baies]** *followed by* and al þe kernel
canc. in red. **12 daies]** *ins. above.* **15 xviii]** *corr. from* xviiii. **16 prac-
tises]** practies. **17** *3-line initial in gold.* **21 stones]** *prec. by* 3erde
canc. in red. **his]** *ins. above.* **24 wiþ]** *ins. above.*

3yue him repercussiues, boþe in oynementis and in plastris,
to smyte a3en þat wyndi mater, boþe aboute þe 3erde, and on
þe sher, and on þe reines. Anoynt þe 3erde, and þe
stones, and þe shar, and þe reines with oile of henbane and
5 oile of mandrake. And let þat membre be waisshid with cold

f. 300v watir or ny3 cold, þat / saleyn leues ben y-soden yn, and
let þe 3erde soke wel þerin. Camphore also is good, boþe
to smel to, and to drinke, and to bere in his hond. And
let him drinke þe sirip of watir-lilies. And strawe his
10 house with cold flouris, and with cold erbis, and þe leues
of cold trees. And make him wake moche, and fast moche,
and wel-akelen hem. And make a plastir of cold erbis
and of vinegre, eiþir of opium and cold erbis. Eiþir
take repercussiues þat shulen be told in swelling of
15 þe stones. And 3iue him diaprunis and diacalamentum
y-medlid togedir. Eiþir-ellis, seeþ rwe or þe iuse in
wyne eiþir comyn, and let him drinke þerof. And let him
ete þe sede of agnus castus and make a plastir of þe leves.

Chapter XVIII, Part 2
Gonorrhea

Gomorra, þat is flowing of a man-is sede a3enis
f. 301 20 his wil, and þis / is of plente of blood, eiþir of palesie
of þe stones, eiþir of grete feblenes of a man þat mai not
withholden his sede, eiþir it comeþ for þe sede is þinne
and flowiþ oute li3tli. And if it comeþ of plente of blode,
þe veynes ouer al a man-is bodi ben ful of blode and to-

---

6 **leues**] *ins. above.* 16 **or þe iuse**] *ins. above.* 17 **comyn**] *prec. by*
in *canc. in red.* 18 **þe** (2)] *ins. above.* 19 *2-line initial in blue.* 23 **it**]
ins. above.

swolowe. And þei han liking whan þe seed passiþ awey fro
hem.   If it comeþ of palesi of þe stones, þei felen not
when her seed passid from hem, as men þat han þe palesi
of þe bladdir felen not when her vrin passiþ fro hem.

5   If it comeþ of feblenes, al þe bodi is feble, and lene,
and of yuel coloure. If it comeþ of þinneship of þe sede,
it wole telle himsilf, and þe complexion of þe man, and
his dieting.   When it comeþ of blood, let him oftesiþis
let blood vndir þe inner ancle, eiþir on þe liuer veine

f. 301v 10   of þe arme. And a/noynte his reines with cold oynementis.
And diete him with suche metis þat gendren litil blood.
Whan he comeþ of palesi of þe stones, 3iue him medicines
þat ben y-told in þe palesi of þe bladdir.   Whan it comeþ
of feblenes, take encense, and mastike, and myntis, and

15   sandris, and storace, in grettir quantite þen of þe oþer,
and medle hem with þe iuse of planteyn and with vinegre.
And make a plastir þerof, and ley vppon his reines, and
aboute his 3erde, and his stones.   And 3iue him oþir
medicines as it ys y-told in diabites. And 3iue him

20   medicines þat ben confortatif and strictories, as diacodion,
[287]   and sugir roset, and þe sirip of roses, for þes quenchen
mi3tili þat appetit þat a man haþ to lecheri. And for þis
sikenes, þou shalt worche with colde medicines as þou
dedist in satiriasis.   Whan it comeþ of þinneship, 3iue him

---

6 þinneship] *corr. from* þinshynnes. **24 3iue him]** *ins. above.*

f. 302   a sirip y-made / of þe iuse of myntis and of sugir. And with þe iuse of myntis anoynt his 3erde and his stones. And diete him with metis þat wolen make þe blode þicke, as white brede, and riys, and 3olkis of eyren, and suche oþer.

Chapter XVIII, Part 3
Pimples and Apostems

5   Pimples and postems ben also in a man-is 3erde. And if þei be not wel y-helid, þei turnen into a canker, eiþir into a festre þat is holowe as a whistil eiþir a pipe. And siche postemes ben eiþirwhilis y-hid withyn þe 3erd, and eiþirwhilis withoute; and eiþirwhilis þei comen of hete, and

10 þan, þeras þei ben, þer is grete hete, and brenyng, and pricking, and ache, and reednes, and eiþirwhilis swelling. Eiþirwhilis þei comen of colde, and þan þei felen heuines þeraboute, and colde, and in boþe is greuaunce whan þei pissen. For boþe enchesons, let hem blede vndir þe ancle

15 and cup hem on þe veines. And make a plastir of gose grece

f. 302v   and of whete meel, and ley it al warme to þe 3erde, / and oftsiþis renew it. And in boþe enchesons, whan þe postemes ben y-turned to quitere, if þei ben withinforþe, 3iue him medicines þat ben duretike to clense þe 3erde of quitere,

20 lest þer wax a festre in þe 3erde. Eiþirwhilis þe 3erde is to-swolle, and þan it must be baþid in warme watir. Eiþir

[287v]   take þe leues of a white þorne and þe smale tendir branchis and seþe hem in wyne, and þerwith waisshe þe 3erde and let him soke þerin. Eiþir seeþ hockis and peritori in wyne

5 2-line initial in blue.

eiþir in watir and þerwiþ waisshe him. And make a plastir
of comyn and of þe rote of holihocke y-soden and y-stampid
togedir, eiþir of peritory and bran, eiþir of drie benes y-
soden in wyn. And let him blede at þe veine þat serueþ to
5   þe lyuer. And if þe ʒerde be y-cankrid, make þis oynement:
Take a pounde of olde swynes grece and medle þerwith oz.
1/2 of vertegrece. And þerwith anoynt his ʒerde. Eiþir
f. 303   bren salte al to poudir, and þat poudir is / good for þe
canker of þe ʒerd. But waisshe þe ʒerd first with vryn
10   eiþir with wyne, but not with watir. And aftir it is wel y-
waisshen, rub it with a cloþe. And þen strawe þeron þe
forseid poudir of salt. Also stampe benes and seeþ hem in
wyn and cast þerto a litil oile and vinegre. And þat is
good þerfore. And if þer be pimples þat wole not breke, let
15   frote hem in hote watir and in sope togedir. And siþ ley on
hem a caul leef, eiþir a lily leef, eiþir þe ʒolke of an ey
and salt. And whan þe quitere brekiþ oute, put þerin þe
poudir of mirre and of aloes, eiþir mastik, eiþir of
pentafilon. And if it soudiþ not togedir as it shuld, medle
20   with þi poudirs þe ʒelev oynement eiþir þe grene þat
surgiens vsen. And þer be þer deed fleisshe, stampe garlike
and ley it on eueriche side þerof, for þat fretiþ awei þe
dede fleisshe and comfortiþ þe good. And whan þe fleisshe
f. 303v   is freten awei, anoynt him with þis oynement: Seþe / benes

and salt togedir, and siþ cast awei þe hollis of þe benes. And medle hem and mastike, and olibanum, and ceruse, and watir of rosis togider, and make an oynement þerof. And þerwith anoynt þe fleisshe, for it wole hele him in two

[?]   5   daies. Forto chaunche kutting or bleding, take bole and salt and medle hem togedir, and ley þeron a litil while. And it wole staunche anoon.

Chapter XVIII, Part 4
Swelling of the Scrotum

[289]   Swelling of þe cod and of þe stones comeþ eiþirwhilis of humours þat fallen doun into þe cod and into þe stones.

10   Eiþirwhilis it comeþ of wynd, eiþirwhilis of a postem, eiþirwhilis of breking of þe inner skyn and of falling doun of þe guttis into þe cod. And if it comeþ of blood, þe veynes of þe bodi be ful of blood, and nameliche þilke þat ben vndir þe ancle. If it comeþ of coler, þe cod is swart

15   rede and brenyng for hete, and þer is greet ache and

f. 304   pricking withinforþ. If it is of fleu/me, þe cod is of a pale coloure, and miche to-swolle, and neisshe, and heuy. If it be of malencoli, þe cod is to-swolle and ful heuy. And if it be of wynd, þe swalme is withouten heuynes. If

20   it be of a postem, it is oon of þe humours and haþ þe same tokenes þat þe oþir swelling haþ, saf þe ache is moche grettir and þe tokenes moche more violent and greuous. Eiþirwhilis þe swelling comeþ of fleisshe þat growiþ in þe cod more þen þer shuld. Whan þis swelling comeþ of humours,

4 hele] *ins. above.* **7 And]** *ins. above.* **8** *2-line initial in blue.* **12 it]** *ins. above.* **24 swelling]** *corr. from* ache.

[289v]

f. 304v

f. 305

of what humour euer it be, let him blede in þe veine þat is vndir þe ancle, and cuppe him aboue þe reines. And siþ make cold plastirs of cold erbis y-soden in vinegre, and ley to þe cod to smyte aȝen þe humours þat ben enchesons of þe

5 swalme. And make a plastir of barly mele, and hennes grece, and oile of violet y-soden togedir and ley þerto. Eiþir make a plastir of henbane and swynes grece y-stampid togedir. Eiþir take þe plastris / þat ben y-told in þe last chaptir, for þe same plastris ben good for postemes of þe

10 cod and of þe stones. Þes medicines and plastris seruen when þe swalme is of hote humours. But if it be of cold humours, make a stufe for þe cod of hote erbis. And siþ anoynt þe cod with hony despumed. And siþ grinde þe piling of garlike and seþe it in watir and plastir it on þe cod.

15 And þat wole drawe oute þe humours bi smoke and by sweting. Eiþir make a plastir of louage y-soden in wyn, eiþir of peritori, eiþir of netlis y-stampid and y-het wel in an erþen pot wel y-stoppid abouen, withouten ony oþir liquor. Eiþir take benes and seþe hem in vinegre and in hony til þei

20 brek. And plastir hem to þe swalme. And if þe man be ful of humours and þe greuaunce be old, if þe swalme comeþ of blode, let him oftsiþes blede vndir / þe ancle. And if it comeþ of ony oþer humour, purge him with a medicin þat acordiþ þerto. And let him be oftsiþes cuppid aboue þe

---

2 reines] veines; *L:* renes. **19 and in hony]** *in l. h. margin.*

278

buttockis.　　And if it be of a posteme, ley þerto þes forseid plastris, first repercussiues to smyte þe mater a3en; and if it wole not, ley þerto dissolutiues, and if þe mater vansissheþ not awei but wexiþ ripe and brekiþ.

5　If þe postem is withoute þe cod, hele it vp as oþer postemes ben y-helid.　And if þe postem be withinne þe cod, 3iue him electuaries and siripis þat ben told herbefore to clense þe cod of quitere, if it wole not be clensid withoute.　And if þe postem wexiþ within, þou must slit þe

10　cod and let out þe quitere.　And siþ hele vp þe wound.　But if þe cod be to-swolle of brusing, make a plastir of oile, and turmentine, and of barli mele and ley þerto.　And if

[290]　þe brusing is olde, make a plastir of benes, and of comyn, and of hony.　Eiþir if þe place is reed, breke benes and

f. 305v　15　seþe hem / in vinegre and ley þerto.　And if þe place is not reed, seþe hem in wyn.

Chapter XIX,
Hemorrhoids

[?]　　　Here beginneþ þe xix chaptir þa conteineþ oo title or practis.

[231]　　　In a mannes ers ben diuerse greuauncis.　Oon is of þe

20　emeroidis.　Oþer þer ben, as figis, and boilis, and cliftes in þe ers.　Emeroidis ben fyue veines þat comen to þe ers to deliuere þe bodi of sori malencoly blode þat wole noye oþir membris.　And eiþirwhilis þes veines bleden to myche, eiþirwhilis þei ben to hard y-stoppid, and eiþirwhilis þei

---

9 wexiþ] wexix. **9-10 þe cod]** *prec. by* þe *canc. in red.* **13 brusing]** *in r. h. margin.* **19** *4-line initial in gold.*

ben to-swolle. And þat swalme is eiþirwhilis withyn, eiþirwhilis without. Swelling of þes veines comeþ eiþirwhilis of drastis of þe blode þat fallen doun to þe veines mouþis and stoppiþ hem, eiþir of þicke blood þat 5 stoppiþ hem, eiþir of þickenes of þe skyn, eiþir for brenyng þat brent hem when þei flowiden to miche. And whan þe blood may not haue / his issu as it shuld haue, it turneþ aȝen to þe lyuer and disposiþ a man to þe dropesi. Stopping and withholding of blode comeþ of þe same enchesons. And 10 eiþirwhilis, þei ben al y-stoppid, and eiþirwhilis sum ben y-stoppid and sum vnstoppid. Moche flowing of þes veines comeþ eiþirwhilis in certeyn tymes, as þe flowing of blode þat comeþ to women ones in a moneþe. Þis flowing comeþ to a man whan he is xl ȝeer olde. And eiþirwhilis þe blood þat 15 renneþ fro a man is reed, and cleer, and hoot in þe flowing. And þes ben þe tokenes of kenesship of þe blode. Eiþirwhilis it is blac and þicke. And þat is a token of malencoly þat is in þe blode. Eiþirwhilis it is þinne and rennyng, and þat is token of sotilte of þe blode. 20 Eiþirwhilis it is ȝelewe, and þat is token of fleume and colere y-medlid togedir. Þes colours of þe blood ben þus y-knowe: Do sum of þe blood on a lynen clooþ and waisshe awei þe blood, / and þe clooþ wole be of such colour as þe blood is. For flowing of þis blode if it comeþ of grete

f. 306

f. 306v

---

6 **whan**] *ins. above.* 7 **haue**] *ins. above.* 9 **comeþ**] *prec. by* cho *canc. in red.* 14 **þat**] þe. 22 **waisshe**] *corr. from* wasshe. 23 **þe** (1)] *ins. above.* 24 **For flowing**] *corr. from* Flowing.

[231v]

plente of blood, let him blede wel at þe lyuer veine at þe
arme.   And if it comeþ of oþer humours, 3iue him a
purgacion.   But 3iue him noon aloes ne oþir medicin þat is
ful openyng, but sum oþir cologoge eiþir fleumagoge.   Siþ

5   make him a baþ as it is y-tolde in dissinterie.   And
aftirward opene þe veine þat is vndir þe vttir ancle.   And
siþ make him suppo[sito]ries and fumigacions as in
dissinterie.   And let him drinke a-morwe and on euen þe iuse
of milfoil y-medlid with warme wyne, and plastir þe erbe

10   to his ers.   Eiþir take an erbe þat is like like and haþ
a white floure and a sauer as garlike.   Stampe it wiþ newe
ale and let him drinke þerof eueriche morevtid.   And make
him a fumigacion of leke and plantein y-soden in wyne.   Lyke
y-eten or y-dronke openeþ þe veines; but if it be emplastrid

f. 307   15   without, he stoppiþ / þe veines.   Also make him a pocion of
white horehoune, and auence, and milfoil, and planteyn y-

[?]   stampid a litil togedir and soden in wyn.   And make him a
poudir to ete of clowes, and femigreke, and canel, and

[231v]   suche oþir comfortable þingis.   An oynement for þe

20   emoroidis: Take þe croppis of ellern and of milbery
tree and stampe hem as þou woldist make sauce of hem.
And siþ tempere hem vp with oile eiþir with 3olkis of
eggis in þe maner of an oynement.   Also take betayn,

[232]   egrimoyn, minte, milfoile, mugwort, plantein, straw-beri

---

4 fleumagoge] *corr. from* fleumage.   **7 suppositories**] suppories.
14 be] *ins. above.*   **22 hem**] *ins. above.*

leues, of eueriche of þes, manipulus i; of pepir, oz. 1/2; of
wyn, quantum sufficit. Seþe þes in wyn and let him drinke
þe wyn ix daies fasting.   Also stampe celidon, and
[231v]   pentafilon, and horehoune, and let him drinke hem with good
5   stale ale.   And medicines þat ben good for dissinterie
and lienterie ben good for þis sikenes.   And let
him absteine him from malencolies metis, ne aforce and
constreyne hem to shite.   And let hem be war of kene /
f. 307v   metis þat wole opene þe endis of þe veynes, and from
10   comyn, and medicines þat ben openyng, as aloes, scamone,
and polipodie, and suche oþer.   For wiþholding of þis blode
and swelling of þe veines, first purge him with sum medicin
[232]   þat is opening, as aloes, eiþir scamone, eiþir with watir
þat polipodi is soden yn.   Siþ make him a baþ of ypericon,
15   and marche, and peritorie, and gorst, and horehoune, and
policarie, and suche oþer erbis y-soden in watir.   Eiþir
make him a purgacion of tyme, and epitime, and sene, and
mirabolani indi, and of lapis lazuli.   Poudir al þes and
let him drinke þe poudir with watir þat borage is soden yn.
20   And siþ let him blede vndir þa ancle in boþe sidis and on
boþe leggis.   And anoon aftir, make him a fumigacion of
comyn salt, and nitre, and of sal gemme, and of piliol,
and of euforbe, and comyn, and of ciler mountein, y-poudrid
and y-soden in wyn in a stoppid vessel.   And let þe fume

---

1 eueriche] *prec. by* þes *canc. in red.* þes] *ins. above.*

f. 308   her-of com þorouȝ a pipe / to þe emeroidis. And þe same dai

let him be cuppid on þe reines. And let him vse

diacalamentum. And eueriche dai in þe morevtid let him

drinke warme wyne þat pepir is soden yn, and on þe euentid

5   also. Eiþir make him a fumigacion of moleyn, and calamynt,

and wormod, and euforbe y-soden in lye and piper þerwiþ.

Eiþir make a plastir of figis, and strawe þe plastir with

poudir of calamynt and of sileris mountein, and ley þerto.

And aboue, ley a lynyn clout y-wet in þe gleir of eiren.

10   And let it lye þerto til it be drie, and þan drawe it

violently awei. Also when þei swellen, wheþir þei aken or

not aken, make a stuf of white wyn þat hote erbis ben

[232v]   soden yn, as wormod, piliol, rwe, sauge, calamynt, and

white horehoune. And let set þer ouer his ers on a stool

15   ful of holes. Eiþir make him a plastir of peritorie y-

stampid a litil and y-fried in his awne iuse. And with þes /

f. 308v   medicines, eiþir þei wolen drye vp eiþir opene. If þe

emeroidis ben to-swol, take þe poudir of bleve cloþe þat is

y-clepid bokerem, y-brent, and of gotis horne y-brent, and

20   psidie y-brent, and springe þe poudir on hem. But let him

first waisshe hem with his avne vrin. Also yonge leke y-

soden and siþ y-stampid with gose grece and leyde to þe

emeroidis wole abate þe swalme of hem. But vndirstonde þat

whan þou shalt staunche þe fluxe of emeroidis, þou muste

4 wyne] *in r. h. margin.*

[233]

[232v]

f. 309

[233]

[?]

[233]

[?]

leue oon or two open, eiþir ellis þe man miȝt fal into a dropesi. Fyges ben white bleynes and neisshe in a man-is ers. And eiþirwhilis þei ben euenlonge, and eiþirwhilis þei ben round. Eiþirwhilis þei ben within þe ers, and

5 eiþirwhilis þei ben without. If þei ben withinforþ, make poudir of alyme and of ooke applen and springe on þe figis. Blacke boilis in þe ers ben incurable as sum men seyn, but if þou wilt bynde hem faste with a selken þrede and / let hem honge til þei fallen awei. Postemes þat ben in a man-is

10 ers ben y-helid with an oynement y-made of oile of roses and of ceruse y-medlid togedir, eiþir of leed y-brent and litarge y-medlid with þe ȝolke of an ey. Brent leed is þus y-made: Melte lede in an erþen vessel and stire it with a grene hasel ȝerde. And it wole turne to blacke

15 poudir. And whoo þat haþ suche postem, aforce he him not to shite. And let him kepe himsilf fro costifnes. And if he be costif, make his wombe neisshe with a mollificatif clisterie. For cleuing of þe ers þat comeþ of hote kene humours, anoynt him with þe oile of roses, eiþir with þe

20 iuse of lily rote, eiþir with freisshe nev bottir, eiþir with þe white of an ey.

Here endiþ þis boke of diuerse sikenessis and of her remedies and of her cures. Deo gracias.

Here folowen medicines þat Y haue ouerpassid for

---

15 he] *ins. above.* **18-19 kene humours]** *marked for reversal.* **21 of]** *ins. above.* **22 sikenessis]** *corr. from* sikessis. **23 her]** *prec. by* his *canc. in red.* **23-24** *A line has been drawn between lines 23 and 24 by a later hand.*

diuerse sekenes.

For þe
morfu

For þe morfu: Take þe floures of lily, of rosmary, and cerfoil, ana (yliche moche of eche). And stille watir of hem. And þerof take a sponeful in þe mornyng.

5 And with þe same watir anoynt þe place withoute þat is infected. For þe colike a proued medicin: Take elena

f. 309v
For þe
colike

campana, bayes, and gynger, / ana, oz. i; and of sugir, thre vncis. And make hem into poudir and ete þerof in þi potage when þou wilte. For þe colike, a good plastir:

For þe
colike

10 Take a quartron of poudir of comyn and xxliiii ȝolkis of eyren, and tempere wel togedir and frye hem. And as hote as þou mai suffre, ley to þe side þat is sore. Then take fenel seed, anise, smalache sede, ana, oz. i. Boyle hem in white wyne and let þe pacient drinke as oft as he wil.

15 Drinke ix daies þre pappis of þe rotis of orpyn y-stampid

For þe
emeroids

A good
plastir
for þe
squinaci

and temperid with good stale ale or wyne, and þou shalt be hool. Þis is provid. Take a gobbet of sorowe dowe, and ii° sponful of þe poudir of comyn, and as moche of oile de olif, and tempere hem wel togedir. Þen frye hem and

20 make a plastir and ley it warm to þe soore. Also make a baþ of hote erbis and of duretike y-soden in watir. And

[264]
A baþ for
þe splene

whan he comeþ oute of þe baþ, anoynt þat place þat is bifore þe spleen with a weþires gal. And ley þer abouen wolle þat is y-shore vnwaisshe and haþ ben y-dried in þe sunne.

10 xxliiii] 34?

f. 310

[226v]

5

A plastir
for þe
colike

10

[?]

Of þe
titil
pissing
of blode

15

f. 310v

20

Aftirward, take hony as it comeþ oute of þe hony-kome and as moche of salt as of hem boþe. And medle þes / togedir. And let him vse of þis confeccion ix daies in waxing of þe mone, on þe moreutid. And let him fast til nown. Take þe iuse of solatre, of hockis, of louage, and vynegre þat hockis, and violet, and anise ben soden yn. And medle þes two togedir. And bete whete in a mortir and medle þerwiþ. Þen seþe it til it be þicke. And þerof make a plastir and ley to his wombe, and it wole cese þe ache. Eiþir seþ þe rote of holihocke and make a plastir þerof. Diete hem and ȝiue hem oþir medicines if it nediþ as it is seide in dissinterie. And with þi medicines, medle eiþir spikenard, eiþir hertistonge, eiþir meidenhere, eiþir þe iiii cold sedis, eiþir dragagant, if þe man be of fleumatike complexion. And if þe spleen be distemperid with hete, put among his oþer medicines lyuerwort, and roses, and violettis, and plumbis, and sandris, boþe þe white and þe rede, and seþe hem in ptisan. / And put þerto oz. i of liquoris. And if þou dredist of drienes of þe breste eiþir of a feuer etike, put to þy medicines gumme arabike and dragagant. And when þe vrin wexiþ cleen, put to þy medicines comferye, and daies-yȝe, and oþir consolidatiues to soude þe veynes þat ben broken. And þus is þe best to doon in al maner siripis þat gumme arabike and gumme

---

4 And] *prec. by* til *canc. in red.*

286

Hou gumme
arabike
and gum
draga[ga]nt
shal be
resoluid

dragagant ben soden yn: To resoluen hem whan þe sirip is colde, for þei wollen moche raþir and bettir be dissoluid in a colde liquore þan in an hote liquor.

To þre þinges God ӡeueþ vertu: to worde, to herbis,
5   and to stonis. Deo gracias.

Commentary

Glossary

Alphabetical List of Plants by Genus

Bibliography

Commentary

1/ In Add 30338 the text begins: "A mon þat woll help men in here sykenesses hym by-houeþ to knowe þe enchesons and þe kyndes of þe sekenesses, þat is to seye, wheþer þey ben hote or colde, oþer drye oþer moyst. And þis ys y-knowe by mony diuerse tokenes, as by þe vryn and by þe pous, by a monnes coloure and by mony diuerse tokenes. And with Goddes grace we wolleþ wryte of summe sykenesses of þe body and of here tokenes and of here cures. And furst we wolleþ by-gynne at þe sykenes of þe hed and furst of þe hede-ache þat may come to a mon þro3 hete oþer colde oþer drynesse oþer moystnosse. And yf hyt comeþ of hete, þese beþ þe tokenesses: hete and redness in þe forhed and a-boute þe yen, and oþerwhyles an hote rewme, red vreyn, and a swyft pous, and luytel slepe, and smoke and hote eyr nuyeþ hym, and hote emplastres, and oþer hote þynges, and he is y-comfortyd with colde þynges, and vnneþes he may suffre ly3t ne bry3tnesse. And yf hit comeþ of colde, he shul fele colde in hys hed, and hys face wol be pale, and hys pous slowe, and hys vryn febelych y-coloured, and he shal slepe muche, and cold þyng nuyeþ hym. And yf hit comeþ of moystnesse, þer beþ mony superfluites, and muche slep ..." (f. 11v).

The Latin begins: "Signa distemperantiarum simplicium. Doloris autem ex simplici distemperentia caloritatis signa sunt calor et rubor in fronte et circa oculos, et aliquando reuma calidum, urina tincta, et pulsus velox, et somnus paucus, et gravatur et leditur a fumo calido, aere, et emplastris, et aliis causis; et iuvatur a frigidis. Et hec adsunt sine gravitate, et ponderositate; lucem et splendorem vix sustinent. Frigiditatis signa sunt

289

frigus sensibile, pallor, et venarum retractus, et minoratio, et aliquando reuma frigidum, et urina discolorata, pulsus tardus, et somnus multus, et gravitur et leditur a frigidis. Signa humiditatis sunt mollicies et superfluitates plurime et hebetudo sensus, et somnus multus ..." (f. 89v). The introductory material found in the Middle English version is not found in the Latin.

1/1   **superfluites.** The Middle English Guy de Chauliac glossed this word as *filþes* (Ogden, *Guy de Chauliac*, p. 57). In this instance, runny nose and eyes are probably what was meant.

1/2   **no grete ache.** Among the four qualities, hot and cold cause pain, moist and dry do not: Bernard Gordon, *Practica seu Lilium medicinae* (Naples, 1480), f. 18v.

1/9   **yuery kombe.** The association of ivory with diseases of the head comes from the belief that elephants "han witte and mynde passynge oþere bestes" (Seymour, p. 1191). The *Secretum secretorum* advised combing the hair so "that fumosities which ascendith fro þe stomake in tyme of slepe by opening of þe poris may depart" (Manzalaoui, *Secretum*, pp. 3-4).

1/ll   **moche waking.** Vigils, thought, the company of women, and bathing, were all thought to be heating: "Isagoge," in *Articella* (Lyons, 1519), ff. 4-4v.

1/14   The recipes for sugar of roses and of violets have been moved forward from a later section of the Latin text, presumably because of their general utility.

2/1   **coler.** Trevisa stated that "þe humoures beþ iclepid þe children of þe elementis, for eueriche of þe humours comeþ of qualite of elementis" (Seymour, p. 147). Here and in many other places, the Middle English text gives an explanation for a term that is not found in L.

2/6   **feuer tercian.** According to *Articella*, "Isagoge," fever is an unnatural heat that proceeds from the heart via the arteries. There were three kinds of fever: *ephimera*, which is described as *in anima*; *ethica*, affecting the solid members of the body; and *putrida*, from the putrefying of the humors. There were four kinds of putrid fevers. *Synocha* was a continual fever caused by blood "burning up" (*comburens*) in the body. *Tertiana* came from rotting choler and occurred every third day (i.e. every other day). A quartan fever was brought on by melancholy and occurred every fourth day (every third day, by modern reckoning): f. 5. The Latin Gilbertus contains a long tract on the various fevers, in which the above doctrine is refined considerably. Because sugar of violets is cold and wet, it would act against choler.

2/13-14 **falling awey of heris.** According to Gilbertus, "capillus est fumus siccus a toto corpore dissolutus per poros capitis exiens ab exteriore aere desiccatus in longum et rotundum productus" (f. 75v). Baldness is caused by "frigiditas intensa constringens et coartans poros ... quare inculcatur . fumus sub cute et suffocatur" (f. 80v). The coldness of this disease would be counteracted by a treatment acting against phlegm.

2/19   **malencolious metis**. Once again, material of general utility has been brought forward from an earlier part of the Latin text the translator has left out.

4/6   **oximel componed**. L: "Oximel compositum sic fit quod dividit, digerit, attenuat, mundificat, vias epatis et splenis aperit. Recipe radicem apii, feni, petrosi, sparagi, brusci, calamenti quod longo usu soluit quartanam, et ypericon, similiter sticados, thimum, camedreos, origanum. Bulliant. Colature mel, addatur circa finem. Addatur capparis, cuscute, epitime, sene, et si fortius volueris facere, addantur xilobalsamum, lapis lazuli, ana dr. ii. Pulveris anacardi, dr. i. Bulliant ad perfectam decoctionem" (f. 48).

4/21   **demegreyn**. L: *emegraneus*. "Who þat haþ þat yuel feliþ in his heed as it were betynge of hamoures and may not suffre noyse, noþir voys, noþir li3t, noþir schinynge" (Seymour, p. 344).

5/20-6/5   This material is not found in other witnesses.

6/11   **postem**. L: *apostema*. An apostem, as Guy explained, comes "from some foule mater, as humoral or reducible to an humour, gadred togedre... . A posteme, a swellynge, a bolnynge, an ingrossacioun, an outsemynge, a lyftynge vp, a growing out ben names as it were signyfieng þe same þing" (Ogden, *Guy de Chauliac*, p. 74).

6/11   **foreparty**. The brain is here seen as divided into three chambers, ventricles, or "principal places." The foremost, according to the Middle English Lanfrank, contained the imagination. The middle part contained the reasoning power. The hindmost part of the brain, harder than the rest, contained the memory, "as a cheste kepiþ tresour": *Lanfrank's Science of Surgery*, ed. Robert von Fleischhacker (1894), EETS 102 (1973), pp. 113-14.

6/24   **difference**. What the difference is between apoplexy and epilepsy is not clear from this explanation. However, Trevisa gave more information: "Epilencia is ny3 of þe kynde of apoplexia, for one is þe place of eiþir. For þe mater of þe whiche þey beþ ibrad is colde and clemy and beþ diuers, in þat apoplexia stoppiþ alle þe chambres of þe brayne wiþ priuacioun and diminucioun of felinge and of meuynge, and epilencia lettiþ but þe principal chambres of þe brayne" (Seymour, p. 353).

7/2   **Scotomye**. The extremely brief treatment of scotomy may be explained by L: "Scothomia et vertigo nomina sinonima sunt" (f. 99).

7/5   **dronken men**. L: "Videns muscas vel corpora nigra ante oculos volitantes ... videtur enim ei quod omnia vertantur in girum" (f. 99).

7/9   **herte lepiþ**. L: "cordis morsus aut saltus."

7/14   **blode**. L: "Ex sanguine cognoscitur per saltum timporum, gravitatem palpebrarum, imaginationem rufam vel rubeam quasi lampadum accensarum, et sanguinis fluxum e naribus et per vrinam intensam et spissam, aut superius spissam et obscuram quasi sanguineam" (f. 99).

7/22-23   **wiþholding of fluxes**. L: "Et ex retentione menstruorum et emorroidarum et aliquo fluxu consueto remisso" (f. 99). Hemorrhoids and the menses were thought to be nature's way of ridding the body of melancholic blood. *Fluxes* is followed in Add 30338 by "þat a man or a womman wos y-wonyd to hafe and on þe efetyd here greuaunce ys muche" (f. 14). Here and in other places, when the Wellcome copyist omitted something from the exemplar, he began again with a new paragraph sign.

8/5-6   **greuaunce, and abhominacion in þe mouþe.** L: "abhominatio et dolor in ore stomachi."

9/7   **A profitable salt**. The Middle English text omits the proper name attached to this preparation: *Sal Marcelli*.

9/9   **akyng of ioyntis**. L: *sciaticis, artheticis, podagricis*.

9/22   **good for þe palesy**. L: *paraliticos curans*.

10/4   **delicat purgacions**. L: *delicatissimas purgationes*.

10/10   **sugir of borage**. L: *dyaboraginimum*.

10/19   **moche waking**. L: "alienationes, vigilie, ira et furia, inquietudo, iacendi inordinatio et proiectio, et erectio subita" (f. 100v).

10/22   **colere**. One of the characteristics of this translation is the careful attention paid to how a disease can be diagnosed according to the signs displayed by the humor causing it. Here, the classic "choleric" symptoms manifest themselves: aggressive behavior, dryness, heating of the spirits causing the heart to leap, pain, swelling, and redness.

11/1   **stering of þe hert**. L: *sincope*.

11/1   **pisse**. Urine could be judged by its textures and colors. Hot diseases were responsible for urine that was judged "rubeam, croceam, auream, citrinam." Cold gave "albam, nigram, plumbeam, lividam." A dry disease yielded thin urine; a wet disease, thick. Whitish urine tokened phlegm; ruddy urine meant blood; reddish-gold, choler; and black or white urine, melancholy: Constantine the African, "De urina," in *Opera* (Basel, 1536), p. 208.

11/3   **tokenes of blood.** L: "Ex sanguine comitatur faciei rubor, flocos et festucas nituntur de pariete extirpare, alienatio est cum minis et opprobriis" (f. 100v).

11/7   **breest.** This is followed in Add 30338 by "oþer in a womman of þe posteme of þat skyn þat a chyld ys y-conceyfed yn" (f. 15), which is canceled from W.

11/8   **grete pouse.** L: "Pulsus est magnus et frequens et velox et spissus." The "Liber Philareti de pulsibus" in *Articella* was widely used as an authority on pulses: "Pulsus est motio cordis et arteriarum qua secundum diastolem et sistolem fit ad infrigidationem caloris innati, et egestionem vel eiectionem fumosarum superfluitatum" (f. 9). Pulse was the primary indicator of fever.

13/16   **flevme is white.** Trevisa explained that "þe brayn is white by kynde for to fonge þe liknes of al colour, ... and haþ but litil of blood, lest he were infecte and ismytted with þe colour þerof; and so al þing þat is apprehendid schulde seme reed" (Seymour, p. 173).

13/24   **dreden.** L: "Timor de re non timenda, cogitatio de re non cogitanda, certificatio rei terribilis et timorose et est sensus rei que non est. Vident enim ante oculos formas terribiles et timorosas et nigras, sicut monachos, homines nigros illos occidentes, demones. Alii surgere celum putant et cadere timent, et deum videndo fatigari, ... sunt medicine desideratissimi et ad medicandum ardentissimi, ut et medicos precentur et preciosiora que habent pollicent, sed medicos ad medicandum venientes non ascultant" (f. 103).

15/11   **fomen.** L: "Si ... spumam per os eiecerint quasi morsibus canis rabidi morsi essent, infra septem dies morientur" (f. 105v).

15/16   **ne he may not slepe.** L: "Dormire non potest et nunquam firmiter dormit."

16/12   **Litargye.** L: "Litargia est passio puppis cerebri oblivionem mentis inducens."

19/22   **slyder.** This is followed in Add 30338 by: "Oþer þow my3t make þy suppositorye of bolles galle, sal gemme, and mose drit y-medled to-gedere. Bot suppositoryes for children shullen be made of lard, or of suger and salt and oyle and vynegre y-soden to-gedere forte hyt be þykke. And þu my3t make suppositoryes for men oþer wymmen of hony y-sode forte hit be þycke. And seþþe cast þerto þe galle of sum beste and namelych of a bole. Whenne þyn hony ys ny3 y-sode y-nowe, oþer cast þer-to sal armoniac oþer sal gemme oþer nitre oþer sal affricanus eiþer euforbe oþer peletre of spayne oþer þe mylk of a fyge tre oþer of tytymalle oþer scamone oþer such oþer þynges. And anoynte þy supposytoryes wyþ oyle" (f. 18v).

20/15   **Epilencie.** L: "Epilempsia est oppilatio principalium ventriculorum cerebri cum diminituione sensus quousque natura se expediat... . Oppilat originem nervorum, et ipsos nervos debilitat" (f. 109).

20/15-21 This section is very similar to Dawson, *A Leechbook*, p. 134, nos. 362-64.

20/19   **accesse.** L: *accessio.*

21/4   **al-togedir y-stoppid.** L: "In maiori oppilantur principales ventriculi cerebri ex toto. Unde non sentiunt patientes, et in accessione spumant, et tremunt per totum corpus, et dificile curantur" (ff. 110-110v).

21/15   **y-heelid.** Followed in Add 30338 by: "And yf a woman hafe þys sekenesse in hir ȝowþe and be not y-heled, whenne heo by-gynneþ to haue hur floures, heo shal neuer be hol" (f. 19).

21/17   **confusion.** L: "Sensuum confusio, clamor, pigricia, tenebrositas oculorum, lingue masticatio; urine, egestionis, et spermatis, involuntaria emissio; et in his cadunt, et insensibiles fiunt precipue in maiori cum dictis signis" (f. 110v).

22/4   **Analempsy.** L: "Analempsia fit ex fumo flegmatico vel melancolico abundante in stomacho corrupto venenoso" (f. 110v).

22/14   **fer.** L: "a remotis partibus ascendente frigido."

22/18   **afraieþ.** L: *conturbationes oculorum.*

24/11   **collaquindida.** This word is not explained in L.

24/16   **hede veyne.** L: *cephalica.* The two principal veins of the arm were the cephalica, evacuating the head and neck, and the basilica, evacuating the rest of the body: Mesue, "Expositio Ioannis de Sancto Amando," in *Opera quae extant omnia* (Venice, 1562), f. 422. For instructions on bloodletting, see Ogden, *Guy de Chauliac,* p. 543.

24/17   **garsid and y-cuppid.** L: "vel si corpus fuerit plectoricum, per ventosas cum scarificatione in collo" (f. 111).

24/21   **castorie.** Followed in Add 30338 by: "of eferych y-liche muche and ȝef hit hym what maner þat þu myȝt. Hit is ful good for children" (f. 20v).

27/14   **Apoplexie.** L: "Apoplexia est oppilatio omnium ventriculorum cerebri cum impedimento vel diminutione sensus et motus universali excepto motu anhelandi" (f. 114).

28/6   **senewes.** "A synow is a symple membre to ȝeue felynge and movyng þat is made to brawnes and to oþer lymmes. ... Alle þe synowes forsoþe spryngen of þe brayne" (Ogden, *Guy de Chauliac,* p. 34). The nerves were hollow, filled with spirit, and could not regenerate once they were cut. Their principal function was to bring "felyng and mouynge to þe oþir membres" (Seymour, p. 278).

28/18   **mysturnyng of þe face.** L: *os distorquetur.*

29/6   **axes.** L: *accessus.*
29/8   **crampe.** L: *spasmus.*
29/10   **vp.** Followed in Add 30338 by: "In wymmen þat beþ y-
          stopped her fallyng ys with muche ache fro the nafel
          donward and with muche hefynesse in here legges by-fore
          þat þey falleþ a-don, and þey straneþ hure wombe with
          here armes and boweþ hure hed to hure knees and
          grynteþ with hure teþ for þe gret ache þat þey hafeþ. And
          when þey falleþ don, summe beteþ þe eorþe wyþ here
          honden and here feet, summe lyggyþ stylle as þey weren
          dede, and al here body ys ful cold, and summe ryseþ vp
          sone, summe lyggeþ in her accesse a day or tweyne" (ff.
          22-22v). A nearly identical passage is found in Rowland,
          Medieval Woman's Guide, pp. 86 and 88 under the
          heading "Suffocation of the Mother."
29/13   **diuerse metis.** L: "Desiderat sibi melancolicos cibos et
          potus afferi diversos, et statim visos abominatur, mortem
          significat. Si non, spes curationis beneficio medicine
          postulabitur" (f. 115).
29/18   **souereigne remedy.** L: *summum remedium.*
30/11   **chyne.** L: *spondiles.*
30/24-31/4 **Blacke soope.** These lines are not in L. Add 30338 gives an
          added explanation of the difference between black soap,
          which is made over a fire out of lye and oil, and white
          soap, which is made of lye and sheep's tallow, using the
          heat of the sun (f. 23).
31/12   **incurable.** According to Guy, there were three times when
          the practitioner should not give treatment: when the
          disease   is   itself   incurable,   when   the   patient   is
          uncooperative or cannot stand the pain of a cure, and
          when the cure would be worse than the disease (Ogden,
          Guy de Chauliac, p. 3).
31/14   **And vndirstonde.** The Middle English version skips a long
          section on palsy and cramp, taking this treatment for
          provoking fever from a section entitled "De provocatione
          febris in apoplexia, paralisi et spasmo," not otherwise
          translated (L, f. 127v).
32/1-3   These lines would appear to be unique to the Wellcome
          Gilbertus translation.
32/5   **wiþynneforþe.** L: "adveniens extrinsece et intrinsece." This
          division of diseases into those caused by external factors
          and those caused by internal factors is often used in the
          Middle English Gilbertus.
32/8   **obtolmye.** The explanation of the meaning of this word is
          not found in L.
32/8   **webbis and cloþes.** L: *ungula sive petia.*
32/14   **Ache.** L: *dolor.*
32/19   **heuynes.** L: *dolor.*

32/24   **redenes of þe y3en.** L: "Ex colera, rubent vel citrinescunt, calent, et sentiunt puncturam quasi acuum" (f. 131).

33/6   **bridlym.** The reference to birdlime is not found in L.

33/6-7   **blere-y3ed.** L: *lippitudo.*

33/22   **pillules of diacastor.** Once again, this translation shows how a panacea has been brought from an untranslated part of the Latin text and placed in the Middle English text.

35/6   **serid clooþ.** L: *cerotum.*

35/8   **cop of þe nose.** L: *de nasi acumine.*

35/9   **stwe.** L: *stupha.*

35/14   **cologoge.** The explanation of the meaning of this word does not appear in L.

36/5   **Special medicyns.** L: *localia remedia.*

38/1   **bowing aweiward.** L: *recedente morbo.*

41/12   **smerte.** L: "Si oculi rubeant et pungant et lucem vel ignem sustinere non possint et non adsit apostematis presentia" (f. 132v).

44/2   **sumwhat bityng.** L: *aliquantulum corrosivum.*

44/3   **Obtalmye.** L: "Obtalmia est apostema nascens supra pelliculam albuginis oculi, id est, supra coniunctivam. Fit autem ex humoribus descendentibus ad oculum" (f. 133v).

44/7   **if þe postum.** L: "Cum vero intra distenditur oculus, et tumet et est durus et non apparet extra et obfuscatur visus, et habet plenitudinem venarum" (f. 133v).

44/21   **y-cuppid.** For instructions on horning and cupping, see Ogden, *Guy de Chauliac*, pp. 545, 549. On how to use leeches, see ibid., pp. 550-51.

45/19-46/1 This material is not found in other witnesses.

47/8   **Esy corosiues.** L: *mediocria corrosiva.*

51/1   This part appears to have been influenced by a source other than the Latin Gilbertus, because in L, web, cloth, and nail are not distinguished in this way. Trevisa explained: "Another euel of þe y3en þat we clepiþ a webbe, and Constantinus clepiþ it albugo oþir pannus, and brediþ in þis manere. Ferst a rewme renneþ to þe y3en and þerof comeþ an yuel þat hatte obtalmia, a schrewed blereynes and ache and a posteme, and if it is euel ikept þerof leueþ a litil mole and infeccioun, and long tyme turneþ and growiþ into a webbe and þicke, and occupieþ more place þan al þe blacke of þe i3e. This webbe turneþ into clooþ by more þicnes and occupieþ more place, for it ocupieþ al þe blacke of þe y3e, and at þe last it turneþ into þe kynde of a naile of þe honde, and so it is more þicke and hard" (Seymour, p. 361).

53/11   **bacyn.** Followed in Add 30338 by several recipes containing a number of unsavory substances, including the blood of hares, worms, flies, gall of eels, bird brains, and powder of shoe soles (f. 32).

53/24-54/3 This recipe is not found in other witnesses. However, see Ogden, *Liber de diversis medicinis*, p. 11.

54/5 **infeccion.** L: "Et si sanguis seu alius humor abundet in viis oculorum ... vocatur infectio" (f. 137v). The presence of certain diseases in other parts of the body would change the color of the eye: "Si autem abundet colera vel melancolia ... ut contingit in yctericia rosea et melachiros et calefactione epatis et oppilatione splenis, secundum humorem abundantem tingitur oculus, et proprie vocatur infectio" (f. 137v).

54/13 **gobet of fleisshe.** Because flesh like blood was hot and moist, blood would be the only humor responsible for this condition.

55/13 **congelid.** L: "Sanguinem autem coagulatum oportet consumere ex quacumque causa et dividere a loco cum succo verbene et plantaginis" (f. 138).

56/7 **Moystnes.** L: "Humiditas oculorum est vitium proveniens ex repletione cerebri quemadmodum lippitudo, aut ex frigiditate, aut ex humiditate, aut debilitate contentive" (ff. 138-138v).

59/11 **spiritis.** Sight was accomplished by a visual spirit communicated between the eye and the brain via the hollow optic nerves: "It byhoueþ þe synowes opitikes to be persed þat þere were the waie of þe spirite and to procede fro two parties, and þat þay beeþ oned wiþynne þe brayne panne" (Ogden, *Guy de Chauliac*, pp. 42-43). These spirits enabled the body to exercise its various functions: "Spiritis beþ instrumentis of vertues to excite hem to here doynge and worchinge" (Seymour, p. 392).

60/8 **yn.** Followed in Add 30338 by a recipe containing goat's livers and spleens (f. 35v).

60/15 **y3e.** Followed in Add 30338 by a recipe that involved blinding a swallow with a needle and then burning it to powder (f. 36).

62/5-6 This material is not found in other witnesses.

64/2 **mylke.** Other witnesses have here *blod*.

64/3 **before.** This is followed in Add 30338 by a recipe using live worms (f. 37v).

64/4-5 This material is not found in other witnesses.

70/14 **festre.** A fistula. For the difference between an apostem and a fistula, see Ogden, *Guy de Chauliac*, pp. 77-78.

71/11 **deefnes.** This is followed in Add 30338 by a recipe from Auycene (Avicenna) using the gall of a crow and a snail (f. 41).

72/5 **þe day þat it shulde flow.** L: *in die cretico*.

74/17 **wol.** Followed in Add 30338 by instructions for how to remove stones from the ear by using a stick (f. 42v).

75/3 **ri3t eere.** Choler came from the gallbladder on the right side; melancholy came from the spleen on the left side.

77/1-2   **yuel dispocicion.** L: *mala complexio.*

78/17-18 This material is not found in other witnesses.

84/12   **emeroides.** Followed in Add 30338 by "oþer in wymmen oþer wyþ-holdynge of hure purgacions and such bledynge in wymmen ys profitabel" (f. 47).

86/17   **myfoil.** Followed in Add 30338 by a recommendation that nosebleed be encouraged by use of swine's bristles on the end of a stick (f. 48).

86/23   **iching.** L: "pruritum et delectationem in pruritu."

87/17-18 **Of cancre.** Although these lines appear in other witnesses, in none are these topics covered.

87/19-20 These lines are not found in other witnesses.

87/23-24 **Cleving of lippis.** L: *scissuras labiorum.*

88/9   **mesel lippis.** L: *ragadia leprosorum.*

88/11   **bledders.** L: *ulceratio.*

88/18   **moist pemplis.** L: *pustula humida.*

89/12   **li3te.** L: *spirituales.*

91/19-20 These lines are not found in other witnesses.

92/14   **swarte rede.** L: *citrinitas.*

92/15   **ful whijt.** L: *albedo.*

92/17   **swart 3elewnes.** L: *lividitas.*

96/9   **hole cheke.** The cheek opposite the affected tooth.

96/9   **cheke.** Followed in Add 30338 by a recipe to be given to children, using hares' brains (f. 52v).

97/7-8   This material is not found in other witnesses.

97/14   **bledders.** L: *vulnera.*

97/17   **blayne.** L: *pustula.*

97/21   **swalme.** L: *tumor.*

98/11   **gargarisms.** L: *gargarismata.*

101/10   Covered in L but not in Middle English are "De ornatu faciei," a chapter for "quedam mulieres pilose et rugose," "De rubefactione faciei," "De pustulis in facie et toto corpore," and "De uva et morbis eius."

101/10   **Squynacy.** L: "Squinantia est apostema gutturis acutum cito suffocationem et sepissime inducens" (f. 177).

101/16   **greet anguisshe.** L: *angustia nimia.*

105/19-20 This material is not found in other witnesses.

105/21   **Hosnes.** L: "raucedo vel asperitas vocis."

111/18   The material that the copyist has crossed out is as follows: "Good pillules for þe cou3: Take dragagante, gumme arabike, seed of portulake, of citonies, and of mellon, and of gourdes, of eueriche, dr.v; of blaunchid almoundes, dr.vi; of þe sede of letuse, of white popy sede, of amide, of eueriche, dr.iiii; of penides, þe same wi3te. Tempere þis with þe musculage of psillie, and make pillulis of þe quantite of a been. Anoþer for þe same: Take þe sede of citonies, of gourdes, of almoundis, and of benes y-blaunchid, and of hockes sede. dr.vii; of gumme arabike, of dragante, iiii dr. Tempere hem with þe musculage of psillie, and make þerof pillules of þe quantite of a bene. Take vinegre and salt, eiþer garlike and vinegre. But let he not þe vinegre goo doun in his þrote." See below, note 132/5.

112/19   **coughe.** L: "Tussis autem est motus animalis et naturalis virtutis iunctus secundum nature cursum circa instrumenta spiritus operantia ad expellenda superflua sibi noctiva" (f. 184).

113/11   **viscous mater.** L: "vel ex inconvenienti materia quam laborat expellere natura, que quia grossa est et viscosa, a pulmonis parietibus nequit separari. Aliquando materia est liquida fluida, et dissolvitur antequam coadunetur" (f. 187).

120/17-18   This material is not found in other witnesses.

120/21   **postem.** L: "Peripleumonia et pleuresis sunt apostemata pectoris, sed peripleumonia pulmonis, pleuresis autem dyafragmatis et costarum" (f. 189v).

120/24   **accorden moche.** L: "Quorum signa concomitantia sunt dolor pectoris et lateris, et tussis, et febris. Accidentia autem subsequentia sepe sunt emoptoycis, empima, ptisis" (f. 189v).

121/16   **diuersite of flevmes.** There were several types of phlegms. According to Trevisa, "kyndeliche fleume is coolde, and moist, and white in colour, and fletinge in substaunce, a litwhat swete in sauour oþir al werisch and unsauoury" (Seymour, p. 156). There were four unnatural phlegms, each taking on a property of the humor it had in excess. Sweet phlegm was so because of blood. Salt phlegm was hot and dry "for infeccioun of rede colera." Glassy phlegm was like natural phlegm except that the coldness and wetness were intensified and it was thicker. Sour or keen phlegm was cold and dry from melancholy (Seymour, pp. 156-57).

122/8   **coler þat is cytryn.** There were several kinds of choler. "Natural is þat þat is kindeliche hote and drye, sotile in substaunce, clere and red in colour, but in sauour bitter wiþ a maner scharpnes" (Seymour, p. 157). "Vnkindeliche colera comeþ of kynde by somme strange humour imedled þerwith. For if rede colera is imedled with wattry fleume, þan is ibred citrina colera, þat is lesse hoot and more noyeful þan oþir coleres. If þe fleume is gret and þicke, þan is bred 3elew3 colera ... þe þridde maner of colera hatte prassina and is grene of colour and bittir" (Seymour, p. 158).

123/5-6   **þoroughe ii° holes.** L: "per foramina palati et eijcitur cum rascatione. Aliquando a faucibus vel guttere cum concussione et titillatione media inter tussim et rascationem. A pulmone autem educitur cum tussi et est spumosum. A stomacho sponte venit" (f. 190).

123/18   **greuaunce.** L: "dolor aggravatius medii pectoris declinans sub sinistra mamillia ante et retro, in spatulis usque ad humeros vel sinistra spatula" (f. 190).

124/14   **experience.** This "experience" and the one following were imported from a later chapter entitled "Signa mortalia in pleurisi et peripleumonia, epimate et ptisi," not otherwise translated.

128/17   **Spitting of blode.** L: "Emoptoys est eiectio sanguinis per os" (f. 194v).

128/20-21 **brusyng of veynes.** L: *ex apertione venarum.*

129/8   **not fomy.** This is followed in Add 30338 by "Oþerwhyles hit comeþ of stoppyng of blod in such places þat shuld flowe as in wymmen þat ne hafeþ noȝt hure purgacyons and in hem þat hafen emmeroydes" (f. 67).

132/5   **mylke.** This is followed in Add 30338 by: "Oþerwhyles sputtynge of blod comeþ of water leches þat a mon swolweþ in water and þey byteþ hys þrote and makeþ hit blede. And forte y-sen hem, take a glasen vessel and set hit by-twene þe sonne and his þrote and þu shalt y-sen hem. Tak hem þenne out wiþ a payre of scheres and seþþe ȝef hym a gargarisme of vynegre and salt oþer garlek, bot ne let he noȝt þe vynegre go doun hys þrote, and seþþe let hym vsen þe forsayd constrycctfes" (f. 68v). See note 111/18 above.

132/7   **Spitting of glat.** L: "Empima est screatus saniei cum infeccione pulmonis" (f. 195).

134/11   **Tisike.** L: "Ptisis est consumptio substantialis humiditatis corporis ex ulcere pulmonis proveniens" (f. 196).

135/8   **contynuel hete.** L: "calor continuus secundum magis et minus in volis manuum et plantis pedum acutior, quia febricitat si parum desistat a calore naturali" (f. 196v).

135/12   **corrupcion of þe nailes.** L: "unguium et extremitatum consumptio."

135/17   **streynyng togider.** L: *constringuntur ungues.*

135/18   **fallyng dovne.** L: *pili cadant.*

135/18-19 **simple fluxe.** L: *diarria.*

135/19   **Suche men shullen speke.** L: "moriendo loquentur, sed loquendo moriuntur."

139/17   **body.** The Wellcome copyist has left out a recipe using snails soaked in spices (Add 30338, f. 72).

140/15   **alle phicisiens.** L: "Concordant autem omnes in hoc quod vulnera pulmonis incurabilia sunt: Vulnus enim non curatur nisi mundetur. Non mundatur nisi cum tussi. Omnis tussis vulnera augmentat, dilatat, et aperit quare necesse est ut putrefiant. Maxime quod mundari non possunt nec curari, quia curculares egritudines non curantur" (f. 197v).

141/22   **defaute in breþing.** L: "Asma et dispnia et orthomia hanelitus et sansugium difficultates sunt hanelandi" (f. 198).

143/4-5   This material is not found in other witnesses.

143/6   **principal membre.** This phrase has been added to the text by the translator. The principal members, according to Guy, were the heart, liver, brain, and testicles (Ogden, *Guy de Chauliac*, p. 30). Trevisa explained that the heart is seated in the middle of the chest, the most noble position, for it is "the welle of lif, and al meuynge and al felinge is þerinne... . No membre is so nedeful to þe lif as þe herte" (Seymour, p. 239). This central position allowed the heart to diffuse "þe spirit of lif ... to þe vttir parties of al þe body" (ibid., p. 238). This spirit was literally air, which was supposed to be contained in the arteries, and abstractly, the vehicle of the innate heat necessary to life. The blood flowed from the heart through a boiling, "of the multitude of spirites beyng in it, for it is a fyry oven of all þe body" (Ogden, *Guy de Chauliac*, p. 31). The blood was consumed by digestion, the superfluities of which were released as sweat, menstrual blood, feces, urine, and mucus. Where this digestion was faulty, undigested humors built up, forming an apostem (ibid., p. 77).

143/7   **cardiacle.** L: "Cardiaca passio est tremor cordis, vel crebra cordis pulsatio ex humiditate coadunata in curcumdantibus cor pelliculis. Et est quandoque cum febribus et sincopi et sudore continuo" (f. 199).

144/3   **compassion.** This compassion on the part of the heart for the plight of other members is added to the text by the Middle English translator.

144/8-9   **passing awei of hete bi poores.** L: *dyaphoresis.*

147/5   **chyn.** L: *spina.*

148/7   **And if.** L: "Item quandoque fit cardiaca de causa flegmatica collecta circa pennulas pulmonis et auriculas cordis, quare comprimitur cor, et ista dicitur cardiaca tremens, quia posita manu supra regionem cordis, non senties motum cordis ordinatum immo tremores" (f. 200v).

149/5   **Sincopis.** L: "Sincopis est defectio cordis unde coadunantur spiritus in ipso superflue et non expelluntur fumi ipsius" (f. 201).

150/12   **humour.** Followed in Add 30338 by: "Oþerwhyles it comeþ to wymmen þro3 beryng of a ded chyld, for þe veynes brekeþ and blod floweþ out more þan hit shuld. Oþerwhyles hit comeþ of to muche strecchynge of þe moder, as whenne it is to muche y-strey3t in-to þe ry3t syde oþer in-to þe lyfte, oþer vpward oþer donward. Oþerwhiles hit comeþ in þe by-gynnynge of conceyfynge, or wyþ-holdyng of blod þat shuld kyndelych flowen ne were hure conceyfynge. Oþerwhiles, hit comeþ in þe

fourþe moneþ, for þe soule of þe child by-gynneþ þen to
worche in his body. Oþerwhyles it comeþ in þe nu3e
moneþe, whenne þe chyld is a-boute to passen out of his
moder wombe. And oþerwhyles þys sekenesse comeþ of
suffocacion of þe moder and oþerwhyles þat duyreþ two
dayes and two ny3ttes" (f. 76v).

151/16   **saleyn leues.** Followed in Add 30338 by: "And 3ef it comeþ
of þe moder þat is y-strau3t vpward oþer donward, oþer a-
syde furþer þan heo shuld be, let þe womman walken on
hure bare foot, forte hit be as hit shuld be. And let seþen
fenel sed and parsyly sed and such oþer þynges þat beþ
goode for þe moder in water and let weten a felte oþer
anoþer wollen cloþ in þe water and leggen þat on þe
moder. And 3ef hit be for berynge of a ded chyld, 3ef
hure suger roset oþer þe syrup of roses, oþer dyapapauer
oþer dyacitonyton. And let hure lyggen vpry3t and hure
feet hy3ere þan hure hed. And let cuppen hure at þe rote
of hure tyttes. And 3ef heo ne hafe no fefer, let hure hafe
a baþ of strictoryes, and elles let weten a cloþ in water þat
strictoryes beþ y-soden yn. And ley þat cloþ on þe moder.
And 3ef hit comeþ to wymmen þat hafe late conceyfed, let
hure vse confortabel electuaryes and wel-smellyng. And
let sprengen hure forhed wyþ water of roses. And 3ef þe
moder be fulle doun and be lower þan heo shuld be, be a-
boute to hefen hure vp by strengþe of medycynes, as lete
hure smelle to hertes horn y-brand and hafe þe fume
þerof in hure nese and fume of storace" (ff. 77-77v).

153/12-13 This material does not appear in other witnesses. The
Middle English translator has skipped over chapters
entitled "De apostematibus generaliter," "De apostemate
mamillarum," "De herisipila," "De vulneribus concavis,"
"De carbunculo," "De vulnere curato," and "De fistula."

153/22   **Greuaunce in swolewing.** L: "Difficultas glutiendi tribus
modis patitur, aut ex mutatione complexionis aut
apostemate aut vulnere. Mutatio complexionis est aut ex
caliditate aut ex frigiditate" (f. 206v).

156/8   **Defaute and lesing.** L: "Appetitus ciborum in stomacho
irrationabiliter diversatur aut enim excedit aut
irrationabiliter fit, aut deficit" (f. 206v).

159/8   **þingis.** The recipe that follows this word in W is
recommended in other MSS "for wymmen þat beþ with
chylde" (Add 30338, f. 80v).

161/16   **þingis.** A recipe follows in Add 30338 for "good pyllules to
holden vnder mennes tonges þat hafeþ gret furst for hete
and þey beþ good for men þat goþ ofer contry and hafeþ
no water to drynke" (f. 81v).

161/19   **citonies.** A recipe follows in Add 30338 for "a good syrup
þat stancheþ a monnes first" (ff. 81v-82).

164/24   **spleen.** Followed in Add 30338 by "and for greuaunce of þe moder."

165/9   **Zosking.** L: "Singultus est violentus sonus commotionis oris stomachi ex spasmosa eius dispositione proveniens" (f. 210).

168/18   **Casting and spuyng.** L: "Fastidium sive anarexia, abominatio sive nausea, et vomitus simbolum habent ad invicem et differentiam. Fiunt autem ex humoribus innaturalibus in ore stomachi abundantibus" (f. 210v).

172/14   **galle.** L: "Si fiat ex aliquo felle quovis ab umbilico superius inunctio provocat secessum. Similiter yera rufa cum amurca olei inuncta in superioribus lacertis brachiorum provocat vomitum. Inuncta lacertis inferioribus provocat secessum" (f. 212).

173/7   **haue sege.** L: *ducit inferius.*

174/7   **But.** There is no direct Latin equivalent to this passage. The sense seems to be "Sometimes it is necessary to allow a man to vomit, for as long as it is good for him, then it is difficult to make him stop."

175/18   **make him leue.** L: "Ab omnibus anime accidentibus preter gaudium abstineant."

176/5   **mouþ of þe stomake.** L: "Anatropha est subversio stomachi superius cum vomitu continuo." The translator has eliminated the name of the disease from his translation and has instead concentrated his attention on the affected part. The mouth of the stomach here refers to the upper opening of the stomach: "The stomak ... haþ twey mouthes, oon bynethe, anoþir aboue" (Seymour, p. 243).

176/10   **feble.** The retentive and expulsive virtues that govern the working of the stomach in medieval physiology are here simplified and made literal. L: "Aliquando ex nimia stomachi debilitatione cum deficit retentio et fortis est expulsio in fundo" (f. 213v).

177/2   **neþir parte.** As was the case with *anatropha* above, the translator has eliminated the name of the disease and has merely explained what that disease was. L: "Catatropha est inferior stomachi subversio seu depositio et est contraria anatrophe. Fit sepe ex crapula."(f. 214).

178/1   **oo maner cure.** That is, both stomach ache from corrupt humors and ache from distempering by hot or cold are cured in one manner, except that in the first case, one must purge the corrupt humors before beginning the treatment (corrupt humors would cause heat by their rotting).

187/20   **Stomaticon.** In other witnesses, recipes for these three stomaticons are given (Add 30338, ff. 94-94v).

187/24   **Colides.** L: "Colerica sive colerides est passio stomachi vel intestinorum a colera furiosa a qua denominatur potissime effecta. Est autem passio acutissima cum ultimato conatu egerendi ut interdum conantur egerere intestina" (f. 217).

188/8-9 **to moche eting.** L: "Fit etiam ex nimia crapula ciborum, vel ex ciborum assumptione immutatibilium, ... vel ex ventre discooperto in somno" (f. 217).

190/3 **ful violent.** L: "Et quia hec passio omnino virtutem contentivam debilitat et mortificat, et impetuose humores educit et humiditatem naturalem, et etiam medullas ossium ad ventrem trahit et per utrumque meatum effundit. Unde omnibus acutis est velocior et unius diei spacio terminatur" (f. 217v).

190/10-11 This material is not found in other witnesses.

190/18 **fluxes.** L: "Dissinteria est fluxus ventris cum excoriatione intestinorum et egestione sanguinolenta. Et non convenit ista diffinitio dissinterie epatice, propterea quia in dissinteria epatica non excoriantur intestina, unde non convenit ei nomen, neque diffinitio data secundum nomen, nisi secundum eam partem que est fluxus sanguineus. Item non convenit lienterie neque dyarrie, quam cum sint de genere fluxus non tamen cum egestione sanguinis. Neque convenit coleride, quam colerides non est fluxus ventris, sed etiam stomachi per superiora et impetuosa humoris et humiditatum a toto corpore eductio" (f. 217v).

191/12 **sori blood.** L: *sanguis adustus.*

191/13 **feble retentif.** L: "a debili retentiva aut forti expulsiva." Nutrition was accomplished by the operation of four "virtues" or abilities: attractive, digestive, retentive, and expulsive (Seymour, p. 104).

191/16 **þre maneris.** L: "Quedam fit in superioribus intestinis, quedam in infimis, quedam in mediis, quia ut dicit Galienus in Tegni" (f. 219).

192/17 **malencoli.** L: "ex melancolia innaturali adusta partim sanguinea, partim nigra ex flegmate salso, partim sanguinea, partim subpalida in sanguinea adusta, est partim sanguinea, partim subnigra" (f. 219).

196/19 **myntis.** Followed in Add 30338 by: "And for þe flowynge of blod þat wymmen hafeþ, hit is good y-dronke wyþ þe iuys of planteyne and hit wol stanche þe bledynge at þe nese 3ef hit be y-cast þer-ynne wyþ þe iuys of sangrinarye" (f. 99v).

197/19 **Blodi flux.** L: "Dissinteria epatica est fluxus ventris sanguinolentus absque excoriatione intestinorum" (f. 223).

199/9 **Diarria.** L: "Dyarria est simplex fluxus ventris sine sanguinolenta egestione et sine excoriatione intestinorum et sine cibi inoperati emissione" (f. 223v).

200/5 **Miclete.** Other witnesses give the recipe for this (Add 30338, f. 101v).

200/6 **Lienterie.** L: "Lienteria est fluxus ventris cum inoperati cibi emissione ex levitate stomachi et intestinorum

progrediens. Dicitur enim a lien vel leiton quid est lenire"
(f. 224v).

201/23   **colon.** There were six guts: "tria gracilia, scilicet duodenum,
ieiunium et yleon; et tria grossa, scilicet orobum, colon et
longaon" (L, f. 225v).

202/7   **ylion.** L: "nunc in dextra, nunc in sinistra vagantes; nunc
acute, nunc graves et ponderose, sepe cum se, sepe sine
se. Et dolores sunt ut parturientis, qui fere ducunt ad
insaniam et quotidie tabescunt" (f. 226). *Stiches* is not in
L.

203/20-21 **winde a 3erde.** This comparison is not made in L.

206/23   **wombe.** Followed in Add 30338 by a recipe using *hote shepes
dryt* (f. 105v).

207/12   **Wormes.** L: "Lumbrici non videntur in stomacho generari
propter fortitudinem caloris digerentis, sed potius in
intestinis propter calorem claudicantem, et eorum
frigiditatem, et hoc videtur dicere Aristoteles in quarto
methaurorum" (f. 228).

208/4   **epilencie.** Followed in Add 30338 by "Summe wymmen
swouneþ as þau3 þey hadden þe suffocacion of þe moder.
Summe grynteþ wyþ þe teþ as þau3 þey hadden goutes" (f.
106).

209/5   **wombe.** Followed in Add 30338 by "Suffocacion of þe moder
comeþ of greuaunce of þe moder, bot þys is of þe wombe
and in suffocacyon, let hure abstene from mete, and he
shal hafe þe more ete" (f. 106v).

211/2   **Tenasmon.** L: "Thenasmon est difficultas egerendi cum
conatu maximo et voluntate et impotentia emitendi et
nimio, et gravi pondere ut propter pondus intestini
videatur patienti quod incessanter debeat assellare cum
nullam habeat potentiam assellandi" (f. 229v).

214/18   **plastir.** Followed in Add 30338 by: "Oþerwhyles boþe þys
sekenesse and thenasmon comeþ of corrupt wynd þat is in
þe gottes and secheþ yssew and may hafe non yssew, and
þat is y-holpe by medycynes þat consumeþ and wasteþ
such wyndes. Oþerwhyles it comeþ of þe greuaunce of
emmoroydes, and þenne it ys y-helid 3ef þey ben y-heled"
(ff. 109v-10).

214/19   **sikenes.** Followed in Add 30338 by "and 3ef heo be a
womman" (f. 110).

216/14   **vnsaueri.** L: "Oris insipiditas aut terrestreitas quasi lutum
vel limum manducaverit sive masticaverit. Occupatio
quasi soporis, et transversus aut tranquillus somnus non
est, sed laboriose dormiunt, ut attoniti, tinnitus etiam
aurium et scotomia adesse consueverunt" (f. 235).

223/10   **Stopping.** L: "Oppilatio epatis sive enfraxis est morbus
officialis. Est enim vitium factum in poro. Quattuor enim
sunt pori epatis in quibus accidit oppilatios: quia aut in

meseraicis aut in gibbo aut in via ad cistim aut in splenem" (f. 237).

224/5   **gibbe.** L: "Oppilationis secunde in gibbo epatis facte ubi sunt exitus capillarium venarum que sunt angustissime sicut dicit Galienus in *Tegni*" (f. 237).

225/1   **3elewe yuel.** L: *ictericia.* This is not discussed in the Middle English. But L described it thus: "Ictericia est mutatio naturalis caloris cutis in innaturalem; ut in croceum, viridem vel nigrum. Crocea vero yctericia fit ex admixtione colere rubee cum sanguine ex cuius deportatione et dispersione per membra ad cutem fit color croceus" (f. 257).

225/19   **noble membre.** The nobility of the liver was, like that of the heart, due to the importance of the organ's function to the entire body: "þe veynes comeþ out of þe lyuour, and souken þerof as it were of here modir, fedinge of blood, and todeleþ and departiþ þat fedinge to eueriche membre as it nediþ" (Seymour, p. 279). On the relative nobility of the heart and liver, see ibid., p. 248.

227/24   **corruption of þe eire.** L: "contra fetentes nebulas matutinales et aerem pestilentialem et fetorem maris" (f. 239v).

231/19-20 This material is not found in other witnesses.

231/21   **spleen.** L: "Splen quandoque est nomen membri quandoque morbi. Secundum quod est membrum, est rarum spongiosum attrahens et conbibens superfluitates humoris melancolici ab epate expulsas ad sui mundificationem. Unde est membrum servile et sine sensu. Quapropter patitur diversas egritudines ut oppilationem et tumorem et duriciem et mollitiem et apostema, et quandoque ventositatem et quandoque repletionem" (ff. 261-61v).

232/2   **from þe lyuer.** The liver drew material digested by the stomach from the veins and "be boylynge of kynde hete" turned the material "into þe kynde of þe foure humours" (Seymour, p. 246).

232/3   **as þe bladdir .** Urine "takeþ begynnynge of þe lyuor" from which "wattry substance of blood is isend by certeyn sotil veynes to fede þe reynes. And so whanne it comeþ to þe reynes, þere it is idreyned and iclensid as wax þat is molte and ipured ... and so it swetiþ and wooseþ forþ by certeyn hooles and poores into þe bladdre" (Seymour, pp. 256-57).

234/12   **Stopping.** The spleen delivered melancholy to the stomach to control the appetite (Seymour, p. 250). The "stoppings" described below, the Latin text makes clear, are of the passages by which melancholy is delivered to or from the spleen.

234/17   **y-sente.** That is, the "backed up" liver would send out its contents through the body instead of to the spleen.

234/18 **þe vrin.** There was no direct connection between the spleen and the urinary tract. The contamination from melancholy would have occurred via the liver.

234/22 **guttis** L: "Et si oppilatur via inter splenem et intestina qua mittitur melancholia ad confortandam virtutem retentivam, cadit retentiva et fluit venter" (ff. 262-262v).

235/1 **al-rounde.** The description given here is of a normal spleen and not the result of disease. The fidelity to L is sketchy and confused in this chapter.

236/23 **þe mater is meving.** L: "Materia movens est et latitans et faciens dolorem manifeste, citius curatur. Non facies dolorem sed latitans vix curatur. Et tamen inveterata melius curatur quam recens" (f. 263).

238/14 **saluitica.** L: "de basilica in sinistro brachio, quandoque de salvatella in sinistra manu que propria est. Galienus dicit quod debet aperiri vena sub aure sinistra retro in hac passione. Item aperitur sophena quandoque sub cavilla sinistri pedis" (f. 263).

244/6 **Agrippa.** Other witnesses give the recipe (Add 30338, f. 124).

244/9-10 This material is not found in other witnesses.

250/1 **Stones.** L: "Lapides et harene nascuntur ex superfluitatibus variis et viscosis in renibus et vesica."

250/23 **oþir place.** L: "Et non solum lapides generantur in renibus et vesica, immo etiam in stomacho, quos quidam per vomitum eijciunt. Et quibusdam accidunt in intestinis, et eijciunt eos per secessum. Et fit plurimum ex eadem causa ex qua fit colica et yliaca. Et fiunt etiam in pectore et aliis locis, ut in iuncturis artheticorum" (f. 268).

253/18 **bladdir** (1). Followed in Add 30338 by a recipe using a live hare burnt with grasshoppers, and another with the legs and heads of grasshoppers and crickets. Finally, there is one with fox's and goat's blood (f. 129).

254/9 **vertu.** Followed in Add 30338 by another recipe "for chyldren þat mowe no3t pysse" (f. 130).

254/19 **Stranguria.** L: "Stranguria ... est morbus per se, quandoque sinthoma aliorum morborum" (f. 274).

256/11-13 **Contra ... verum.** This material is not found in other witnesses.

256/24 **stoon.** Followed in Add 30338 by a recipe "for soukynge chyldren, both whenne þe chyld ys two 3eres old oþer more" (f. 131v).

260/24 **Diabites.** L: "Dyabetes est immoderatus transitus vel attractus urine ab epate ad renes, et per renes transitus. Fit enim ex calida et sicca distemperantia renum; ... renes ad se trahant per uritides poros et capillares venas humiditatem ab epate, et epar a meseraicis, et meseraici ab intestinis, et intestina a fundo stomachi, et fundus ab ore" (f. 278).

265/22 **bladdir**. Followed in Add 30338 by "and of þe moder" (f. 137).

267/17 **difference**. L: "Discernitur autem ab hernia quoniam in hernia sentitur dolor in profundo testiculi et ligamentis ipsius usque ad renes. Et in crepatura siphac vel omenti manifestatur inflatio ab altera parte pectinis usque ad bursam, et in ipsa bursa est tumor non in testiculis" (f. 280v).

271/7-14 **Anoþir good ... of God**. This recipe is in Sl 5 but not in Add 30338.

271/15-16 This material is not found in other witnesses.

271/20 **Satiriasis**. L: "Satyriasis est immoderata virge erectio, cuius causam abundantiam spirituum esse commemoravimus. Fit igitur ex calida fumositate et grossa descendente ad testiculos et virgam ipsam distendente et erigente. Unde fit sine delectatione aliqua, quia non est cum appetitu, sed cum dolore et extensione" (f. 287v).

272/19 **Gomorra**. The flowing of pus associated with gonorrhea was confused with that of sperm, hence the name. There also seems to be an association with the city of Gomorrah.

272/20 **plente of blood**. Sperm was said to be engendered from blood. L: "Gomorrea est involuntaria spermatis emissio, et fit ex superabundantia sanguinis, et quandoque ex paralisi testiculorum, et quandoque ex debilitate virtutis contuntive eorundem, quandoque ex liquiditate spermatis" (f. 287v).

274/2 **stones**. Followed in Add 30338 by: "And þys same ys good to make þe mylke þykke þat is in a wommanes tyttes" (f. 142).

274/5 **Pimples and postemes**. L: "Pustule et apostemata fiunt sepissime in virga ex reumatismo humorum vel mala complexione ipsius. Unde accidit quandoque in ea cancer vel fistula si pustule curare non fuerint" (f. 287).

274/7 **festre**. The comparison to a whistle or a pipe is provided by the Middle English translator.

275/9 **3erd**. Followed in Add 30338 by "and for þe cancre of a wommanes pryfe membre" (f. 143).

276/5 **daies**. Followed in Add 30338 by: "And 3ef þe cancer wol no3t ben y-heled wyþ medycynes, cutte a-wey as muche as ys y-cancred and brenne þe remenant with a hot yre. And 3ef þer be a festre and an hol oþer mony holes in þe 3erde, hele it with þe oynement ruptory and with oþer medycynes þat beþ y-told in þe festre" (f. 143v).

276/5-7 **Forto ... anoon**. This material is not found in other witnesses.

278/10 **quitere**. The Wellcome copyist has removed yet another surgical operation here: "And 3ef þer be postume oþer flesch growynge on any of þe stones, schafe it a-way with a rasor and 3ef þe ston be hard and sond, let hym a-byde stylle, and ȝef he rote any-þinge, cutte hym of and seþþe hele up þe wonde" (Add 30338, f. 145).

278/17-18 This material not found in other witnesses. The chapter on hemorrhoids appears in L after the chapter on prolapsed rectum.

278/21 **Emeroidis.** L: "Emoroyde sunt v. vene circa pudibundum circulum cum longaone terminantes, quas natura creavit in quibusdam viris et mulieribus. Quibus propter purgationem grossi et melancolici sanguinis atque superflui quam natura odio habens illuc mandat, per illas v. venas ut tempore congregationis talis superfluitatis aperiantur, et sanguis ille expellatur. Et post expulsionem claudantur, quemadmodum accidit ex menstruo sanguine in mulieribus. Per illas ergo corpus a nocivis humoribus purgatur" (f. 231).

279/5-6 **for brenyng.** L: "Interdum eas nimis fluentes urunt cyrurgici, postea cicatrizant, et tunc vix aut nunquam aperiuntur, sed redit sanguis feculentus super epar et virtutem ipsius corrumpit, unde sequitur ydropisis" (f. 231).

279/13 **moneþe.** It would seem that the Wellcome copyist believed that he was about to encounter material about women and routinely skipped a few lines as a consequence. In fact, the material he left out or summarized is as follows: "Such flowynge of þese veynes ne schal noȝt ben y-stanched by medycynes, for þey wolleþ hem-selfen cesen of bledynge, and bleden also whenne it is nede. Bot whenne þe bledynge ys to muche, hit is good to stanchen it and such fluxe comeþ of gret plente of blod oþer of keneschyp of þe blod, oþer of þinneschyp of þe blod, oþer of febelnesse as oþer fluxes comeþ. And þys flowynge comeþ to a mon whenne he ys xl ȝere old, to suche men þat han y-lyfed esylych in hure body and oþerwhyles þe blod þat floweþ from hem ys red" (Add 30338 f. 146).

279/24 **is.** This is followed in Add 30338 by: "ȝet he bledeþ muche at on tyme and bledeþ oftesyþes and þe veynes of hys legges and of hys þyes ben ful of blod, þenne þys flowynge comeþ of plente of blod, bote ȝef hit comeþ contynewelych, and luytel and febeleþ a mon and grefeþ hym in þe flowynge, þenne it comeþ of febelnesse. Tokenes of wyþholdyng of blod þat schuld flowe beþ hefynesse a-boute þe reynes and ycchynge of þe bottokes and of þe rugge and of þe schere, and greuaunce þey han to schyte, and hedache þey hafeþ, and pale colour of face" (ff. 146-146v).

282/23-283/2

But vndirstonde ... dropesi. Next to *ars longa, vita brevis*, this was the most popular Hippocratic quotation in the

Middle Ages. See also Seymour, p. 408 and Ogden, *Guy de Chauliac*, p. 323.

283/21   **ey.** This is followed in Add 30338 but not in Sl 5 by: "In al þys book þer-as þu seest vyolet y-don in electuaryes, oþer in syrupes, þu schalt take þe flour of violet and noȝt þe lefes. Ofer al in þys bok þer-as þu y-findest in electuaryes þys word "cytre" þus y-wryte oþer þus "cytr," it shuld be safren. Roust of yren ys y-don in electuaryes bot þat ne is noȝt of old rousted yren, bot it ys þat scrofe þat ys y-beten a-wey at þe anfeld and me clepeþ þat in summe places smyþes colm. Bot er þan me do it in medycynes, it schal be furst smale y-poudred and seþþe ben y-soden in vynegre þryes oþer four syþes. And þenne it ys profitabel in medycynes, for hyt restoreþ colere and consumeþ malencolye, and it sleeþ þe cancre and þe festre and it druyeþ qwyture and a-bateþ a monnes fatnesse. Deo gracias" (f. 149).

283/22-23   This material is not found in other witnesses.

283/24   The text that follows here is divided from what comes before by a line drawn horizontally across the page. Some of it seems to have been added by the Wellcome copyist, some is taken from sections of the Latin not otherwise translated, and some comes from sections of the text that the Wellcome copyist has left out. The sections from the Latin are marked in the edited text.

286/4-5   **To þre þinges.** This phrase ends one version of the Middle English John of Arderne as well (Power, *John of Arderne*, p. 104), and may have belonged to the less learned or religious practitioners. When Guy de Chauliac was dividing various methods of medical practice into sects, he cited this phrase also, but not with approval. The fourth, and next to worst sect, he said, was "Alle knyȝtes of Saxoun and of men folowynge batailles, þe whiche procuren or helen alle woundes wiþ coniurisouns and drynkes and with oyle and wolle and a cole leef, foundynge ham þerfore vppon þat, þat God putte his vertu in herbes, wordes and stones" (Ogden, *Guy de Chauliac*, p. 10).

Glossary

The purpose of this glossary is to define all major words used in the text of this edition and to give the location in the text of these words. Definitions are necessarily brief; the citations to folio numbers with each word will give a better idea of nuance and in many cases point out the care with which the translator has explained his Latin material. Within a word, the letters 3 and þ are alphabetized like g and th respectively. When they are initial, 3 has been placed after w and þ after t. The letter y is treated as if it were i. First usages not found in the *Middle English Dictionary* (MED) are marked with a single asterisk. Unique usages that are found neither in the MED nor in the *Oxford English Dictionary* (OED) are marked with two asterisks. Plants are classified where possible by botanical family, genus, and species. A list of these plants arranged in alphabetical order according to genus and species follows the glossary. It has been necessary to limit the number of folio references to certain words. Selected references attempt to reflect among other things the variety of ways in which a substance was used in medicine, how a compound was prepared, which plants were used both in pharmacy and in diet, how various colors and qualities were aids to diagnosis, and how the translator defined the terms. Particular attention is paid to glossary entries that will throw light on aspects of medieval medicine such as diet (ex. **mete**), physiology (ex. **melancholy**), phlebotomy (ex. **blede**), regimen (ex. **fasting, angir**), anatomy (ex. **membre**), and pharmaceutical practice (ex. **clarifie**). Folio references on occasion will not be in numerical order within an entry. This is due to the replacement of misplaced folios by the editor.

The following is a list of the fifty most commonly used herbal remedies in this text:

almondis, aloes, anet, anyse, barliche, betis, calamynt, canel, cardamomum, carewey, castor, clowes, comyn, dragagant, encense, euforbe, eufrace, femygreke, fenel, galles, gynger, gorde, gum arabike, hock, ysop, liquoris, lorer, marche, mastik, meiden-her, mynt, mirre, notemyg, olibanum, parseli, pepir, piretre, planteyn, roses, rw, safron, sage, sandragon, sandris, sarcacol, scamony, sene, syneuey, storax, tyme.

aaron *n.* Araceae, *Arum maculatum*, cuckoo-pint 76v.

abhominacion (*to*/*of*) *n.* feeling of disgust (toward) 53v, 66, 72v, 221v, 224, 234v, 235v.

abst(e)yne *v.* (*refl.*) hold (oneself) back from 48, 49v, 67v, 78, 131v, 132, 260v, 261, 268v, 289v, 307.

abstinence *n.* fasting, self-denial 240v-242v. See **fasting**[1].

acacia, acacie, acasie *n.* gum of Rosaceae, *Prunus spinosa*, green sloes 80, 85, 87v-88v, 108v, 109, 171, 186, 240, 257, 298v, 299. See **sloo(n), þorne.**

accarnes, ackernes *n. pl.* acorns 275v, 298. See **oke.**

acces(se), axes *n.* attack, onset (of illness) 64v-65v, 66v, 67, 72, 191-192, 270. Cf. below **axes.**

accorun see **yreos.**

ache *n.*, -s *pl.* pain 48, 49, 49v, 50v, 51v, 52, 53, 53v, 54v, 55v, 75-76, 77v-79, 80, 80v, 81, etc.; *hede- a.* 48, 48v, 50v, 51, 53v, 59, 84, 85v, 128; *toþe- a.* 135v, 137, 138.

acori see **cicori.**

ademant stoon see **magnes.**

adiantos see **meiden-her(e).**

aferde *ppl. adj.* frightened 234v.

affodille *n.* Liliaceae, *Allium ursinum*, ramsons 62v, 104; *a. rotis* 123.

afraieþ *pr. 3 sg.* turns aside 66v.

agarike, agaricum, agarici *n.* Polyporaceae, *Polyporus officinalis*, bracket fungus 54, 62, 76v, 261v, 262v, 201, 201v, 209v.

agaste *adj.* surprised 232.

agnus castus *n.* Verbenaceae, *Vitex agnus-castus*; *sede of a. c.* 300v.

agrimonie see **egrimoyn(e).**

agrippa *n.* ointment used by Agrippa, King of the Jews 221. See MED **marciatoun.

ake *v.* ache 107, 120v, 191; **akiþ, akeþ** *pr. 3 sg.* 49, 79, 85v, 106v, 136v, 244v; **aken** *3 pl.* 120v, 133v, 308; **akeþ** *subj.* 107, 246; **aking** *pr. p.* 139.

akyng *vbl. n.* pain 54v, 70v, 71v, 117v, 124v, 231, 236, 270.

ale *n.* ale 51v, 87, 299-300; *newe a.* 306v; *smale a.* 127; *stale a.* 74v, 307, 309v; *strong a.* 53v.

alym(e) *n.* aluminum potassium sulfate 89, 112v, 137v, 308v.

alipiados see **lauriole.

almondis *n. pl.* Rosaceae, *Prunus amygdalus*, almonds 150v, 161, 183v; *a. mylke* 166v, 167, 222v, 249, 249v, 258; *bitter a.* 115, 117, 174; *blanchid a.* 152, 156. See **oyl(e).**

al(l)oes *n. pl.* dried juice of Liliaceae, *Aloe* spp., aloes 54, 62, 68, 70, 73, 76v, 80, 89-90, 91v, 92, 93, 94, 103v, 105, 115, 132v, 145, 234, etc., also 271, 290, 306v, 307v; *a. cicotryn, A. perryi* 100v; *a. epatike, A. vera* 51. Cf. **lignum al(l)oes.**

amachites see **emachite(s).**

a(u)mbir *n.* ambergris, gray substance in intestines of sperm whales 80, 88v.

ameos *n.* Umbelliferae, *Aegopodium podagraria*, gout weed 55, 102v, 167, 174v, 225v, 230, 230v, 231v, 234v, 246v, 247, 274; *a. sede* 197v. Cf. MED.

amyde *n.* wheat starch 83v, 85, 87v, 88, 91v, 92v, 94v, 130, 146, 148, 150-151, 152, 153, 156, 167, 171v, 177v, 178v, etc.

amomum, amoni(e) *n.* seed of Zingiberaceae, *Amomum cardamomum*, amomum 70, 141v, 225v, 230, 231v, 241. See **cardamomum**.

amoniac, amoniake *n.* gum of Umbelliferae, *Dorema ammoniacum*, gum ammoniac tree 136v, 242, 218v-219v, 298v.

ampte eiren *n. pl.* ant eggs 119.

ana *adv.* of each the same amount 51v, 54, 54v, 63, 70v, 87v, 88, 103v, 123, 123v, 141v-142v, 149v, 152, 153, 155v-157, etc.

anacardi *n.* Anacardiaceae, *Semecarpus anacardium*, marking nut 77.

analempsi(e) *n.* type of epilepsy caused by disease of the stomach 65, 66, 67, 69v-70v.

anentiship *pr. 3 sg.* wastes 226; **anentishid** *p. p.* 258.

anentising, a-nyntishing *vbl. n.* wasting 190v, 191v, 193v, 232v, 233.

anet(um) *n.* Umbelliferae, *Anethum graveolens*, dill 59v, 69, 73v, 103, 139v, 145, 167, 173, 174, 226, 234v, 241, 247, 250; *a. sede* 197v.

angir *n.* anger 50v, 98v, 151. See **wrap(þe)**.

anguisshe *n.* constriction 142v.

anyse, anees, anese, anisi *n.* Umbelliferae, *Pimpinella anisum*, anise 51, 54v, 55, 60, 76v, 81, 102v, 117, 119, 161, 172v, 178, 189, 225v, 234; *a. sede* 197v.

anoynte(n) *v.* apply an ointment to 69v, 149, 157v; **anointist** *pr. 2 subj.* 238v; **anoynt(e)** *imp.* 49, 57v, 62, 62v, 63v, 64, 69v-70v, 74v, 77v, 80, 84, 92, 98v, 100v, 104v, 105, 109, 111, etc.; **anoyntid** *p. p.* 73, 73v, 139v, 151v, 168v, 187v, 225, 245v, 252, 252v.

anoynting *vbl. n.*, **-is** *pl.* application of ointment 173v, 187, 229v, 234, 239v, 291.

antimony(e) *n.* ore of antimony, stibnite 68v, 69, 70, 76v, 88v, 89v.

*ant(h)os see **ros(e)maryn**.

apium ranarum *n.* Ranunculaceae, *Ranunculus sceleratus*, celery-leafed crowfoot 174.

ap(p)oplexi(e), appoplixie *n.*, **-is** *pl.* impairment of the brain's function with symptoms similar to epilepsy 52v, 65v, 70v-72v, 74, 147, 270v.

apostolicon *n.* an ointment 100v.

appeiren *v.* harm 58; **apperiþ** *pr. 3 sg.* 132, 175v; **appe(i)rid** *p. p.* 59v, 259, 195v; **appeiring** *vbl. n.* deterioration 51.

appetit(e) *(to)* *n.*, **-is** *pl.* desire (for/to), appetite 221, 224v-227, 230, 235, 236, 203v, 213, 291v, 301v; *houndes a.* disorder characterized by excessive desire for food followed by vomiting 224v, 270.

appil *n.*, **applis** *pl.* fruit of Rosaceae, *Malus* spp., apple 49, 67v, 115v, 151, 249. See **erþe appel, galles, pynes.**

aqua see **watir.**

arage *n.* Chenopodiaceae, *Atriplex* spp., orache 59v, 146v, 222, 283; *seed of a.* 237.

aristologia, aristologie *n.* the "root" of Aristolochiaceae, *Aristolochia* spp., birthwort; *long(e) a.* or *a. longa, A. clematitis* 76v, 178, 246v, 298v-299v; *a. rotunda* or *a. þe rounde, A. rotunda* 76v, 130, 174v, 178, 192v, 230v, 298-299v.

arme *n.*, **-s** *pl.* arm 170v, 249, 260v, 215v, 216, 277, 281v, 289v, 301, 306v; **arme-pittis** 74v. See **veyne.**

armoniac see **sal(t) armoniac.**

aromatike *adj.* sweet-smelling 51, 159v, 187, 187v.

arrogon *n.* an ointment 267, 295v.

asarum, asari, azarum *n.* Aristolochiaceae, *Asarum europaeum*, hazelwort 76v, 182, 225v, 201, 204v, 217, 230, 250. MED **azarabacca(ra).**

**ase *n.* gum of Umbelliferae, *Ferula* spp., asafetida (L *asa*) 76v.

ashamid *ppl. adj.* ashamed 232, 234v.

aspalte *n.* naturally occurring asphalt 193.

a(i)ssh(e) *n.*, **-is** *pl.* Oleaceae, *Fraxinus excelsior*, English ash; *bowes of gren a.* 119; *rynde of an a.* 218v, 299v; *rote of a. tree* 271v; *seed of a.* 284v. See **oyl(e).**

asshis see **axes.**

a-stonyen *pr. pl.* make numb 80v; **(a)-stonied** *p. p.* 248v, 195v, 281v.

**athanasia *n.* an electuary 256v, 257, 259, 263.

attir-coppe *n.* spider 115v.

attrament *n.* 90v, 128; ***calcant** 192v; **coperos** 88v, 128; ***lapis armenicus** 61, 68, 90, 220v. All refer to various hydrated metallic sulfates, usually of iron or copper. **Calcant** and **lapis armenicus** are probably copper sulfate. **Coperos** may be ferrous sulfate. **Attrament** is a general term for any kind of metallic sulfate or vitriol. The word also refers to the black pigment used by painters, made of soot and black wine burned on coals.

a-twyny *adv.* having gaps between 133v.

auence *n.* Rosaceae, *Geum urbanum*, herb bennet 51v, 64v, 68, 97, 122v, 123, 141v, 192v, 290v, 298, 307; *iuse of a.* 93; *rotis of a.* 246.

axes, axen, ass(h)is *n. pl.* ashes of a fire 49, 110, 110v, 111v, 115, 117, 219, 281; *smyþþes a.* ashes from a forge 188v. See **acces(se).**

axiþ *pr. 3 sg.* demands 143v, 148.

bag(ge) *n.*, **baggis** *pl.* bag 85, 92, 136, 136v, 182v, 187, 250v, 273v, 275, 200.

baies see **iuniper, lorer.**

balaustia see **pomgarnard.**

balkeþ *pr. 3 sg.* belches 243, 207v, 210v; **balken** *pr. pl.* 243v.

balking *vbl. n.*, **-is** *pl.* belching 221v, 223v, 224, 229-231, 236, 242v, 243, 246, 248v, 211.

ballis *n. pl.* pills 135v, 178v, 179, 280v.

barliche, barl(e)y *n.* Gramineae, *Hordeum distichon*, barley 145-146v, 149, 150v, 157, 167-168, 171v, 180v, 250v, 267, 275, 280v; *smale chaf of b.* barley chaff 107v, 129. See **bred(e), mele[1], (p)tisane.**

basilica see **veyne**.

basilicon *n.* Labiatae, *Ocimum* spp., basil 80, 187; *seed of b.* 182; ****oz(i)mi, ozimum** *n.* 76v, 230, 250; **basilicon** meant the herb and **ozimi** its seeds.

baþ(e), baþ(þe) *n.*, **-es** *pl.* bath, esp. a medicinal bath 69v, 82v, 98, 194, 229v, 252, 257, 263, 263v, 266v, 216, 277v, 282v, 283-284v, 286-287, etc.

baþe, baþen *v.* (*refl.*) bathe, esp. in a medicinal bath 60v, 77v, 98, 142v, 193v, 252, 263, 199, 205, 286; **baþid** *p. p.* 82v, 266v, 273, 287v, 299, 302v.

baþing, baþeng *vbl. n.* bathing, esp. in a medicinal bath 48, 49v, 67v, 86, 92, 172, 260v, 284v.

bawme (þat is an herbe), bavme *n.* Labiatae, *Melissa officinalis*, balm 64v, 76v, 109v, 183v, 187, 250, 267v, 269; *croppis of b.* 51v; **melisse** *n.* balm 141v.

bawme (þat is an onment), bavme *n.* an ointment, esp. one made with resin from Burseraceae, *Balsamodendron opobalsamum*, balsam of Gilead 79v, 88v, 245v, 278v. See ****carpobalsamum, opobalsamum, zilobalsamum.**

bdellie, bdellium *n.* resin from Burseraceae, *Balsamodendron* spp., bdellium tree 68, 76v, 258, 298v.

bean, been *n.*, **be(e)nes, benen** *pl.* Leguminosae, *Vicia faba*, broad bean 53v, 64v, 67v, 110, 117, 125, 130, 268v, 202v, 302-303v, 304v, 305; *b. stalkis/stelis* bean stalks 110, 117, 119; *floure of b.* 263v; *hollis of b.* 303v; *quantite of a b.* 123. See **mele[1].**

beche, biche *n.* Fagaceae, *Fagus sylvatica*, beech tree; *leues of a b. tre* 271, 271v.

bed *n.* bed 108, 108v, 123, 123v, 283, 294, 295v; *bringe to b.* put to bed 107v.

bedegar *n.* the gall growing on **þistil** 290v.

beef *n.* beef 67v.

bellerici see **mirabolani(s)**.

berberis *n.* Cruciferae, *Berberis vulgaris*, winter-cress 182.

*berdane *n.* Compositae, *Arctium lappa*, great burdock; *rote of b.* 286v, 287.

berde *n.* beard 191v.

betayn, betein, betony *n.* Labiatae, *Betonica officinalis*, betony 84, 98, 110, 122v, 295v, 307; *asshis of b.* 49.

be(e)tis, bletis, blitis *n. pl.* Chenopodiaceae, *Beta* spp., beets 59v, 63v, 67v, 69v, 73v, 76v, 111, 111v, 146v, 183v, 228v, 237v, 249, 250v, 266v, 267, 273, 273v, 218, 278, etc.

biche see **beche**.

byle *n.*, **boilis** *pl.* kind of apostem, esp. one that can be seen 124v, 305v; *blacke b.* thrombosed pile 308v.

bipissen see **pisse**.

birche *n.* Betulaceae, *Betula* spp., birch 131. See **oyl(e)**.

bismalue see **holy-hock**.

biteþ *pr. 3 sg.* bites 125; **biten** *pl.* 270; **biten** *p. p.* 193; **biting** *ppl. adj.* keen, penetrating 69, 73v, 85v, 114, 118, 267, 293. See **mete**.

bitinge *vbl. n.* biting, a gnawing feeling 65v, 244v.

bitter *adj.* severe 55v; bitter-tasting, esp. from choler 70, 115, 143, 149v, 155v, 225, 226, 228, 236, 243, 248, 270v, 271, 203v, 206v, 211v, 212v. See **almondis, lupynes**.

bitternes *n.* bitter taste 53, 116v, 142v, 163v, 224.

black(e), blac *adj.* colored black 52v, 58v, 89, 89v, 92v, 95, 255v, 281, 284v, 289, 309; having a blackish color caused by melancholy 67, 71v, 139v, 164, 244, 244v, 255v, 203v, 210v, 212, 306. See **byle, pepir, plumb, popi, so(o)pe, þorne, vyne**.

blacknes *n.* blackness 55v.

bladdir *n.* urinary bladder 201, 210v, 215, 277v, 280v, 281v, 282, 282v, 284-285v, 287-288v, 289v, 291-292, etc.; the gall bladder 210v. See **necke**.

bledders *n. pl.* types of apostem (L *ulceratio*) 130, 138v.

blede, bleed *v.* bleed 60, 68, 72v, 77v, 84, 86, 96v, 99, 126v, 128-129, 134, 134v, 136, 139v, 140v, 143, 143v, 147v, etc.; **blediþ** *pr. 3 sg.* 126, 127; **bleden** *pl.* 105, 131, 305v; **blede** *subj. sing.* 57v, 126v, 193v. See **bleding, blode, blode-letting, let(e) blood**.

bleding *vbl. n.* emission of blood 126, 169v, 170v, 171, 193v, 290, 303v; phlebotomy 122, 125v; *nose b.* nose bleed 53, 126, 172, 172v, 193, 288v. See **blede, blode, blode-letting, let(e) blood**.

bleynes, blayne(s) *n. pl.* types of apostem, blains (L *pustulae*) 100v, 124, 139, 139v, 179, 308v.

blereship *n.* bleariness 97v.

blerid *p. p.* made bleary 86; *blere-y3ed* 75v, 86. See **y3e**.

bletis, blitis see **be(e)tis**.

blode, blood *n.* blood 53-54, 55v, 57-58, 59, 59v, 62, 66v, 68, 70, 71, 71v, 72v, 74v-75v, 77v, etc., also 78v, 95v, 97, 126, 127, 139, 191v, 270v, 206v, 279v, 306; *b. of a boor* 91; *b. of a capon* 91; *b. of a cheken* 80, 100; *b. of a coluir* 80, 100; *b. of an hare* 91; *b. of an hen* 80, 94v; *b. of a lapwynge* 91; *b. of a ramme* 91; *b. of a swalewe* 91; *manis b.* 297, 298v; *leting of b.* phlebotomy 53v, 96v. See **blede, bleding, blode-letting, let(e) blood**.

blode-letting *n.,* -gis *pl.* phlebotomy 57v, 84v, 93, 145, 147, 192. See **blede, bleding, blode, let(e) blood**.

blodi *adj.* bloody 279, 289. See **flux(e)**.

boc(c)he *n.,* -s *pl.* apostem, esp. whose swelling can be felt 124, 124v, 144v, 165v, 170, 178.

body *n.,* **bodies** *pl.* human body, esp. the trunk apart from the head and limbs 61v, 64v-66v, 72, 72v, 74v, 79, 82, 86, 96, 102v, 121, 126, 132, 134, 144v, 147v, etc.; **bodies** physical masses 101, 289v.

boile *v.* boil 63v.

boistesnes *n.* coarseness 116. See **mete**.

boistous, boisteis, boistrois *adj*. coarse 53v, 219v, 256, 300. See **mete**.

boke *n*. book 74v, 105v, 120, 129, 133, 138v, 184, 221, 253v, 194, 210, 275v, 309.

bokerem *n*. type of cloth, buckram 308v.

bo(o)le *n*. Armenian bole, type of clay made red by iron oxide 99, 135, 161v, 171v, 178v, 179v, 186, 223, 240v, 256v, 257v, 259, 260, 275v, 290, 290v, 297, 298, 298v, 303v; *b. armoniac* 171, 178v, 258v. See **gal(le), talowe**.

bolte *imp*. strain 91; **y-bultid** *p. p*. 83v.

bo(o)n þat is in an herte-is hert(e) *n*. cartilage inside a hart's heart 182, 187v, 189v.

borage *n*. Boraginaceae, *Borago officinalis*, borage 59v, 64v, 67v, 68, 171v, 186v, 187, 220v, 307v; *b. floures* 55, 141v, 215v; *iuse of b*. 186, 220. See **sirip, sugur**.

boras, borace *n*. borax, hydrated sodium borate, once thought to be a vegetable gum, 100v, 140v.

bottir, buttir *n*. butter 49, 63v, 64, 111, 111v, 119v, 123v, 145, 146v, 150, 151, 157v, 161, 161v, 223, 266, 266v, 267v, 271, 272, etc.

y-braied *p. p*. broken into small bits 97, 123.

brayn *n*. brain 50v, 51v-52v, 55v, 56v, 58, 64, 71, 71v, 77v, 98, 98v, 99v, 106, 106v, 120v, 169, 220; *foreparty of þe b*. brain's front ventricle 52; *myddel of þe b*. middle ventricle 52, 58; *principal places of þe b*. ventricles 65, 70v, 71; *turnyng (up) of þe b*. vertigo 51, 52, 52v, 71v, 231, 236.

brake *v*. vomit 76.

bran(ne) *n*. bran 85, 104, 170v, 267, 273v, 198, 302v; *barliche b*. 267; *clensing of b*. liquid from bran that has been washed and strained 146v, 150v, 166v, 170v, 249, 249v; *whete b*. 63v, 73, 123, 266v, 273, 287v, 288.

bras *n*. copper, either metallic or in an alloy with other metals 84v, 88v, 89v; *lymail of b*. brass filings 89.

brasen *adj*. made of brass 102, 104v.

bred(e), breed *n*. bread 258, 202v, 206; *barliche b*. 67v, 240; *crommes of (whete) b*. 80, 111v, 166v; *rye b*. 67v; *soure (whete) b*. 83, 239v, 240; *tostid b*. 74, 206; *whete b*. 181; *white b*. 302; **loof** *n*. loaf of bread; *croust of a l*. 97; *crummes of an hote l*. 82v.

brede *n*. breadth 85.

breem *n*. bream 181v. See **fysshe**.

brenyng *vbl n*. burning 53, 73v, 90v, 248, 194v, 206v, 212v, 214, 276, 279, 285, 302, 305v; *ppl. adj*. 55v, 66v, 257v, 281v, 303v.

brenneþ *pr. 3 sg*. burns 242v; **bren(n)e** *imp*. 101v, 105v, 258, 298, 302v; **brent** *p. p*. 305v; **(y)-brent(e)** *ppl. adj*. 63, 64v, 74, 88v, 89v-90v, 127v, 128, 129v, 130, 133, 178v, 192v, 271, 275, 220v, 308v, 309.

breris þat growen in þe fildis *n. pl*. prob. Rosaceae, *Rubus caesius*, dewberries 283v.

brest(e), breest *n.*, **brestis** *pl.* chest 48v, 56, 121, 122, 122v, 123v, 134v, 144v, 147, 147v, 149, 150-151v, 153, 154, 154v, 157v, 158v, etc.

breþe, breeþ *n.* breath 67, 144v, 148, 155, 162v, 164v, 169, 176v, 182v, 228, 234, 248, 207.

breþen *v.* breathe 162v, 163; **breþiþ** *pr. 3 sg.* 154; **breþen** *3 pl.* 153; *narow-y-breþid* short of breath 164.

breþing *vbl. n.* 52v, 61v, 66v, 71, 71v, 143v, 155v, 158v, 163v, 164, 164v, 173v, 182v, 183, 185v, 231.

bridlym *n.* birdlime 75v, 154v.

bries *n. pl.* eyelashes 99v, 103v, 104v-105v.

brymston, brenston *n.* sulphur 69v, 136v.

brionie see **go(u)rde.**

broke (ballokid) *adj.* having a scrotal hernia, ruptured 296v, 299v.

brome *n.* Leguminosae, *Sarothamnus scoparius*, broom 51.

broþþes *n. pl.* broths 170, 257v.

brovn *adj.* brown 76. See **rede.**

browes *n. pl.* brows, forehead 53, 76, 176v.

bruse *imp.* crush, bruise 128, 146; **y-brusid** *p. p.* 98; **brusyng** *vbl. n.* crushing 169, 305.

burnet *n.* Rosaceae, *Sanguisorba officinalis*, great burnet (L *bruneta*) 282v, 283v, 284.

buttockis *n. pl.* buttocks 305.

calamina *n.* prob. calamine, a hydrated zinc silicate ore, or zinc carbonate 88v, 89v, 90v, 92, 94.

calamynt(e) calament(e) *n.* Labiatae, *Calamintha officinalis*, calamint 50, 59v, 63v, 85, 103, 115, 141v, 142, 148v, 149v, 151v, 160v, 174v, 183, 189v, 222v, 226v, 231, 234, 234v, etc.; *floures of c.* 273v, 298; *iuse of c.* 239.

calamus aromaticus/aramaticus *n.* Araceae, *Acorus calamus*, sweet flag 76v, 122v, 160v, 161, 230, 230v, 241, 250.

*****calcant** see **attrament.**

****camapiteos** *n.* Labiatae, *Ajuga chamaepitys*, ground pine 219v.

camedreos *n.* Labiatae, *Teucrium chamaedrys*, wall germander 76v, 192v, 219v; *iuse of c.* 105; *rotes of c.* 138.

camomil(le), camemyl(le), camamille *n.* Compositae, *Chamaemelum nobile*, chamomile 69, 73v, 122v, 123v, 139v, 140, 250, 259, 290v; *c. floures* 84.

camphor(e), campher(e), camfer *n.* gum from juice of Lauraceae, *Cinnamomum camphora*, camphor tree 80, 88v, 91v, 94, 103v, 104v, 109, 152, 153, 182, 245, 261, 216, 300v.

cancre, canker *n.* apostem that appears as an external open sore 75, 99v, 101v, 120v, 129, 129v, 300, 302, 303. See **crabbe.**

y-cancrid, y-cankrid *p. p.* afflicted with **cancre** 139v, 302v.

canel *n.* bark of Lauraceae, *Cinnamomum zeylancium,* cinnamon tree 54v, 62, 64v, 76v, 124v, 125, 131v, 132v, 138, 141v, 142v, 152, 153v, 162, 173, 178, 182, 186v, 187, 225v, etc.

cap(p)aris, caperis *n. pl.* Capparidaceae, *Capparis spinosa,* caper bushes 77, 250, 217, 218v, 219; *leues of c.* 271; *stalkis of c.* 216v.

carabe *n.* Leguminosae, *Ceratonia siliqua,* St. John's bread 171v, 179, 179v.

cardamomum, cardamomi *n.* seeds of Zingiberaceae, *Elettaria cardamomum,* cardamom 54v, 55, 60, 64v, 103, 113, 132v, 141, 182, 187, 225v, 226v, 230v-231v, 234v, 250, 200v, 201, 220v, etc.; *c. boþe of þe more and of þe lasse* larger cardamoms are from *Elettaria,* smaller from **amomum** 76v.

cardiacle *n.* general term for heart disease 48v, 101v, 182, 184, 187, 187v, 188v-190, 191, 193v, 200v.

carewey, carewai *n.* Umbelliferae, *Carum carvi,* caraway 54v, 60, 103, 167, 174, 230v, 231v, 241, 246v, 199v, 278v, 283, 284; *seed of c.* 117, 123, 234.

carloke *n.* Cruciferae, *Sinapis arvensis,* charlock (L *eruco*) 59v.

carpobalsamum *n.* fruit of Burseraceae, *Balsamodendron opobalsamum,* balsam of Gilead 189v, 230v, 246v, 201. See **bawme (þat is an onment), opobalsamum, zilobalsamum.

carses, carsen *n. pl.* Cruciferae, *Lepidum sativum,* garden cress (L *nasturcium*) 59v, 68, 141v, 142, 263, 268v, 269, 199v, 206, 278; **carsede, carse sede** 83, 273v, 214v, 298v; *iuse of c.* 73, 137v; *watir* **c.** *n. Rorippa nasturtium-aquaticum,* watercress (L *nasturcium aquaticum*) 267; *3erde* **c.** *n. Lepidium sativum* (L *nasturcium ortolanum*) 267. See **oyl(e).**

cassia fistula *n.* pudding-like substance inside pods of Leguminosae, *Cassia fistula,* purging cassia 146, 178, 181, 188v, 221v, 233v, 249, 261v, 201v.

cassie, cassia lignea *n.* 62, 225v, 230, 250; **zilocassia, zilocassie** *n.* 201, 201v; both terms mean the bark of Lauraceae, *Cinnamomum cassia,* cassia bark tree.

cast(e), casten, kast (*up*) *v.* vomit 50, 53v, 61, 76, 188v, 192, 221v, 225, 226, 226v, 228v, 234v-235v, 236v-239, etc.; **castiþ** *pr. 3 sg.* 60, 224v, 231, 243, 270v, 207v; **casten** *pl.* 191; **cast** *pr. subj. sg.* 247v; **cast(e)** *imp.* throw 50v, 54, 54v, 56v, 152v, 176v, 177v, 188v, 194, 233v, 246v, 249, 260, 267, 275, 197, 197v, 290, 293, 298, etc; **(y)-cast(e)** *p. p.* thrown 160v, 170v, 275. See **spue, volaten.**

casting *vbl. n.* vomiting 226v, 232, 234v, 236v, 239v-240v, 242, 247, 247v, 251v, 203v, 281v.

castor(e), castory(e) *n.* dried perineal glands of beaver or their secretions 62, 62v, 63v, 68v-70, 73, 73v, 76, 88v, 112v, 117v, 119v, 124v, 136, 140v, 141, 142, 173, etc. See **oyl(e).**

cat(h)alempsie *n.* epilepsy caused by illness of organs other than the brain or stomach 65, 66v, 67v, 68, 69v, 70v, 270v.

cathmie, cathmia *n.* ore containing gold or silver 88, 88v, 89v; *c. argente* 87v.

caul(e) *n.* Cruciferae, *Brassica* spp., cabbage (L *caulis*); *c. leef* 110, 115, 303; *c. seed* 141; *c.-wortis* 53v, 67v; *iuse of c.* 51; *iuse of wilde c., B. oleracea,* wild cabbage 140v; ** **macematicon** ? = *mabethematicon,* cabbage juice 76v.

cause *n.*, **-s** *pl.* case 86, 92, 110, 124, 134v; cause 56, 71v, 78v, 95v, 96, 99, 103, 105v, 109v, 110, 122, 122v, 125, 139, 142, 147, 153, 158v, 159, 162v, etc.

celidon(e) *n.* Papaveraceae, *Chelidonium majus,* greater celandine (L *celidonia*) 79v, 102, 102v, 103v, 209, 214, 307; *iuse of c.* 90, 94, 94v, 102v.

cene see **sene.**

centori(e) *n.* Gentianaceae, *Centaurium erythraea,* lesser centaury or poss. *Blackstonia perfoliata,* greater centaury 69, 97, 113, 174, 271, 209, 217; *iuse of c.* 73v, 115v, 116, 130, 271v, 272; *iuse of les c.* 238, 271v, 205v. Cf. MED.

centrum-galli *n.* 69v, 88v; **gallitricum** *n.* 103 both terms mean Labiatae, *Salvia horminoides,* wild clary.

cerfoil *n.* Umbelliferae, *Anthriscus cerefolium,* chervil 309.

ceruse *n.* lead carbonate, a white powder 83v, 87v-88v, 91v, 92, 99v, 130v, 275, 303v, 309; *c. þat is clepid blank plum and white lede* 81.

ceterake, ceterac *n.* Polypodiaceae, *Ceterach officinarum,* rusty-back fern or spleenwort 150v, 197v, 219.

chacc(h)ing *vbl. n. c. of colde* becoming chilled 149; *c. of grete hete* becoming too warm 172, 291.

chache *v.* absorb 169v; *c. a coughe* contract a cough 122; *pr. subj. sg.* 170v; **y-cau3t** *p. p., y-c. his rote* taken root 247v; *c. cold* become chilled 251v, 254v.

chaptir, chapt(i)re *n.* chapter 74v, 83v, 86, 92, 103v, 105v, 110v, 111v, 120, 129, 133, 138v, 146v, 155, 162, 170v, 172v, 181, 184, 221, etc.

cheyne, chyn[1] *n.* chin 73v, 128v, 188.

cheke *n.*, **-s, chechis** *pl.* cheek 106v, 120v, 133v, 134, 135v, 137, 137v, 164v, 165, 231.

chekenes *n. pl.* chickens 59v. See **blode.**

chekenmete, chikenmete, chikenweed *n.* Caryophyllaceae, *Stellaria media,* chickweed (L *ypia*) 89; *iuse of c.* 93v; *iuse of c. þat haþ a rede flour* Primulacea, *Anagallis arvensis,* scarlet pimpernel 82v; **oculus Christi** *n.* ? *S. media* 100; *iuse of o. c.* 87; *mussilage of o. c.* 91v.

che(e)s, chese *n.* cheese 49, 97v, 258.

chesteyn *n.*, **-es** *pl.* Fagaceae, *Castanea sativa,* chestnut tree 167, 173, 249, 257, 206; *iuse of c.* 115v; *quantite of a c.* size of a chestnut 283, 290, 292; *rindes of c.* 298.

chiboillis *n. pl.* spring onion (L *cepula*) 110. See **onyon.**

child(e) *n.* **children** *pl.* child 68v, 271, 294, 296v; *knave c.* 98v; *man c.* 119v; *meide c.* 57; *with c.* in childbirth 264; *childis vryn* 89v.

**chymole *n.* "erþe þat is founden vnder a gryndyng stone" (Ogden, *Guy de Chauliac,* p. 619) 171.

chyn(n)e, chyn(e)[2] *n.* spine 73v, 135, 277v, 279.

chiry *n.*, **-es, cheries** *pl.* Rosaceae, *Prunus avium,* wild cherry 233; *iuse of c.* 220v; *kirnels of c. stones* seeds inside cherry stones 284v.

ciceres *n. pl.* Leguminosae, *Cicer arietinum,* chick peas; *rede c.* 167.

cicori *n.* Compositae, *Cichorium intybus*, chicory 197v, 205v, 284v; **acori** error for *c*. 216v.

ciler see **siler**.

cineuei see **syneuey**.

ciperi *n.* Cyperaceae, *Cyperus longus*, galingale 64v. Cf. **galengal(e)**.

ciphac see **siphac**.

citernes *n. pl.* Rutaceae, *Citrus medica*, citron; *iuse of c.* 205v.

citonie *n.*, **-s** *pl.* Rosaceae, *Cydonia oblonga*, quince 148, 240, 247; *iuse of c.* 179, 188v; *seed of c.* 149v-150v, 156-157, 167, 168, 171v, 177v, 182v, 186v, 228v, 232v.

citre see **saffron**.

cytryn *adj.* dark red, esp. as a symptom of choleric illness 139, 158v, 163v, 177, 244, 264v, 194v, 211v, 212v.

clay þat is baked in an ouene *n.* oven-baked clay 62v.

clarifie *v.* cause foreign matter to settle out of liquid using egg whites and shells 69; *imp.* 69; **y-clarified** *ppl. adj.* 239v.

clene, cleen *adj.* pure 48, 58, 87, 106, 119v, 153v; healthy 56, 288v, 310v; not dirty 94, 130v, 141v, 170v, 192v, 251, 258, 259, 274v, 290v; with inedible matter removed 117, 144, 157, 162, 177, 183, 247; *c. of* free from 113.

clense(n) *v.* cleanse 50, 77v, 96, 96v, 112, 113, 114, 114v, 116, 138v, 174, 181, 250v, 208v, 302v, 305; **clenseþ** *pr. 3 sg.* 99, 171v, 179, 280v; **clensen** *3 pl.* 112, 113, 180, 225v; **clense** *imp.* 97, 108v, 130, 144, 153v, 156, 161, 161v, 171, 178, 182v, 222v, 231, 250v, 251, 256v, 258, 262v, 266v, 218v, etc.; **(y-)clensid** *p. p.* 63v, 69, 113, 124v, 146v, 152, 157, 167-168, 170v, 171v, 178v, 179, 181, 181v, 183v, 259v, 275, 213, etc.; **clensing** *vbl. n.* 181v, 256v.

cliftes *n. pl.* clefts (L *ragadie*) 305v.

clisterie, clesterie, clistre, clistir, clistring *n.*, **clisters** *pl.* enema 56v, 60v, 63v, 64, 69, 73v, 178, 192, 259-260, 266-267, 268v, 272, 273, 274v, 275, 198, etc.

clooþ, cloute, cloþ(e) *n.*, **-s** *pl.* growth covering the eye 75, 87, 92v; a piece of cloth 81v, 83, 87, 91, 91v, 93v, 95v, 102v, 109, 110v, 111v, 135v, 137, 170v, 233, 242, 245, 261, 275v, 277, etc.; *lynen c.* 77v, 83v-84v, 98v, 100v, 101v, 117, 127, 131, 132, 138v, 188, 192v, 249v, 266, 198, 306, 306v, 308. See **bokerem, horned c., serid c.**

clowes *n. pl.* dried flower buds of Myrtaceae, *Syzygium aromaticum*, clove tree 49v, 51, 54v, 60, 62, 64v, 103, 132v, 136v, 141, 152, 153v, 182, 189v, 192, 225v, 226v, 230, 240, 241, etc.

coconidie see **lauriole**.

cod *n.* scrotum 296v, 297, 303v-305.

cokil see **nigil(le)**.

colagoge, cologoge *n.* medicine acting to purge choler 77v, 136, 148, 155v, 186, 228v, 239, 266v, 196v, 216, 277, 292, 295, 306v.

co(o)lde[1], coold, cold *n.* physiological quality of coldness, opposite of heat 49v, 51v, 63, 70v, 80v, 82v, 83v-85, 85v, 92, 106-107, 109v, 110v, 111v, 116, 117v, 121v, etc.; atmospheric or environmental coldness 49v, 57v, 97, 99, 106, 106v, 121v, 129v, 130v, 133v, 147, 149, 151, 159, 164, 170v, 185v, 190, 190v, 194, etc.

co(o)lde[2], **cold** *adj.* having the physiological quality of coldness, opposite of heat 48, 50, 56v, 57v, 61v, 63, 67, 70, 70v, 76, 77, 78-79v, 82, 92, 101v, 106v, 108, etc.; *cold flouris* 300v; *c. herbis* 56v, 57v, 78v, 109, 129, 134v, 136, 157v, 167v, 187, 188, 230v, 245v, 266, 197, 208, 222, 277, 277v, 286, etc.; *c. seedis* 150, 197, 208v, 216v, 221, 282v, 283, 310; *seedis of c. herbis* 245; cold to touch, having atmospheric or environmental coldness 51v, 56v-57v, 64, 83, 85, 91v, 97v, 99, 108v, 127, 130, 133v, 135, 139, 143v, 144v, 150, 153v, etc. See **mete, oyn(e)ment, pillules, sirip.**

co(o)ldenes, co(o)ldnes *n.* physiological quality of coldness, opposite of heat 48v, 98, 224v, 229v-230v, 232, 269v, 198v, 291v; coldness to touch 139, 147.

coler(e), coller *n.* choler 48v, 52, 53, 54, 55v, 58-59, 61v, 66v, 67, 75, 76, 77v, 78v, 85v, 99v, 107, 116v, etc.; *cytryn c.* dark red choler 163v; *rede c.* red or egg-yolk-colored choler 163v, 203.

col(l)erik(e) *adj.* containing choler 56, 189, 224, 227, 229, 232v, 237, 237v, 241v, 252, 252v, 261v, 266, 272v, 203v, 294v; having a choleric complexion 235v.

colet *n.* collect 51v.

coliandre *n.* Umbelliferae, *Coriandrum sativum,* coriander 60; *c. seed* 246; *iuse of c.* 107v.

colides *n.* illness of the stomach or guts characterized by violent contraction of the guts 251v.

colike *n.* colic 309, 309v.

coli(i)s, coolis, collis *n.* broth 166v; *c. of a capon* 170v; *c. of a cheke* 151; *c. of fisshe* 180v; *c. of an (olde) hen* 126, 151, 170v.

collaquindida see **go(u)rde.**

collica passio *n.* illness of the colon 244, 253v, 263v, 269v, 273, 274v, 279v, 297. Cf. **colike.**

colliry(e), *n.*, -s *pl.* eye medicine 83, 83v, 85, 87v, 88, 90-93v, 96, 96v, 97v, 98v, 99v, 100, etc.; also 114v, 117v.

colofoyne, colofonie, colofyne *n.* resin from residue of distillation of pine tar, Greek pitch 130v, 144, 257v, 298v.

colon *n.* large intestine 263v, 264.

y-colo(u)rid *p. p.* colored 255v, 195, 203.

colour(e) *n.* color 56, 76, 139, 147v, 151, 158v, 160, 163v, 164, 185, 243, 255v, 265, 270, 274v, 194v, 195v, 202v, 203, 203v, etc.

columbine *n.* Ranunculaceae, *Aquilegia vulgaris,* columbine 137v, 290v, 298.

comfery(e) *n.* Boraginaceae, *Symphytum officinale,* comfrey (L *consolida*) 97, 240, 257, 290v, 297, 298v, 299, 299v, 310v; *iuse of c.* 298; **symphite** *n.* Boraginaceae, *Symphytum officinale,* comfrey (L *simphitus*) 171; **myddel c. n.* Labiatae, *Ajuga reptans,* bugle 97. See **daies-i3e.**

comyn *n.* seeds of Umbelliferae, *Cuminum cyminum,* cumin 51, 54v, 55, 60, 84v, 87, 89, 97, 102, 103, 110, 112v, 117, 135v, 160, 229v, 230, 231v, 233, 240v, etc.

compassion *n.* sympathy 185.

complexion *n.* balance of humors or qualities within a member or the body 59v, 140, 155, 227, 252v, 310; bodily constitution 64, 72v, 143v, 256, 301.

componed *ppl. adj.* (of a medicine) made of two or more ingredients 79v, 81. See **oximel.**

confortatif *adj.* (of a medicine) having a comforting effect 98v, 293v, 301v.

confortatives, confortatifis *n. pl.* medicines having a comforting effect 78v, 79, 86v, 90v, 91v, 93, 98v, 100, 100v, 276v.

(y)-congelid *ppl. adj.* (of blood) hardened and thickened by cold, clotted 96, 97, 171v.

congir *n.* large eel, conger 49.

conglutinatif *adj.* (of a medicine) having a restorative effect 181.

consolidatif *adj.* (of a medicine) having a soothing effect 296v.

consolidatiues *n. pl.* medicines having a soothing effect 93, 96v, 100, 100v, 114, 114v, 116, 127, 177, 251, 310v.

constrictif *adj.* (of a medicine) strictory 240. See **strictory.**

contageous *adj.* noxious 130v.

contrari *n.* an opposite 227.

contrary(e) *adj.* opposite 50v, 116v; *c. to* (of a medicine) acting against 108.

cop of þe nose *n.* tip of the nose 77v, 128v.

coperos see **attrament.**

coral *n.* coral 64v, 127, 189v; *reed c.* 103v, 171; *whijt c.* 103v, 171, 186v.

corigiole *n.* prob. Polygonaceae, *Polygonum aviculare*, knotgrass (L *corigiola*) 171.

cor(r)isif, corosif *adj.* (of a medicine) consuming flesh 80, 88, 89v, 96.

cor(r)osiues, corrisyues *n. pl.* medicines consuming flesh 89-90v, 93, 95, 95v, 96v, 118v; *esy c.* mild corrosives 88v, 95v; *stronge c.* harsh corrosives 88v, 95v, 96v. See **freteris.**

corrup(te) *adj.* tainted, putrid 55v, 59v, 61, 70v, 71, 85v, 92v, 102v, 106-107v, 112, 116, 116v, 119, 120, 120v, 124, 129v, etc.

corruption *n.,* **-s** *pl.* putrefaction, deterioration 114v, 130v, 132, 135, 138v, 154, 175, 176-177, 224, 227v, 264v, 208v; *c. of þe eire* polluted air 206v.

co(o)st, coste *n.* Compositae, *Chrysanthemum balsamita*, costmary 54v, 88, 112v, 137v, 141v, 142v, 178, 225v, 242, 204v.

costif(fe) *adj.* constipated, constipating 64, 69, 73v, 86, 166v, 178, 185, 238v, 239v, 240, 241v, 242v, 243, 249, 257v, 258, 194v, 198, 210, 212 etc. See **mete.**

costifnes *n.* constipation 176, 309.

coton *n.* Malvaceae, *Gossypium* spp., material from cotton bush 84, 108v, 111, 249v, 273, 278v; *seed of c.* 223.

coughe, co(u)3h(e), coghe *n.*, *-s pl.* disease whose primary symptom is cough, cough as a symptom of another disease 122, 149, 151v, 154-155, 156v, 157, 159, 160, 161-163, 165, 165v, 166v, 170v, 169v, etc.; *colde c.* a cough caused by cold humors 153, 159, 173v, 174, 177, 247; *drye c.* cough producing little sputum 148, 149v, 151, 154v, 161v, 163v, 168; *hoot c.* cough caused by hot humors 149v, 151, 177; *moyst c.* cough producing sputum 147, 147v.

coughe see **mylke.**

cou3hing, coughing, cowghing *vbl. n.* act of coughing 151v, 159, 164v, 165v, 166, 168v, 169v, 181v, 297v.

crabbe *n.*, *-s pl.* crab 173, 174v, 177v, 178v, 180v; **watir cankre** 90v.

crampe *n.* disease causing spasm 70v, 74v; spasm 72, 232, 195v.

cucumer *n.* Cucurbitaceae, *Cucumis sativus*, cucumber; *sedis of c.* 197.

cup(pe) *imp.* phlebotomize with a cupping device 84v, 302, 304; **(y)-cuppid** *p. p.* 60v, 68v, 77v, 84, 86, 112v, 125, 128v, 134v, 193, 278v, 305, 308.

cuppe *n.* bleeding glass or similar device 245v.

curable *adj.* treatable 87. See **incurable.**

cure *n.*, *-s pl.* cure 51v, 53v, 56v, 57, 116v, 174, 243, 263v, 276v, 309.

cuscute *n.* Convolvulaceae, *Cuscuta epithymum*, dodder of thyme 54, 68, 201v, 204v, 218v; *iuse of c.* 205v.

day, *n.*, *-es pl.* day 48, 48v, 60, 68, 71, 72, 81v, 86v, 87, 94, 95v, 101v, 102, 104v, 113, 113v, 125v, 132, 132v, 144, etc.

daies-i3e, daiesy *n.* Compositae, *Bellis perennis*, daisy 97, 257, 290v, 298v, 299, 310v; *iuse of d.* 298. Poss. same as **myddel* **comferey.**

damasenes *n. pl.* fruit of Rosaceae, *Prunus domestica* ssp. *insititia*, damson 167v.

datis *n. pl.* fruit of Palmae, *Phoenix dactylifera*, date palm 168v, 233v, 280; *fleisshe of d.* 250.

dauke *n.* Umbelliferae, *Daucus carota*, wild carrot 76v, 167, 172v, 231v, 246v, 250, 199v, 209, 278v, 283, 283v, 284; *seed of d.* 117.

decoccion *n.*, *-s pl.* liquid medicine made by cooking 61, 189v, 209v.

deed, dede *adj.* dead 53, 59, 67, 72, 303. See **dye, token.**

    deef *adj.* deaf 112, 120.

deefnes, def(e)nes *n.* deafness 105v, 113, 118-119, 120.

    deeþ see **dye, token.**

defie, defien *v.* digest, (of a medicine) consume and disburse harmful matter 67v, 128v, 142, 159, 165v, 186v, 225, 231v, 235, 242v, 251, 198v, 212, 214, 215, 277, 291v, 292, 295; **defieþ** *pr. 3 sg.* 50, 224, 224v, 195; **defien** *pl.* 203, 211; **defie** *imp.* 237v, 238, 196v, 218; **defied** *p. p.* 53v, 54, 78, 145v, 158v, 160, 163v, 190, 254, 261v, 199, 205v; **defieng** *vbl. n.* 190. See **digestion.**

demegreyn *n.* ache on one side of the head 50v-51v.

desiccatiues *n. pl.* drying medicines 125.

deute *n.* an ointment 143v, 144, 149, 157v, 168, 168v, 237v, 267, 209v, 218, 218v, 278, 280.

develis *n. pl.* devils 58v.

***diaanisum** *n.* electuary based on anise 188v, 209v.

diabetes *n.* disease of the kidneys causing excessive urination 285, 291, 291v, 294v, 301v.

diacalamentum *n.* electuary based on calamint 151v, 160v, 225, 246v, 198v, 206, 209v, 300v, 308.

diacameron *n.* costly electuary 186v, 199.

***diacap(p)aris** *n.* electuary based on capers 217, 218.

diacene *n.* electuary based on senna 225, 239, 218, 220, 220v.

****diaceraseos** *n.* electuary based on cherries 216v, 220v.

diacinimum *n.* electuary based on cumin 160v, 225, 246, 263, 198v.

diacitoniton *n.* electuary based on quinces 188v, 196v; *d. muscata* d. with musk added 186v; *d. pat is cold* cooling d. 229, 247; *d. pat is hoot* heating d. 247, 198v.

diacodion *n.* electuary based on poppies 170, 256v, 257, 260v, 290, 301v; *d. pat is* **diapapauer** 170; **diapapauer** 149v, 173v, 186v; *colde dp.* cooling d. 155v.

diadragagantum *n.* electuary based on gum tragacanth 159v, 167, 170, 232v, 215v; *colde d.* cooling d. 153, 173v, 263v, 286; *d. pat is hote* heating d. 153, 153v.

diagalange *n.* electuary based on galingale 225v. Cf. MED.

diagredii, diagredium *n.* electuary based on scammony 55, 201v, 216, 221.

diamargariton *n.* electuary based on pearls 186v, 246, 269, 199.

diameron *n.* electuary based on mulberries 143v.

****diampnes** *n.* disease of the urinary bladder causing excessive urination 285, 291v, 293v, 294v.

diantos *n.* electuary based on rosemary 252, 269, 198v, 200v; *d. muscate* d. with musk added 186v.

****diapagamum, diapigamum** *n.* electuary based on rue 160v, 225.

diapapauer see **diacodion**.

diapenidion *n.* electuary based on barley sugar 148, 149, 149v, 151v, 167, 170, 173v, 232v, 215v, 286.

****diaperetron, diapiretrum** *n.* electuary based on pellitory 160v, 162.

****diaprassium** *n.* electuary based on horehound 151v, 225.

diaprunis *n.* electuary based on plums 196v, 208v, 277, 282, 283, 292, 292v, 300v.

diarodon *n.* electuary based on roses 186v, 218; *d. abbatis* 182, 229, 252, 196v; *d. of Galien's making* 199; *d. of Iulien's making* 199.

diarria *n.* disease characterized by diarrhea containing no blood or sloughing from the guts 261v. Cf. **dissinterie**. See **flux(e)**.

****diarris** *n.* electuary based on iris 148, 151v.

diaspermaticon *n.* electuary based on various kinds of seeds 189, 231, 231v, 246, 268, 218.

diatrionpiperion *n.* electuary based on three kinds of pepper 151v, 225, 225v, 227, 263, 199, 206.

diazinziber *n.* electuary based on ginger 225v.

dye *v.* die 172, 176v, 190v. See **deed, token**.

dieten *v.* adjust the diet 232v, (*refl.*) 53v; **diete** *subj.* 283; **diete** *imp.* 172v, 240, 260v, 198v, 199v, 206, 293v, 297v, 301v, 302, 310; **dietid** *p. p.* 64, 67, 74, 173v, 226v, 241, 242, 249. See **reule.**

dieting *vbl. n.,* **-is** *pl.* diet 63, 78, 86, 109, 110v, 127, 150v, 155v, 160, 166v, 170, 173, 181, 181v, 186v, 229, 229v, 257v, 267, 216v, etc.

digestion *n.* digestion 153v, 169, 230v, 208v, 211.

dissinterie, dissenterie *n.* disease characterized by diarrhea containing blood and sloughing from the guts 252v, 253v-254v, 255v, 256, 260v, 261v, 262, 263, 273, 274, 201v, 289v, 292v, 293v, 295, 306v, 307, 310. Cf. **diarria.** See **flux(e).**

dissolutiues, dissolatiues *n. pl.* heating medicines that dissolve harmful matter 78v-80, 82, 86v, 121v, 183, 189, 225v, 208, 209, 305.

dissolutif *adj.* (of a medicine) heating to dissolve harmful matter 214v, 215; *d. herbis* 59v.

dissolue *v.* (of a medicine) dissolve harmful matter 78v, 82, 139v, 189, 214v; **dissolueþ** *pr. 3 sg.* 77v, 78v; **dissoluen** *pl.* 132; **dissolue** *imp.* 97, 105v; **dissolued** *p. p.* 109, 153, 156v, 157v, 161, 310v.

distempre *n.,* **distemprances** *pl.* disturbance of humoral balance 237v.

distemp(e)rid *ppl. adj.* having the humoral balance disturbed 236, 252v, 204-205, 217v, 277v, 292, 310; blended (with) 240v.

distemp(e)ring *n.,* **-s** *pl.* disturbance of humoral balance 235v, 242v, 194-195, 196, 196v, 198v, 199v, 200, 204v-205v, 277v, 278, 291, 292. See **tempriþ.**

distille *imp.* instill 55; **distillid** *p. p.* formed into droplets 137; **stille** *imp.* gather droplets from 309.

ditteny, ditandre *n.* Labiatae, *Amaracus dictamnus,* crete dittany (L *diptamus*) 76v, 192v.

dodden *imp.* trim the hair short 124.

doun-ri3t *adv.* face down 60.

dragagant(um) *n.* gum tragacanth from the tree Leguminosae, *Astragalus* spp. 64v, 76v, 83v, 87v, 88, 91v, 97v, 99v, 130, 145v-146v, 148, 150, 150v, 152, 153, 153v, 155v, 156, etc., also 156v, 161, 310v.

dragance see **serpentarie.**

dramme, dr. *n.,* **drammes** *pl.* drachm 51v, 54-55, 57, 57v, 62, 62v, 64, 73v, 76v, 83v, 87v, 88, 91v, 94v, 99v, 103, 103v, 117v, etc.

drastis *n. pl.* dregs 279, 305v. See **oyl(e), wyn(e).**

drede *n.* dread 58v; *for d. of* for fear of 86v, 113v, 178, 252, 267.

drede *v.* be wary 58v, 283; **dredist** *pr. 2 sg.* are afraid 310v; **dreden** *3 pl.* fear 58v.

dredeful *adj.* fearful 58v, 203v.

dreem *v.* dream 106v.

dremes *n. pl.* dreams 203v.

drye *adj.* having the physiological quality of dryness, opposite of moistness 78v, 95v, 179, 181v, 227, 291, 293; lacking in moisture 48, 95, 113, 138v, 140, 141, 141v, 149, 154v, 155v, 159v, 161, 166v, 167v-168v, 178v, 181, 183v, 228v, etc. See **coughe, mete.**

drye *v.* dry 112v, 125, 138v, 308v; **drieþ** *pr. 3 sg.* 77v, 95, 178v, 264v; **(y)-dried** *p. p.* 95, 144v, 179, 212, 309v; **drie** *subj.* 178; **drye** *imp.* 85, 91, 94v, 102v; **drieng** *vbl. n.* 85. See **sirip**.

dry(e)nes *n.* physiological quality of dryness, opposite of moistness 48, 48v, 49v, 55v, 106, 148, 149v, 151, 151v, 155, 176, 194, 195v, 196, 200, 207, 291, 310v; dryness to the touch 55v, 194v.

drinke, drinking *n.*, **-is** *pl.* that which is drunk 60, 66, 69, 74, 78, 101v, 122, 138v, 159v, 162, 163v, 171, 187v, 221, 221v, 224v, 226v, 228-229, etc.; drinking 122, 151, 224v, 228, 231v, 234, 246, 265, 228v, 250, 251v, 262, 291v, 293.

drinke, drinken *v.* drink 55, 68v, 69, 74v, 82v, 122v, 128v, 131v, 150, 150v, 151v, 161v, 171, 172v, 181, 182, 189v, 193-194, etc.; **drinkeþ** *pr. 3 sg.* 219; **drinken** *3 pl.* 71v, 147, 294v; **drinke** *pr. 3 subj.* 256v, 205v; **drinke** *imp.* 51v, 54v, 87, 102, 142, 251, 309v; **(y-)dronke(n), drunken** *p. p.* 52v, 68v, 193, 228, 259, 263v, 271v, 272, 217, 291v, 294, 295v, 306v.

drit(te) *n.* feces 65v, 243, 244, 244v, 255, 255v, 262, 264v-266, 195v, 196, 203v, 211v; *d. of a man* 88v, 244, 256v; *d. of euery beste* 88v; *ganderis d.* 145v; *swynes d.* 127v.

drope *n.*, **-is** *pl.* drop 105, 108v, 111v, 115, 117, 119v, 270, 272v, 281.

dropesy *n.* dropsy 54v, 244v, 195, 195v, 306, 308v.

duretike *adj.* (of medicines) opening the pores 197v, 215, 218v, 219v, 279v, 302v; *d. herbis* 197, 200; *colde d. erbis* 197; *hote d. erbis* 197v, 218v, 309v; *d. sedes* 200, 209v; *cold d. sedis* 197; *hote d. sedes* 197v, 200, 209v. See **oximel**.

duretikes *n. pl.* medicines opening the pores, diuretics 208v; *cold d.* cooling d. 197v, 279v; *hoot d.* heating d. 208v, 279v.

echyng see **yc(c)hyng**.

egrimoyn(e), agrimonie *n.* Rosaceae, *Agrimonia eupatoria*, agrimony 49, 94v, 99v, 102, 102v, 103v, 111v, 138, 217, 307.

ey(e), eg(ge) *n.*, **eggis, eiren** *pl.* egg 149, 161, 173, 183v, 241v, 296; *crowes e.* 68v; *gleyr of e.* beaten egg whites 81v-82v, 91v, 97v, 105, 109v, 265, 197v, 290, 297v, 308; *quantite of an e.* size of an egg 62; *quantite of an e.-shelful* 161v; *shellis of e.* 69, 128; *white of e.* 51v, 69, 81, 81v, 83v, 87v, 93, 97v, 99, 109, 111, 127, 135, 137, 157v, 167v, 186, 188v, 240v, 253, etc.; *ʒolkis/ʒelkis of e.* 80, 126v, 127, 146, 149, 163v, 173, 249v, 290v, 299v, 302, 303, 309. See **ampte**.

eyer *n.* air 52v, 226, 227v, 228. See **corruption**.

elde see **o(o)lde**.

el(l)eborus niger *n.* Ranunculaceae, *Helleborus niger*, Christmas rose 55, 68, 115v, 238v, 239.

*electarie *n.* Cucurbitaceae, *Ecballium elaterium*, squirting cucumber; *rote of e.* 238v.

electuari, electuare, lectuarie *n.*, **-s** *pl.* pastelike medicine usually having a sugar base 64, 78, 103, 148, 149, 150v, 156, 161, 167, 170, 172v, 171v, 174, 177, 177v, 179v, 180, 187v, 222, 225v, etc; *coolde e.* 186v, 188v, 229, 278, 289v; *hote e.* 160v, 186v, 194, 222, 225, 227, 233v, 234, 263.

elena campana see **hors(e)hel.**

el(l)ern *n.* Caryophyllaceae, *Sambucus nigra*, elder tree *iuse of e.* 271v; *e. bowes* 49; *croppis of e.* 307. See **oyl(e).**

(e)elis *n. pl.* eels 49, 257v. See **fat(nes), grees.**

elme *n.* Ulmaceae, *Ulmus glabra*, wych elm; *rynde of e.* 127v.

emachite(s), amachites *n.* prob. red hematite, iron ore with impurities 88v, 93, 96v, 97, 127, 179v, 256v, 275v, 298v.

emblici see **mirabolani(s).**

emeroides *n. pl.* hemorrhoids 126, 295, 305v, 308, 308v; the 5 hemorrhoidal veins 305v.

encense, incense *n.* incense, whose main component was **olibanum** q.v. 76v, 82, 85, 87v, 88v, 90, 91v, 92, 93, 96v, 97v, 99, 99v, 114, 114v, 122v, 127, 134v, 136v, 137, etc.

encheson *n.*, **-s** *pl.* cause (of disease) 71v, 98v, 107, 118, 119, 138, 154v, 166v, 169v, 175v, 181, 183, 183v, 221v, 232, 235, 242, 252, 254, 261v, etc.

endyue *n.* Compositae, *Lactuca virosa*, wild lettuce 48, 80, 180, 233, 249, 198, 204v, 208, 208v, 282v, 286; *iuse of e.* 81v, 87v, 94v, 97.

enkis *n. pl.* inks 150. See **galles.**

epilencie, epilence *n.* disease caused by moist humors congesting the brain 52, 52v, 64v-66, 67, 69v, 70, 70v, 72, 147, 269v, 270v. See **falling yvel.**

epityme see **tyme.**

erbis see **herbe.**

(e)ere, 3eer(e) *n.*, **(e)eris, eren, 3e(e)res** *pl.* ear 54v, 105v-114v, etc.

ers *n.* anus 253v, 272, 272v, 274, 275, 274v, 282, 284v, 289v, 305v, 306v, 308-309; *e.-hole* 294v, 296.

erþe appel *n. iuse of e. a.* Primulaceae, *Cyclamen neapolitanum*, sow bread 140v; **siclamen** *n.* sow bread 238v.

erþe þat liyþ bifore an oxe stalle *n.* 268.

esula *n.* Euphorbiaceae, *Euphorbia uralensis*, esula 55, 263.

ete, eten *v.* eat 49, 51, 53v, 68v, 70, 74v, 127, 131, 133, 149, 166v, 222, 224v, 225v, 226, 238, 241v, 245v, 249, 256, etc.; **etiþ** *pr. 3 sg.* 133v, 223, 224v, 227v, 254, 262, 220; **eten** *pl.* 71v, 202v; **ete** *subj.* 53v, 256v; **ete** *imp.* 309v; **(y)-ete, (y)-eten** *p. p.* 68v, 141, 161, 163, 183v, 224v, 227v, 234v, 236-237, 247v, 265, 196, 205v, 216v, 295v, 306v.

etike see **feuer.**

eting *vbl. n.* eating 122, 151, 231v, 234, 240v, 244v, 251v, 262.

euen(tide), euening *n.* evening 48v, 84v, 85v, 131v, 132v, 149, 152v, 161v, 162, 173, 174, 174v, 179v, 182, 189v, 251, 260v, 197, 215, 282, etc.

euforb(i)e *n.* gum from Euphorbiaceae, *Euphorbia resinifera*, officinal spurge 55, 62, 62v, 68, 69v, 73, 76v, 115v, 117v, 136, 136v, 287, 290, 307v, 308.

eufrace, eufras(e) *n.* Scrophulariaceae, *Euphrasia officinalis*, eyebright 80, 83v, 87, 88v, 92, 95v, 98v, 100v, 102-103v, 230v; *iuse of e.* 85, 91, 94v.

**exage *n.* 12 pennyweight, 6 oz. Troy (L *exagium*) 178v, 179.

experience *n.* test 166.

expulsif *n.* ability of the body to rid itself of something, a tendency to do so 254v. Cf. **retentif.**

extenuatif *adj.* (of a medicine) making something rarefied 219v.

falling yvel *n.* 64v, 68v epilepsy. See **epilencie.**

faste *v.* fast 70, 221, 300v, 310.

fasting[1] *vbl. n.* fasting 49v, 50v, 70, 147v, 151, 172, 188v, 225, 241, 270v. See **abstinence.**

fasting[2] *ppl. adj.* fasting 60, 87, 131, 228v, 237, 198v, 220, 307.

fat(nes) *n.* fat 108, 226, 287; *f. of bestis* 111v; *f. of a calfe* 111; *f. of an eel* 119v, 120; *f. of a goot* 160v; *f. of an henne* 100v; *f. of a qwaal* 88v.

fat *adj.* fatty 276. See **fysshe, mete.**

feisantis *n. pl.* pheasants 67.

felte *n.* piece of felt 267v.

femygreke *n.* Leguminosae, *Trigonella foenum-graecum*, fenugreek 63v, 73, 81v, 88, 93v, 144, 148v, 168v, 174, 183, 193, 223, 231v, 232v, 250, 258, 216v, 307. See **mele**[1].

fenel *n.* Umbelliferae, *Foeniculum vulgare*, fennel 49, 50, 54v, 55, 56v, 59v, 67v, 69v, 76v, 83v, 84, 92, 98, 98v, 99v, 102-103, 109v, 140, etc., also 197v; *f. root* 69, 81, 156v, 161, 167-168, 233, 197v, 219, 278, 283; *iuse of f.* 51, 54, 63v, 80, 84v, 85, 89, 89v, 91, 93v-94v, 102, 102v, 110, 246v, 290v; *seed of f.* 117, 123, 159v, 182, 183, 225v, 228v, 230, 231v, 234v, 246, 246v, 250, 262v, 197v, 199v, 208v, 209v, 280, 283, etc.

feren leues *n. pl.* fronds from a plant of the order Filicales: ferns 187.

festre, festring *n.* fistula, a hollow sinus 112, 112v, 114v, 302, 302v.

fete, feet *n. pl.* feet 48, 48v, 56v, 63, 121v, 170v, 187v, 238v, 245, 254v, 257, 211.

feuer *n.*, **-is** *pl.* fever, unnatural heat of the body 62v, 63, 64, 66v, 71v, 74v, 107, 121, 121v, 170, 170v, 173v, 174v, 175, 176, 176v, 178, 179v, 180v, 181, *etc.*; *f. cotidian* fever peaking daily 100v, 193; *(f.).* **etike** hectic fever 90v, 175v, 180v, 182, 182v, 185, 253v, 310v; *f. quarteyn* fever peaking every third day 60v, 193; *f. tercian* fever peaking every other day 48v, 78, 109, 126v, 248; *continuel f.* continuous fever 61, 165, 214; *kene f.* acute fever 170; *sharpe f.* acute fever 162v.

fich *n. quantite of a f.* size of a pea 174v.

fyer(e) *n.*, **-s** *pl.* fire 60, 69, 74v, 83, 89, 95, 100v, 104v, 115v, 119, 136v, 140v, 141v, 144, 144v, 153v, 167v, 180, 193v, 222, etc.

fyg(g)e *n.*, **-)is** *pl.* fruit of Moraceae, *Ficus carica*, fig tree 113, 140, 146, 149, 157, 159v, 160v, 161, 166v, 167v-168v, 183, 183v, 280, 308; *gretnesse of a f.* size of a fig 54, 132v, 157; *mylke of a f. tre* 140v.

figis *n. pl.* piles 305v, 308v.

filago *n.* prob. Compositae, *Gnaphalium uliginosum*, marsh cudweed 88v; *iuse of f.* 94v.

filbert *n.*; *quantite of a f.* size of a filbert nut 135v.

filipendula *n.* Rosaceae, *Filipendula vulgaris*, dropwort 219.

fyngir *n.*, **fyngris** *pl.* finger 64, 99, 131, 136, 173v, 191v, 232, 212, 215, 281v, 293, 299.

fysshe *n.*, **-s** *pl.* fish 59v, 132, 173, 180v; *f. not fat* 59v; *f. of myry watris* 67v; *f. of ryvers* 59v; *f. of stony placis* 59v; *fresshe f.* 49, 226; *freisshe-watir f.* 181v; *salt f.* 49; *scalid f.* 181v; *shalid f.* 67v, 229v. See **breem, fat(nes), perche, pike, roche.**

fleissheli, flesshili *adj.* fleshy 105; *f. desire* carnal desire 300.

fle(i)sshe *n.* flesh as food 101v, 132, 178v; *f. of dates* 250; *hertis f.* 67v; *oxe f.* 49; *shepes f.* 67v; *swynes f.* 67v; animal skin 158v, 254v, 255; human flesh 96, 118, 118v, 120v, 131, 131v, 178v, 303-304.

flevmagoge *n.* medicine purging phlegm 143, 148v, 159v, 199, 239, 295, 306v.

fleumatike *adj.* containing or characteristic of phlegm 49, 178, 189, 243, 285v; (of a person) with a complexion dominated by phlegm 71v, 235v, 310. See **mete.**

flevme *n.* the humor phlegm 48v, 49v, 53, 54, 58, 61, 61v, 66-67, 71, 71v, 73, 75, 75v, 77v, 83v, 84, 85v, 86, etc.; mucus, spittle 137; *clene f.* untainted phlegm 58; *glasy f.* intensely cold, wet phlegm 163, 244, 269, 272v, 273v; *kene f.* thin, sour phlegm 163v; *kyndeliche f.* natural, untainted phlegm 163, 244, 269; *salte f.* salty phlegm 143, 163, 175v, 228, 228v, 244, 254v, 255v, 265, 269, 272v; *soure f.* keen phlegm 244, 269; *swete f.* phlegm that is not salty 244, 269; *þynne f.* thin, cold phlegm 154v, 294v; *viscouse f.* thick, sticky phlegm 143, 154v, 161, 264v, 212, 294v; *herbis þat maken moche f.* 132.

flux(e) *n.*, **-is** *pl.* diarrhea 48v, 122v, 126v, 127, 147v, 170v, 176v, 178, 190v, 232v, 236, 240, 242v, 244, 248v, 251-253v, etc.; *bloodi f.* 224, 244v, 254, 260, 288v; *simple f.* diarrhea with barely digested food 176, 254; emissions from the body that purge it of harmful matter 53; a flowing 112v, 161v, 295, 308v. See **diarria, dissinterie, lienteri(e).**

**folii, folium *n.* leaves of trees of the cinnamon family, Lauraceae (L *folium*) 64v, 76v, 98v, 99v, 230v, 234v.

forbrent *ppl. adj.* burnt up (L *colericus*) 243.

foreheed *n.* forehead 56v-57v, 75, 77v, 81v, 83, 85v, 99, 106v.

fote *n.*, **fete, feet** *pl.* foot 48, 48v, 56v, 63, 121v, 170v, 187v, 238v, 239, 245, 254v, 257, 211, 214; **barfote** 294.

frenesy(e) *n.* apostem in the brain's front ventricle or in its skins caused by blood or choler 52, 55v, 56, 57v, 59, 118, 128; *coold f.* a kind of lethargy 61v.

frentike *adj.* afflicted with frenzy 57v, 224, 269v, 270; having an illness similar to frenzy 56.

frete, freten (*awei*) *v.* fret or corrode 96, 96v, 118v, 131; **fretiþ** *pr. 3 sg.* 94, 99v, 103v, 303; **freten** *p. p.* 94, 96v, 303; **freting** *ppl. adj.* freting, corrosive 80, 88.

freteris *n. pl.* corrosive medicines 94. See **cor(r)osiues**.

fru(y)t *n.*, **-is** *pl.* fruit 127, 172v, 181v, 238, 241v, 260v, 268v, 270v, 289v; *cold f.* 229v; *parles of f.* fruit peels 271; *ripe f.* 59v. See **mandrake**.

fume *n.*, **-s** *pl.* hot gases within the body 52, 65, 66, 154, 159, 191v, 209; smoke or vapor 123v, 307v.

fumigation *n.*, **-s** *pl.* treatment using smoke or vapors 108, 122v, 123, 134v, 136, 136v, 139v, 151v, 160v, 161v, 257v, 268, 273, 273v, 275, 306v, 307v, 308. See **stufe**.

fumiter *n.* Fumariaceae, *Fumaria officinalis*, fumitory 129. See **sirip**.

fundement, fondement *n.* anus, rectum 56v, 64, 73v, 243, 253v, 257v, 265v-266v, 270, 273, 273v.

furmenti, frumenti *n.* frumenty 249v, 258.

gal(le) *n.* substance in the gall bladder 272, 202v, 210v; gall bladder 202, 202v; *g. of eueriche beste* 80, 88v, 238; *g. of rauenge briddis* 88v; *bol(l)es g.* 73v, 88v, 100, 238, 271v, 272; *dogge g.* 68v; *swynes g.* 104; *weiþeres g.* 309v.

galbanum *n.* gum from Umbelliferae, *Ferula galbaniflua* 49, 76v, 135, 135v, 137, 144, 145v, 174v, 183v, 242, 298v.

galengal(e), galingal, galange *n.* Zingiberaceae, *Alpina officinarum*, galingale 54v, 64v, 76v, 103, 141, 160, 186v, 230, 230v, 241, 200-201, 220v. Cf. **ciperi**.

galles *n. pl.* oak galls, excrescence of an oak leaf caused by the action of insect larvae; ink was made from crushed galls, iron salts, and often carbon black and a gum 114, 135v, 145, 171, 186, 240, 242v, 251, 257, 258v, 259, 260, 275, 297, 298-299v; *g. þat enke is made of* 138; **oken apples, ooke applen** galls 55, 308v. See **enkis**.

**gallia muscata, gallie muscate *n.* medicine containing musk 132v, 182.

gallitricum see **centrum-galli**.

gardens *n. pl.* gardens 59.

gargarisme *n.*, **gargarisms** *pl.* liquid or semisolid medicine held in the mouth or chewed but not swallowed, a gargle 136v, 139v, 140, 141, 142v, 143v, 145, 146, 148v, 149, 173, 180, 180v, 189, 189v.

garlik(e), garleke *n.* Liliaceae, *Allium sativum*, garlic 49v, 74v, 263, 274v, 275v, 303, 306v; *iuse of g.* 110, 137v; *piling of g.* garlic peels 304v.

garsen *v.* scarify 185v; **(y)-garsid** *p. p.* 68v, 77v, 155v, 278v.

garsyng *vbl. n.* scarification 193, 245v.

gencian *n.* Gentianaceae, *Gentiana lutea*, yellow gentian 77, 183v, 192v, 193, 271v, 204v.

generatif *n.* (of medicine) generating 170v.

gibbe *n.* hump of the liver 202, 203, 207.

gynger *n.* Zingiberaceae, *Zingiber officinale*, ginger root plant 49v, 54v, 55, 60, 62, 64v, 76v, 84v, 88v, 92, 100v, 102v, 103, 135v, 137v, 141, 141v, 142v, 148v, 149, etc.

gipsum *n.* naturally occurring hydrated calcium sulfate 298v.

gith, gite *n.* Ranunculaceae, *Nigella damascena*, fennel flower (L *gith*) 70, 217. See **nigel(le)**.

glad *adj.* glad 51, 232.

gladnes *n.* joy 190, 241.

glat, glet(te) *n.* mucus, phlegm 162v, 165v, 173, 174, 176, 179.

**(y)-gloderid *p. p.* coagulated (L *coagulatus*) 260v, 276, 285v, 289.

God *n.* 299v, 310v.

gold(e) *n.* 84v, 95, 189v, 193v, 240, 242, 216; *lymail of g.* gold filings 80, 88v, 187v, 241v.

*gomorra *n.* involuntary flowing of sperm 300v.

go(u)rde *n.*, **gourdes** *pl.* Cucurbitaceae, *Bryonia dioica*, bryony (L *cucurbita*) 146v, 194, 222, 222v, 228v, 249, 201, 205v; *herbe g.* leaves of bryony 150; *iuse of g.* juice inside bryony 146, 178v, 221v, 238, 262v; *seed of g.* 148, 150v, 152, 153, 156, 156v, 168, 171v, 179v, 180, 182, 182v, 197, 295; *shap of a g.* 269; **brionie** *n.* 239; *wilde g.* (*þat is* **collaquindida**) *n. Citrullus colocynthis*, colocynth 68, 201; *iuse of wielde g.* 116. See **sirip**.

gorst *n.* Leguminosae, *Ulex europaeus*, gorse 307v.

goute *n.*, **govtis** *pl.* gout (L *arthetica*) 281v; *colde g.* gout from cold (L *arthetica frigida*) 70v, 287; *rosi g.* 128v; **gutta rosacea** illness of the nose with redness and pimples 120, 128. See **potagre**.

grapes *n. pl.* Vitaceae, *Vitis vinifera*, grapes; *iuse of g. þat ben not ripe* verjuice 82v, 105; *iuse of soure g.* 89. See **onyfacie, reisen(e)s, vyne**.

gras *n.* Leguminosae, *Trifolium pratense*, red clover; *iuse of iii-leuyd g. þat haþ white spekis* 95.

grauel *n.* small urinary calculi 281-282, 286; a small stone 75v.

grees, grece *n.* melted or rendered fat, grease 111v, 145, 183v, 233v, 237v; *g. of a cat* 287; *g. of an eel* 111, 119v; *g. of an eyron* 111; *g. of a foxe* 287; *g. of a gandir* 111, 287; *g. of an henne* 111, 280, 304; *gose g.* 280, 302, 308v; *oold sowes g.* 69v; *swynes g.* 239, 284, 302v, 304.

greyne *n.*, **-s** *pl.* Zingiberaceae, *Amomum melegueta*, grains of paradise 76v, 137; 1/480th of an ounce Troy 76v, 77, 85, 108v, 153v, 182, 192v, 274, 274v.

grene, green *adj.* green in color, esp. from choler 95, 110, 119, 139v, 163v, 177, 244, 255v, 194v, 203, 281, 309.

greneþ *pr. 3 sg.* gnashes the teeth 74; **grinnen** *pl.* 269v.

greuaunce *n.*, **-s** *pl.* illness, pain 52v-53v, 55, 58, 65, 73v, 74v-76, 77, 82v, 92, 92v, 93v, 94v-95v, 99v, etc.

greue *v.* cause pain 83v; **greueþ** *pr. 3 sg.* 66v, 123v, 160, 169, 184v, 239v, 251, 253v, 256, 276v, 291v, 292, 294; **greuen** *3 pl.* 243, 276v; **(y)-greued** *p. p.* 75, 107, 126, 185, 193, 239v, 243v, 260v, 267, 220, 276v, 281v, 282.

greuous *adj.* severe, difficult 61v, 72v, 79, 106v, 107, 109, 111, 135v, 149v, 160, 163, 165v, 171v, 172, 221v, 264, 208, 304.

gromel *n.* 284v; ***mil(i)um solis** *n.* 283v; **palma Christi** *n.* 286v all three terms mean Boraginaceae, *Lithospermum officinale,* gromwell. See MED **palma christi.**

groundswili *n.* Compositae, *Senecio vulgaris,* groundsel 258, 266v.

gruel *n.* gruel 258, 260.

gum(me) *n.,* **-s** *pl.* natural gums, exudates from trees and shrubs, water-soluble 79v, 130v, 150, 310v; resin 161v; *g. arabike, gummi a.* Leguminosae, *Acacia senegal,* gum arabic 68, 81v, 83v, 87v, 88, 91v, 99v, 148, 150, 150v, 152, 153, 153v, 155v-156v, 171, 171v, 177v, 182, etc., also 310v; *g. edere/of yuy* ivy gum 119v, 135v, 144, 192v, 245v. See **dragagant(um), yue.**

gumme *n.,* **-s** *pl.* the gingivae 130v-132, 135v, 141v.

gut(te) *n.,* **guttis** *pl.* intestinal tract, internal organs 56v, 101v, 121, 184v, 191, 192, 192v, 224v, 225v, 228, 243v-244v, 251v, 253v-255, 256, 259, etc., also 269, 202v, 281v, 291; *middel g.* 254v, 255, 259; *neþirmost g.* 254v, 255, 259; *ouer g.* 192, 251v, 254v, 255, 259, 272. See **ilion, longaon.**

gutta rosacea see **goute.**

hayhoue, heyne-houe *n.* Labiatae, *Glechoma hederaceae,* ground ivy 49, 80; *iuse of h.* 102.

hande, hond(e) *n.,* **-s** *pl.* hand 48v, 63, 67, 68v, 128, 146, 170v, 187v, 189, 191v, 238v, 239, 245, 207, 207v, 211, 212, 216, 218v, 297v, 300v.

handful *n.* handful (as a measure) 63v, 77, 103v, 199.

harueste, heruest *n.* autumn 160, 164.

hasil *n.* Fagaceae, *Corylus avellana,* hazel nut; *quantite of an h.-not* 182v; *grene haselne stick* 95, 309. See **not(t)e.**

hede, heed *n.,* **-s** *pl.* head 48-49, 50v-52, 53v-54v, 55v-57, 60v-63, etc. See **ache, veyne.**

heel *n.* recovery 172.

heel, helen *v.* heal 65, 83, 95v, 110v, 116, 124, 191, 221v, 262, 262v, 204, 204v, 279v, 303v; **heliþ** *pr. 3 sg.* 85, 85v, 129v, 170, 285v; **helen** *3 pl.* 261v, 217v 285v; **heel, hele** *imp.* 50v, 76, 83v, 86, 96v, 124v, 131, 133, 262, 268v, 269, 277, 305; **(y)-he(e)lid** *p. p.* 65v, 86v, 87, 92v, 93, 100, 104, 114, 118v, 119, 124, 124v, 129v, 132v, 135v, 140, 151, 151v, 155, 162v, etc.; **helyng** *vbl. n.* 101, 110v, 118v, 124v, 185v. See **heel.**

heer *n.* **heris** *pl.* hair 49, 89, 104-105, 124, 127v, 173v, 176v, 191v, 297; *h. of an hare* 127v; *manis h.* 63.

hemloc *n.* Umbelliferae, *Conium maculatum,* hemlock 246v.

hempe, henipe *n.* Cannabiaceae, *Cannabis sativa*, Indian hemp; *h. sede* 100, 181; *inner pilyng of h.* hemp fiber 207v.

henbane *n.* Solanaceae, *Hyoscyamus niger*, henbane 57, 80v, 123, 134v-136, 138, 157, 239, 304; *h. sede* 129v. See **oyl(e)**.

hennes *n. pl.* flesh of hens 59v, 67. See **blode, coli(i)s, fat(nes), grees, mawe**.

herbe *n.*, **(h)erbis** *pl.* green plant, herb 50v, 55, 59v, 68v, 69, 79v, 91, 95, 98, 102, 102v, 103v, 105, 108v, 109v, 124, 124v, 127, 131v, 136v, etc., also 237v; plants in general 310v. See **bawme (þat is an herbe), co(o)lde²**, **dissolutif, duretike, flevme, hote, inscisif, moist(e), root, seed¹, strictory**.

herbe of þe palesy *n.* prob. Primulaceae, *Primula veris*, cowslip 141v, 142.

hering *vbl. n.* sense of hearing 54, 71, 111v, 118v.

hermodactalis *n.* Liliaceae, *Colchicum autumnale*, meadow saffron 239, 262v.

hert(e) *n.* heart 52v, 53, 55v, 66, 72, 144v, 184-186, 187v, 189, 190, 190v, 191v, 192v, 193v, 248. See **bo(o)n, veyne**.

hertistonge *n.* Polypodiaceae, *Phyllitis scolopendrium*, harts-tongue fern 233, 197, 204v, 219, 282v, 283, 284v, 286, 310.

hete, heet *n.*, **hetis** *pl.* physiological quality of hotness, opposite of coldness 48, 48v, 59, 75, 78, 81, 82, 82v, 84v, 86, 89v, 92, 99, 99v, 106, 107, 108v, 109, 110v, 111v, etc.; atmospheric or environmental heat 60, 78v, 106, 172, 190, 190v, 192v, 227v, 291. See **hote, kyndeli, vnkynde**.

hete(n) *v.* make hot 89, 172, 178, 192v, 193v; **heteþ** *pr. 3 sg.* heats up 121; **heten** *3 pl.* 172; **hete** *imp.* 84v, 145v, 268, 273v.

hock(e) *n.*, **hockis** *pl.* Malvaceae, *Malva sylvestris*, common mallow 56v, 63v, 84, 93v, 107v, 111, 111v, 129, 146, 146v, 150v, 156, 157, 233, 237v, 266v, 267, 273, 198, 216, etc., also 277; *h. leeues* 73v, 168; *h. rootis* 63v, 110v; *blosme of h.* 298; *flovres of h.* 156v; *iuse of h.* 148v; *sede of h.* 150, 156v, 168, 171v, 177v, 293; **malue** *n.*, **mallewis** *pl.* common mallow 63v, 183v; *leues of m.* 168v; *rote of m.* 144v.

holy-hock *n.*, **-is** *pl.* Malvaceae, *Althaea officinalis*, marsh mallow 56v, 93v, 237v, 266, 273, 218, 280; *rote of h.* 168, 216v, 302v, 310; *rotis of* **bismalue** *þat is þe h.* marsh mallow 143v; **bismalue** *n.* 183v; *rote of b.* 144v, 168.

honde see **hande**.

hony *n.* honey 49v-51, 56v, 64, 73v, 77v, 79v, 80, 88v, 92, 100v, 102, 102v, 104v, 105v, 112v, 119v, 130, etc., also 167v, 223v; *h. kome* 309v; *h. roset* electuary made of honey and roses 222, 230; *cleen/purid h.* clarified honey 130, 160v, 292v; *despumed/dispumed h.* cooked and skimmed honey 123v, 129, 140, 263, 200, 220v, 278v, 304v; **mel(lis)** 60v, 150v; *m. roset* honey roset 189v, 199.

horeho(u)ne, horhovne *n.* Labiatae, *Marrubium vulgare*, white horehound 68, 69, 115v, 142, 159v, 160v, 161, 174v, 183, 189v, 222v, 267v, 199, 214, 307, 307v; *iuse of h.* 68; *white h.* 160v, 307, 308. See **sirip**.

horne *n.*, **-s** *pl.* horn used in phlebotomy 84v, 245v; musical instrument 116; animal horn 127v; *gootis h.* 74, 308v; *hertis h.* 63, 133, 188v, 271, 275, 197v; *two h. þat ioynen to þe necke* collarbone 86.

y-horned *p. p.* phlebotomized using a horn 125.

horned cloþ *n.* cornea 100.

hors(e)hel *n.* 148v, 151v, 174v, 186v, 250, 250v; **elena campana** *n.* 309; both terms mean Compositae, *Inula helenium*, horseheal.

horsing *vbl. n.* rushing about noisily 213v. Cf. MED.

hote, hoot(e) *adj.* having the physiological quality of hotness 50, 56, 64, 73, 74, 75v, 78v-79v, 82, 99, 106v, 133, 138, 139v, 153, 153v, 154v, 158v, 160, etc.; *h. herbis* 51v, 62v, 77v, 122v, 159v, 160v, 252v, 215, 278, 286v, 292v, 295, 304v, 308; *h. sedis* 123; hot-feeling 56v, 57, 66v, 67, 69v, 75v, 80, 82v, 83, 84v, 100, 106, 106v, 111v, 114v, 117, 122, 123v, 125, 128, etc. See **duretike, hete, mete, oyl(e), oyn(e)ment, sirip**.

houndistonge *n.* Boraginaceae, *Cynoglossum officinale*, hound's tongue 69, 69v, 103, 123; *iuse of h.* 120; *rote of h.* 157.

humour *n.*, **-s** *pl.* one of the four bodily humors: blood, choler, phlegm, and melancholy 50v-52v, 53v, 54, 54v, 55v, 58v, 65v, 66v, 70-71, 72v, 75, 76, 78v, 82, 83, etc.; moist superfluous substance found in various places of the body 64v, 65, 75v, 98v; *salt h.* moist substance in the nose 121v.

hurling *vbl. n.* (in the digestive tract) gurgling or growling noise 243v, 244v, 265, 269v, 196, 296.

iacinctus *n.* jacinth, a blue stone 189v.

yche *v.* itch 100.

yc(c)hyng, echyng *vbl. n.* itching 82v, 83, 97v, 103v, 104v, 114v, 115v, 128v, 269v, 270, 272v, 194v, 203v, 289v.

ydelnes *n.* idleness 49v.

iera *n.* group of bitter, purging electuaries, often containing aloes 189v; *i. alogodion* with aloes 72v; ** *i. fortissima Galieni* recipe of Galen 187v; ** *i. yreas* ? with iris 230v; *i. pigra* a bitter medicine 72v, 239, 272; *i. pigra of Galienis making* 201, 214, 218; ** *i. pigra of Constantine's making* recipe of Constantine the African 201v; ** *i. rufa* ? i. ruffini 238v.

y3e *n.*, **y3en, yen**, *pl.* eye 54v-55v, 57v, 65v, 66v, 67, 72, 74v-76, 77-79, 80v-81v, etc., also 165, 173v, 176, 191, 260, 194v, 203, 211; *y3eliddis* 75v, 103v, 104, 105; *whijt of þe y.* 75, 96v, 100, 206v; **liddes** eyelids 75. See **blerid**.

yis *n.* ice 78v.

ilion *n.* one of the small guts, ilium 263v, 264.

yllica passio *n.* disease of the ilium 263v.

incense see **encense**.

incurable, vncurable *adj.* incurable 71, 72v, 74, 118v, 119, 124v, 176v, 181v, 182, 227v, 255, 214v, 215, 296, 308v. See **curable**.

infeccion *n.*, **-s** *pl.* tainting, esp. by a humor other than blood 95v, 96, 128, 173.

infecte(d) *ppl. adj.* tainted, esp. by a humor other than blood, 95v, 126, 194v, 309.

inscisif *adj.* incisive, penetrating; *i. herbis* 59v.

inubes, innibes *n. pl.* fruit of Rhamnaceae, *Zizyphus jujuba*, common jujube 156, 157, 167, 168, 181, 221v. See **sirip**.

ioy(e) *n.* joy 98v, 190v.

ioynt *n.*, **-is** *pl.* joint 54v, 277v, 281v.

ypericon *n.* Hypericaceae, *Hypericum androsaemum*, tutsan 68, 290v, 307v.

ypoquistidos *n.* Cytinaceae, *Cytinus hypocistis*, hypocistis 172v, 171, 186, 257, 297, 297, 298.

yren *n.* iron 128, 145v, 273.

yreos *n.* Iridaceae, *Iris* spp., iris 77, 148v, 189v, 250, 251; **accorun** *n.* iris 239.

ysop(e) *n.* Labiatae, *Hyssopus officinalis*, hyssop 54v, 68v, 76v, 97v, 103, 131v, 136v, 141, 141v, 142v, 148v, 150v, 153v, 159v, 160, 161v, 167v, 174v, 177, 183, etc., also 209; *flouris of y.* 273v; *iuse of y.* 87. See **sirip**.

yue *n.* Araliaceae, *Hedera helix*, true ivy 204v, 284v; *iuse of y.* 110v, 119v. See **gum(me)**.

yuel *n.*, **-is** *pl.* illness 48v, 52v. See **falling yvel, 3elew(e)**.

yuel *adj.* harmful 54, 70, 129v, 227; inauspicious 57, 65v; bad 70, 118v, 227, 301; difficult 142, 165v, 169, 198v.

yuery *n.* ivory 48, 49, 188v.

iunctis of þe chyn *n. pl.* vertebrae 277v.

iuniper *n.* Cupressaceae, *Juniperus communis*, juniper; *baies of i.* juniper berries 142.

kebulis see **mirabolani(s)**.

keke *v.* preserve 51.

kiddis *n. pl.* goat kids 59v.

kidney *n.*, **kidneiren** *pl.* kidney 275v; *k. of a goot* 160v. See **reynes**[1].

kynde *n.*, **-s** *pl.* type 65, 71, 78, 78v, 87, 89, 94v, 115v, 119, 172v, 188v, 191, 192, 224v, 239, 239v, 242v, 253v, 261, 203v, 215v, 218; natural state 265v; virtue 180, 197v, 204, 219v; sperm 65v.

kyndeli, kyndeliche *adj.* natural 162v, 189, 190, 211; *k. hete* heat necessary to life 184v, 190v, 247, 278v; *k. moistnes* moisture necessary to life 175, 179v, 180v, 253v, 253v. See **flevme, vnkynde**.

kyndli *adv.* naturally 190, 225.

kisse *v.* kiss 191v.

kit *imp.* cut 50, 57v, 299; **(y-)kitte, kut** *p. p.* 96v, 97, 282.

kutting *vbl. n.* surgery 297; a cut 303v. See **surgery**.

lacertis *n. pl.* muscles 294; *neþir l.* lower arm muscles 238v; *ouer l.* upper arm muscles 238v.

lambren *n. pl.* lampreys 59v.

lanceola þat groweþ in water *n.* Ranunculaceae, *Ranunculus lingua*, greater spearwort (L *lanceola aquatica*) 89.

langdebef *n.* Boraginaceae, *Anchusa officinalis*, ox tongue 104, 283v, 284.

lapdanum *n.* gum of Cistaceae, *Cistus* spp., rock rose 122v, 123.

***lapis armenicus** see **attrament.**

lapis lazuli *n.* lapis lazuli 90, 218v, 220v, 307v.

lapwynge see **blode.**

larde *n.* fat cured in brine or by smoking 266.

Latin *n.* the Latin language 50, 68.

laton *n.* latten, a metallic alloy resembling brass 95.

lauendre *n.* Labiatae, *Lavandula officinalis*, lavender (L *lavandula*) 68, 117, 141v.

lauriole *n.* Thymelaeceae, *Daphne laureola*, spurge laurel 70v, 174; ****alipiados** *n.* spurge laurel 77; **coconidie** *n.* spurge laurel seed 238v. Cf. MED.

lawgheþ *pr. 3 sg.* laughs 58v; **lawghing** *vbl. n.* 58.

laxatif, laxe *n.* laxative 54v, 86, 122, 233, 251v, 267v.

laxatif *adj.* laxative 54, 90, 238v, 254, 268v, 215. See **mete.**

laxe *adj.* laxative 109; flaccid 121, 139, 285v, 294, 294v.

leche *n.* water leech 57v, 112v, 289.

lecheri *n.* lust 301v.

lechis *n. pl.* medical practitioners 58v.

lectuarie see **electuari.**

lede, leed *n.* lead 95, 297v, 298v, 309; *coloure of l.* 265, 203v. See **ceruse.**

le(e)ke, like *n.* Liliaceae, *Allium porrum*, leek 142, 263, 306v, 308v; *l. seed* 134v; *iuse of l.* 73, 110, 113-114v, 117v; *leues of l.* 273; *erbe þat is like l. and haþ a white flour* prob. *A. ampeloprasum*, wild leek 306v.

lendis *n. pl.* loins 288.

lenetif *n.,* **lenetiues** *pl.* medicine having a softening and moistening effect 149v, 161.

lenetif *adj.* (of a medicine) having a softening and moistening effect 155.

lentes *n. pl.* Leguminosae, *Lens* spp., lentils 145, 202v.

let(e) blood *v.* cause blood to be purged 114, 215, 301; *p. p.* phlebotomized 57, 70, 73. See **blede, bleding, blode, blode-letting.**

leþer, leder *n.* leather 49, 104v, 296, 297v.

letuse *n.* Compositae, *Lactuca sativa*, garden lettuce 59v, 179v, 222, 228v, 233, 249, 258, 204v, 292; *iuse of l.* 57v, 108v, 158, 249; *sedis of l.* 156, 157, 247, 197, 293, 295.

leues *n. pl.* leaves or petals 188; *l. of cold trees* 300v; *cold l.* 188, 193v.

licium *n.* dried leaves of Caprifoliaceae, *Lonicera* spp., honeysuckle 80, 82v, 85, 88v, 91v, 94, 108v, 130, 145.

liddes see **y3e.**

lye *n.* lye 49, 105, 199, 208, 308.

lienteri(e) *n.* illness characterized by diarrhea containing undigested food 254, 262, 273v, 203, 307. See **flux(e).**

lift(e) *adj.* left (side of the body), esp. with reference to diseases involving the spleen 116v, 126, 165, 166, 169, 176, 193, 264, 210v, 211, 212, 212v, 214, 215v, 216, 218v, 288v, 289v. Cf. **ri3t.**

lignum al(l)oes, ligni aloe(s) *n.* 103, 122v, 132v, 186v, 230, 240, 241, 200v, 220v; **ziloaloes** 201v; Thymelaeaceae, *Aquilaria agallocha*, lignum aloes.

li3t(e), lungis *n. pl.* lungs 48v, 121, 126, 131, 133, 144v, 147, 147v, 151v, 153, 154, 154v, 158v, 160v, 162, 162v, 164-165, 166, etc.

lijff *n.* life 125v.

lyking *vbl. n.* pleasure, relief 128v.

lily(e) *n.*, **lilies** *pl.* the family Nymphaeaceae, the lilies; *l. leef* 303; *l. roots* 84v, 104, 144v, 183v, 250v, 218; *iuse of l. rotis* 237, 309; *floures of l.* 309; *watir l.* 135, 197v, 284, 292v; *watir l. leues* 156, 157v, 177v, 187; *sedis of watir l.* 197. See **sirip.**

lymail see **bras.**

lyme *n.*; *unslekid l.* calcium oxide 128.

limes *n. pl.* limbs of the body 295v.

lynseed, lynen seed *n.* Linaceae, *Linum* spp., flax seed 63v, 81, 88v, 93v, 144, 148v, 160v, 161, 168, 168v, 174, 183, 223, 232v, 237v, 250, 267, 198, 218. See **clooþ, mele**[1].

lippis *n. pl.* lips 130v, 269v, 195v; *cleving of l.* cracked l. 129-130v, 140. See **mesel.**

liquoris, licoris *n.* Leguminosae, *Glycyrrhiza* spp., licorice 64v, 76v, 103, 146, 146v, 150, 150v, 153, 156-157, 159v, 161, 166v, 167, 177v, 178v, 180v, 182v, 183, etc.; *iuse of l.* 148, 152, 153v, 155v, 167v, 179v, 182, 189, 200v; *rote of l.* 167v.

litarge *n.* litharge, prob. protoxide of lead 100, 130v, 275, 298v, 309.

litargie *n.* disease of the brain from an apostem in the rear ventricle causing forgetfulness, lethargy 52, 57v, 61, 62v, 63, 64, 118, 248v, 269v, 270v.

lyver *n.* liver 48v, 77, 95v, 126, 127v, 154, 169, 173v, 175v, 184v, 188v, 193, 194, 195-196, 198, 199, 199v, 200v, etc., also 204, 210, 210v, 213, 291; *distempering of þe l.* disruption of the liver's complexion 252v, 194, 195, 196v, 199v, 204-205, 217v, 277v, 278; *stopping of þe l.* blockage of the liver's ducts 50, 194, 196v, 202, 203, 205, 216v. See **veyne.**

lyuer-worte *n.* Marchantacieae, *Marchantia polymorpha*, liverwort 197, 216, 216v, 219, 310.

longaon *n.* longanon or rectum 272v, 274. See **gut(te).**

loof see **bred(e).**

lorer *n.* Lauraceae, *Laurus nobilis*, laurel tree; *l. leues* 70v, 98, 119, 122v, 199; *baies of l.* laurel berries 51, 141v, 142, 192v, 240v, 245v, 246, 273v, 295v; *shalis of baies* prob. shells of laurel berries 299v; **bayes** prob. laurel berries 309. See **oyl(e)**.

louage *n.* Umbelliferae, *Levisticum officinale*, lovage 49, 54v, 69v, 102v, 189, 229v, 230, 231v, 247, 258, 258v, 266, 197v, 287v, 288, 304, 310; *l. leues* 290v; *l. seed* 258v, 290.

loueþ *pr. 3 sg.* loves 191v, 224.

luys *n. pl.* lice 104, 105.

lungis see **ly3t(e)**.

lupynes *n. pl.* Leguminosae, *Lupinus albus*, white lupines 105, 272; *bitter l.* 271; *iuse of l.* 116.

**macedo *n.* Umbelliferae, *Smyrnium olusatrum*, alexanders 231v.

macematicon see **caul(e)**.

macis see **notemyg(e)**.

madir *n.* Caprifoliaceae, *Rubia tinctorum*, madder 129; *iuse of m.* 100v; *leues of m.* 80.

magnes *n.* 88v; **ademant stoon** 104v; loadstone.

maioran, maiorone *n.* Labiatae, *Marjorana hortensis*, sweet marjoram 64v, 142, 230, 230v, 250, 267, 269; **san(g)suke** *n.* sweet marjoram 73v, 80, 139v, 141v, 142v, 233v; *iuse of s.* 62v .

*malagoge *n.* medicine acting to purge melancholy 159v, 239, 199, 295.

malencoly(e) *n.* melancholy 49v-50v, 53, 54, 55, 58-59, 66-67, 71v, 73, 75, 75v, 83v, 84, 85v, 86, etc., also 134, 139, 160, 164, 185v, 224v, 225, 244v, 255v, 196, 207, 210v, 213v, 294v.

malencolious, malencolike, melencoly *adj.* containing or characteristic of melancholy 66, 288v, 305v. See **mete**.

malmesyn *n.* **malmsey** 82v, 83v.

mandrake *n.* Solanaceae, *Mandragora officinalis*, mandrake; *fruyt of m.* 80v; *ryndes of m.* 77, 80v. See **oyl(e)**.

mania *n.* disease of middle ventricle of the brain 58.

manna *n.* soft, white, sweet substance found on or near plants and produced by the actions of certain insects; honeydew 188v, 249.

marche *n.* Umbelliferae, *Apium graveolens,* wild celery 49, 54v, 55, 67v, 76v, 83, 84, 102v, 142, 157, 161, 167, 174v, 183, 225v, 231v, 267, 271v, 197v, 199, 204v, 209, etc.; *m. seed* 159v, 229, 231v, 250, 197v, 199v, 209, 297v; *iuse of m.* 57, 63v, 73, 97v, 222, 280; *leues of m.* 105v; *rote of m.* 50, 105v, 156v, 283, 283v; **smalache sede** *n.* 309v wild celery seed.

marciaton *n.* an ointment 142, 149, 151v, 267, 295v.

margery peerles, margaritis *n. pl.* pearls 103v, 182, 187v, 189v.

mary(e), merie *n.* bone marrow 253; *m. of a calf* 280; *m. of an herte* 111; *m. of hennes boones* 100v.

mastik(e) *n.* resin from Anacardiaceae, *Pistacia lentiscus*, mastic 51, 54, 62, 64v, 76v-77v, 83, 96v, 97v, 99, 103, 105v, 108v, 110v, 114v, 125, 127v, 130v, 135, etc.

maturatif *n.*, **maturatiues** *pl.* medicine causing an apostem to mature 110v, 111v, 208, 209.

maturatif *adj.* (of a medicine) causing an apostem to mature 168v.

mawe *n.* stomach; *m. of an hare* 113; *inner skynne of an hennes m.* 89.

medicinable *adj.* medicinal 55v, 173.

medisyn(e) *n.*, **-s** *pl.* medicine 51, 51v, 58, 59, 60v, 61, 70, 72v, 74, 77v-79v, 81, 90, 90v, 92, 94v, 107v, etc. See **componed, souereyn(e), special, simple.**

meeting *vbl. n.* dreaming 53.

meiden-her(e) *n.* Polypodiaceae, *Adiantum capillus-veneris*, maidenhair fern 150v, 156v, 157, 183, 197v, 204v, 206v, 216v, 219, 282v, 310.

y-meynd *p. p.* mixed 223, 260v. MED **mengen.**

mel see **hony.**

mele[1], **meel** *n.* grain meal 183v, 240v; *barley m.* 81v, 82, 85, 127, 129, 168v, 188v, 245, 249v, 253, 261, 273, 197v, 208, 219, 290v, 292v, 299v, 304, 305; *been m.* 92, 100, 104, 171v; *femygreke m.* 85, 145, 273, 208; *lynen-sede m.* 85, 145, 273, 208; *rye m.* 83; *whete m.* 49, 82, 173, 253, 257v, 258v, 261, 208, 209, 302.

mele[2] *n.* meal of food 131v, 262.

melisse see **bawme (þat is an herbe).**

mellicratum, mellicrate *n.* drink made of two parts wine and one of honey 223v, 229, 237. Cf. MED.

mellilot(e), mellilotum *n.* Leguminosae, *Melilotus officinalis*, common melilot 69, 73v, 81v, 84v, 85, 139v; *m. floures* 84; *iuse of m.* 104.

mel(l)one *n.*, **-s** *pl.* Cucurbitaceae, *Cucumis melo*, muskmelon 205v; *seed of m.* 148, 150v, 152, 153, 156, 157, 167, 171v, 179v, 180, 182, 182v, 197. See **seed**[1].

membre *n.*, **-s** *pl.* body part 50v, 65, 69v, 79, 80v, 121, 144v, 184, 185, 185v, 204-205, 276v, 300, 305v; = *priue(y) m.* 233; *priue(y) m.* penis 127v, 253; *spirituel m-s* organs above the diaphragm 144v, 147.

memyth(e) *n.* Papaveraceae, *Glaucium flavum*, yellow horned poppy 88, 88v, 103v, 145.

mentastre *n.* Labiatae, *Mentha longifolia*, horsemint 136v.

mercury(e) *n.* Chenopodiaceae, *Chenopodium bonus-henricus*, all-good 56v, 63v, 266v, 267, 216v, 282v; *iuse of m.* 283.

mesel *n.* leper 128; *m. lippis* 129v.

mete *n.*, **-s** *pl.* food 53v, 54v, 59v, 60, 66, 67, 72v, 74, 76, 78, 101v, 103, 107, 122, 127, 133v, 138v, 142, 142v, 151, etc.; **mete** a meal 52v, 53, 76, 138v, 232, 236v-238, 247v, 270, 195-196, 205, 211, 211v, 215, 216v, 297v; *biting m.* 78; *boistous m.* coarse foods 53v; *colde m.* 133v, 227, 233v, 243; *comfortable m.* 166v, 239v, 241, 242; *corrupte m.* 133v; *costif m.* 240, 242v, 264v, 268v; *drie m.* 227; *fat m.* 226; *fleumatike m.* 49, 66, 142, 159; *fried m.* 67v, 78, 151; *good m.* 187v, 226v, 229, 232, 249; *grete m.* foods difficult to digest 53v, 131v, 170, 224, 198v, 216v; *hoot m.* 74, 133v, 190, 227v, 242v, 243; *inflatif m.* 202v; *yuel y-sauorid m.* 131v; *keen m.* 133v, 172, 233, 234, 263, 293, 307; *laxatif m.* 254, 275v; *malencolious m.* 49, 59v, 66, 67v, 159, 196, 216v, 307; *moiste m.* 59v, 131v, 227, 261; *rostid m.* 67v, 78, 151, 240, 257v, 198v; *salte m.* 67v, 78, 148, 151, 172, 223, 263; *sharpe m.* 151; *sory m.* 244v; *sotil m.* 198v, 293; *soure m.* 78, 133v, 148, 167, 172, 223, 226, 227; *souping m.* 275v; *swete m.* 270v, 205v; *temperat m.* 216v; *temperat coolde m.* 67; *temperat hoot m.* 249v, 293v; *vnctuous m.* 226; *viscouse m.* 198v; *white m.* 49, 67v; *windi m.* 268v, 198v, 220. See **oyl(e)**.

meþ(e), meeþ *n.* mead 54v, 55, 148v, 181v, 189v, 251, 252v.

**miclete *n.* an electuary 256v, 257, 262, 263, 263v.

middai *n.* noon 182v.

mydrif *n.* diaphragm 144v, 154, 162v, 164v, 165v, 168v, 169, 169v, 173, 201v.

mylbery *n.* Artocapeae, *Morus* spp., mulberry tree; *croppis of a m. tree* 307; *rynde of a m. tree* 145; **mores** *n. pl.* 143v mulberries.

myl(l)efoyle, mylfoil(e) *n.* Compositae, *Achillea millefolium*, yarrow 51v, 258, 307; *iuse of m.* 306v; *leef of m.* 128.

mylke *n.* milk 49, 67v, 131v, 140, 145, 173, 223, 271, 282; *m. of a coughe/cow* 258v-259v, 261, 280v; *m. of a woman* 57, 80v-81v, 82v, 89v, 91, 93v, 98v, 100, 107v, 109, 109v, 110v, 112v, 114, 114v, 117v, 119v, 157v, 274v; *asse m.* 81, 89v, 146; *gotis m.* 89v, 105v, 146, 150v, 187, 222v, 240v, 250v, 280, 280v; *whey of gotis m.* 180v; *shepis m.* 150v; *swete m.* 271. See **almondis, fyg(g)e**.

mil(i)um solis see **gromel**.

mynde *n.*, **-s** *pl.* mind, consciousness 51, 52, 61, 64, 269v.

mynt(e), *n.* **-s**, **meyntis** *pl.* Labiatae, *Mentha* spp., mint 49v, 59v, 60v, 63v, 103, 109v, 122v, 131, 131v, 135, 137v, 138, 142, 160, 171, 226v, 227, 231, 233v, 239v, etc., also 293v; *iuse of m.* 74, 80, 132v, 193, 239v, 240v, 252v, 253, 258v, 259, 261, 263, 263v, 199v, 286v, 295, 302. See **sirip**.

mirabolani(s) *n.* 76, 244v, 256v, 209v; (*m.*) *bellrici* 256, 201v; *m. citri(ni)* 77v, 188v, 239, 256, 261v, 263v, 197, 201v; (*m.*) *emblici* 256, 201v; *m. indie/indorum* 54, 187, 239, 256, 262, 201v, 218v, 307v; (*m.*) *kebulis/keber* 54, 239, 256, 261v, 262v, 201v; *fyue kyndes of m.* 78, 218; *ryndes of m.* 103v; fruits of similar-looking plants yield the 5 kinds of mirobalans; four belong to the family Combretaceae; *m. indi* and *m. citri* come from the same plant: *Terminalia citrina*; the former is the ripe fruit, the latter the green fruit; *T. chebula* yields *m. keber*; Euphorbiaceae gives *Phyllanthus emblica*: *m. emblici*.

mirre *n.* resin from Burseraceae, *Balsamodendron myrrha* 76v, 88v, 91v, 92, 93, 94, 112, 112v, 115, 117v, 119v, 123, 123v, 135, 138, 140, 157, 159v, 160v, 170, etc., also 278v.

myrþe *n.* mirth 59, 60, 241.

mirtille *n.* Myrtaceae, *Myrtus communis*, myrtle tree; *rynde of m.* 64v; **mirtillis** *pl.* myrtle seeds 251, 258, 258v; **mirte**, *n.*, -**s** *pl.* myrtle leaves 258v; *leues of m.* 188, 216v. See **oyl(e)**.

myssein *pr. 3 pl.* menace, verbally abuse 56.

mysturnyng *vbl. n.* distortion 72.

mitigatif *adj.* (of medicine) acting to lessen pain 89, 89v, 168v.

mytigatiue, mitigacion *n.*, **mytigatiues** *pl.* medicine acting to lessen pain 78v, 79v, 80, 80v, 82, 86v, 90v, 91v, 93, 100, 110v, 118.

moist(e) *adj.* having the physiological quality of moistness, opposite of dryness 48, 64, 64v, 78v, 86v, 93, 95, 100, 130, 181, 227, 232v, 292v, 298; moist to touch 75, 82, 95v, 163v, 186; *m. herbis* 233, 267. See **mete**.

moyst(e)nes *n.* physiological quality of moistness, opposite of dryness 48, 48v, 98, 106, 133v, 149, 194, 195v-196v, 200, 202v, 210, 212v, 291, 291v, 295, 296; moisture, precipitation 97v, 120, 169v. See **kyndeli**.

moleyn *n.* Scrophulariaceae, *Verbascum thapsus*, Aaron's rod 308.

mollificatif *adj.* having a softening effect 155, 267, 209v, 214v, 297v, 299, 309.

mollificatiues *n. pl.* softening medicines 88, 93, 93v, 94v, 105v, 149v, 178, 267, 215, 218v.

mo(o)ne *n.* moon 72v, 310.

monkis *n. pl.* monks 58v.

mon(e)þe *n.*, -**s** *pl.* month 86v, 120, 277v, 283v, 293, 293v, 306.

morel *n.* Solanaceae, *Solanum nigrum*, black nightshade 80v, 198, 216v.

mores see **mylbery**.

morewe, mor(e)w(e)tide, mornyng *n.*, -**s** *pl.* morning 48v, 55, 84v, 85, 95v, 115v, 132v, 152v, 161v, 162, 173, 174, 174v, 176v, 182, 182v, 189v, 221, 228v, 251, etc.; *m. dew* 102v.

morfu *n.* morphew, a morbid eruption on the skin 128v, 309.

mormale *n.* necrotic sore (L *malum mortuum*) 203v.

mortir *n.* mortar 250v, 310.

mouþ(e), mooþ(e) *n.* mouth 53, 53v, 55v, 60, 61v, 62, 65, 67, 72, 74, 77, 87, 98v, 116v, 129, 130-132, etc.; -s openings 305v. See **stomak(e)**.

mugwort(e) *n.* Compositae, *Artemisia vulgaris*, mugwort 110, 199, 199v, 307; **mug-wede or worte** 142.

mummie *n.* gum prepared from mummies 171, 259, 290, 297, 298-299v.

mundificatif *n.*, **mundificatiues** *pl.* cleansing medicine 97, 112, 114, 114v, 116, 170, 170v, 177, 250v, 208v.

mundificatif *adj.* having a cleansing effect 63v, 96, 259v, 209v.

musculages, muscilagis *n. pl.* viscous substances 272v, 211, 276, 294. See **ps(c)illie**.

muske *n.* secretions of the preputial follicles of the musk deer 76v, 80, 88v, 182.

mustard *n.* Cruciferae, *Sinapis alba*, mustard 263.

nayl, vngula *n.* fingernail-like growth over the eye 87, 92v; **nailes** *pl.* fingernails or toenails 173v, 176.

nausea *n.* disease of the stomach characterized by a desire to vomit but without result 235. Cf. MED.

nauel *n.* navel 238v, 255, 255v, 257v, 264, 271v, 283v, 284, 287v, 290, 290v, 292, 297v.

necke *n.*, -s *pl.* neck 57, 60v, 68v, 86, 112v, 128v, 173v, 176, 188; *n. of þe bladdir* 285v, 287, 294; *n.-pitte* 60, 77v, 86, 125, 134v.

neep *n.* Cruciferae, *Brassica rapa*, turnip; *iuse of n.* 115.

nepte *n.* Labiatae, *Nepeta cataria*, cat-mint 231.

ne(i)sshe *adj.* soft, esp. from phlegm or blood 63v, 83, 88, 125v, 139, 143, 149v, 239v, 247, 248, 249, 254, 267, 274v, 196, 201, 203, 210, 211v, 212, etc.

nesshenes, ne(is)ship *n.* softness 145v, 210, 211v, 214, 296.

net(t)le *n.*, -s *pl.* Urticaceae, *Urtica* spp., nettle 67v, 69, 73v, 110, 203, 206, 214, 304v; *n. seed* 83, 102, 230v; *iuse of n.* 114, 137; *rotis of n.* 137v; *reed n.* Labiatae, *Lamium purpureum*, red dead-nettle 79v, 127v, 137; *croppis of rede n.* 135v, 149.

nigel(le), cokil *n.* Gramineae, *Lolium temulentum*, darnel (L *nigella*) 62, 141v, 142v, 193, 271. See **gith**.

ny3t(e) *n.*, -s *pl.* night 48v, 81, 83, 109v, 115v, 147v, 160, 163, 163v, 169, 228v, 229, 231, 242, 262v, 265, 220v; *ny3tis-tyme* 75v.

ny3tingale *n.* nightingale 141.

(sal) nitre, nitrum *n.* sodium carbonate 69v, 73v, 76v, 89, 112-113, 117v, 138, 141, 173, 272, 201, 298, 307v.

noble *adj.* important, noble 93v, 204.

noli me tangere *n.* disease of the skin causing sensitivity to touch 120v, 129.

nolle of þe heed *n.* back of the neck, nape (L *nucha*) 149.

nose *n.* nose 57v, 98, 120, 120v, 121v, 123v, 124v-125v, 126v-129, 147, 191v, 193v, 269v. See **cop, bleding**.

noseþirl(e) see (nose)þirl(e).

not(t)e *n.*, **-s** *pl.* Fagaceae, *Corylus avellana*, hazelnut (L *nux*) or some other type of nut 49, 67v, 93v, 220v; *kernels of n.* 93v; *quantite of a n.* 77; *rynde of a n. tree* 145; *saap of a n. tre* 145, 145v. See **hasil**, **oyl(e)**, **walle-notte**.

notemyg(e) *n.*, **-gis** *pl.* 103, 132v, 141, 161v, 226v, 230v, 240, 242, 200v, 201, 220v; **macis** *n. pl.* 103, 132v, 186v, 225v, 226v, 230, 230v, 241, 246v, 259, 200v, 220v; Myristicaceae, *Myristica fragrans*, nutmeg tree; the kernel of the seed provides nutmeg, its hull, mace.

obtolmye, obtalmye *n.* apostem in the white of the eye, ophthalmia 75, 85v, 87v, 88, 92v, 93.

oculus Christi see **chekenmete**.

oyl(e) *n.*, **-s** *pl.* medicine with an olive oil base; olive oil itself 56v, 57, 62, 64, 69, 70, 70v, 73v, 90, 100v, 108, 110, 111v, 115v, 117v, 119, 119v, 123, 129v, 144v, etc., also 226, 278v; *o. of almondis* 145v, 146v; *o. of asshes* 218; *o. de bay* oil of laurel berry 69v, 74v; *o. de olijf* 63v, 79v, 130v, 188, 309v; *o. of birches* 218; *o. of bitter almondis* 110, 117; *o. of carses* 174; *o. of castorie* 62v; *o. of ellern* 49, 62v, 219v; *o. of henbane* 300; *o. of lorer* 74v, 77v, 109v, 110, 115, 119, 122v, 142, 151v, 233v, 234, 240v, 246v, 284, 295v; *o. of mandrake* 300; *o. of mirtis* 188, 249, 216v; *o. of notes* 93v, 110, 115v; *o. of piliol* 77v, 110, 159v, 246v; *o. of piretre* 62v; *o. of roses* 57, 57v, 81, 97v, 107v, 108v, 109, 110v, 111, 112, 114v, 117v, 124v, 129v, 168v, 188, 226, 233, 241, 245, etc.; *o. of rwe* 62, 110, 122v, 246v; *o. of saleyne* 188; *o. of syneuey* 49; *o. of violet* 57v, 63v, 81, 107v, 108v, 109, 110v, 111, 123v, 124v, 129v, 130v, 145v-146v, 157v, 159v, 168, 168v, 188, etc.; *comen o.* olive oil 168v, 188, 199v, 266v; *drastis of o.* dregs of oil 238v; *hote o.* 62, 122v, 187v, 233v, 234, 199v; *mete o.* olive oil 64, 188, 237.

oyn(e)ment, onement, onyment *n.*, **-is** *pl.* ointment 62, 69v, 73v, 100v, 111, 111v, 117v, 120, 124, 129-130v, 139v, 142, 146v, 149, 157v, 193, 222, etc.; *colde o.* 239v, 218, 301v; *hote o.* 73, 139v, 187v, 225, 229v, 234, 239v, 245v, 252v, 199v, 284v, 287, 291, 295v; *ʒelev o. eiþir þe grene þat surgiens vsen* ointment of sulphur and verdigris 303. See **bawme (þat is an onment)**.

oke *n.*, **-s** *pl.* Fagaceae, *Quercus* spp., oak; *blosmis of o.* 258v; *rynde of an o.* 240, 257; ****roris ciriaci** oak flowers (L. *ros syriacus*) 171. See **accarnes**.

oken apples see **galles**.

o(o)lde, elde *adj.* old 82v, 88v, 94v, 95v, 108, 115v, 118v, 120, 164, 174, 223, 247, 258, 267v, 273, 197, 217, 281, 296, 297, etc. See **coli(i)s**, **grees**, **skyn(ne)**.

olibanum *n.* resin of Burseraceae, *Boswellia* spp., frankincense (L *olibanum*) 69, 77v, 83, 84v, 105v, 112v, 123, 130v, 138, 140v, 174v, 240v, 242, 245v, 246, 274, 298v, 303v. See **encense**.

onyfacie *n.* juice of green white grapes (L *omfacinum*) 171. See **grapes**.

onyon, oynon, onoun, oynen *n.*, **-s** *pl.* Liliaceae, *Allium cepa*, onion 49, 59v, 110, 110v, 111v, 142, 250v, 263, 218; *iuse of o.* 107v, 119, 129, 145v. See **squill(i)e**.

opium *n.* dried juice of green poppy heads 57, 57v, 83v, 85, 87v, 88, 91v, 92v, 99v, 109, 111, 123, 123v, 135, 138, 171, 172v, 183v, 274, 278v, 300v. See **popi**.

opobalsamum *n.* juice of Burseraceae, *Balsamodendron opobalsamum*, balsam of Gilead 77. See **bawme (þat is an onment), **carpobalsamum, opobalsamum**.

opoponac, opopinac *n.* Umbelliferae, *Opoponax chironium*, opopanax 68, 68v, 76v, 242.

origanum, origane *n.* Labiatae, *Origanum vulgare*, marjoram (L *origanum*) 54v, 63v, 76v, 103, 122v, 131v, 136v, 137v, 138, 141-142v, 148v, 161, 189v, 226v, 233v, 234v, 246, etc., also 209, 214; *flouris of o.* 273v.

orobus *n.* Leguminosae, *Vicia orobus*, bitter vetch 174v, 250v; *sede of o.* 178.

orpement, or(y)pyment *n.* arsenic trisulphide 149, 151v, 160v-161v, 183v.

orpyn *n.* Crassulaceae, *Sedum telephium*, orpine 80v; *iuse of o.* 272; *rotis of o.* 309v.

os sepie *n.* cuttlefish bone 94, 140v.

otis, oten *n. pl.* Gramineae, *Avena* spp., oats 275, 277; *smale chaf of o.* oat chaff 107v, 129.

oxifistula see **tamarindi(s)**.

oxi3e *n.* Compositae, *Chrysanthemum leucanthemum*, marguerite 298.

oximel *n.*, **-lis** *pl.* medicine made of two parts vinegar and one of honey, sometimes used as a base 49v, 67v, 68, 78, 128v, 141v, 142v, 145v, 148v, 160v, 226, 197, 200, 214, 215, 215v, 277, 278, 282v, 292, 295; *o. compouned* 49v, 50, 50v, 233v; *o. duretike* 160, 199, 283, 286v; *o. of radiche* 49v, 50, 67v, 160, 238, 218; *o. squillitike* 49v, 50, 67v, 159v, 183, 238, 199, 218, 283; *simple o.* 49v, 50, 183, 245.

oz., vnce *n.*, **vncis** *pl.* ounce 51, 54-55, 57, 60, 60v, 62, 62v, 64v, 68, 69v, 73v, 103, 117v, 131v, 132v, 140v, 141v, 142, etc., also 299v.

****oz(i)mi** see **basilicon**.

pacient *n.* patient 87, 172v, 171, 181, 185v, 265, 266, 274, 220v, 292, 299v, 309v.

pale *adj.* pale, esp. from phlegm 71v, 106v, 147v, 151, 163, 185, 244, 255v, 265, 272v, 274v, 211, 211v, 304.

palenes *n.* paleness, esp. from phlegm 133v.

palesy(e) *n.* paralysis, weakness 55, 65v, 70v, 71, 74v, 77v, 121, 140v, 293v; *p. of þe bladdir p.* 295v, 301; *p. of þe ers* 274; *p. of þe stones* 301, 301v; *p. of þe tunge* 139, 140, 142. See ***herbe**.

palma Christi see **gromel**.

pappe *n.* breast 165.

pappis *n. pl.* pap, soft food for invalids 309v.

parchemyn *n.* parchment 254v.

parseli, parsil(y), parcil *n.* Umbelliferae, *Petroselinum* spp., parsley 50, 54v, 55, 59v, 67v, 76v, 103, 161, 167, 167v, 174v, 231v, 247, 197v, 199v, 278v, 290v, 298; *rotis of p.* 233, 219, 283v; *seed of p.* 117, 246, 197v, 208v, 282v, 283, 284, 297v.

partriche *n.*, **-s** *pl.* partridge 59v, 67.

pasnep, pastnepe *n.* Umbelliferae, *Pastinaca sativa*, parsnip 167; *iuse of p. leues* 130v.

pavmes, pawmes *n. pl.* palms of the hand 187v, 245, 211.

pees *n.*, **pe(e)sen, peses** *pl.* Papilionaceae, *Pisum sativum*, garden pea 53v, 67v, 268v, 202v; *quantite of a p.* size of a pea 123v, 245v.

peyne *n.* pain 264.

penides *n.* barley sugar, pennet 130, 146v, 148, 150v-152, 153, 156-157, 167, 183, 250v.

penyworte *n.* Crassulaceae, *Umbilicus rupestris*, pennywort 244v.

pentafilon *n.* Rosaceae, *Potentilla reptans*, creeping cinquefoil 171, 219, 283v, 290, 303, 307; *iuse of p.* 298; *rotes of p.* 137v.

pepir, pipir *n.* Piperaceae, *Piper nigrum*; berries yield various types of pepper 49v, 55, 60, 62, 69v, 74v, 89, 103, 122, 131v, 136, 136v, 137v, 141, 148v, 149v, 161v, 174v, 183v, 231v, etc.; *p. cornes* 104v, 135v; *black p.* 54v, 141v, 225v, 230, 231; *long p.* 62v, 103, 117v, 141v, 142v, 161v, 174v, 178, 225v, 230-231v, 200v, 220v; *macro p.* long pepper 64v; *melano p.* black pepper 247; *white p.* 54v, 103v, 140v, 141v, 142v, 225v.

perche *n.* European perch 181v. See **fysshe**.

(re)percussyues *n. pl.* cold medicines repelling or expelling harmful matter 78v, 79v-81, 82, 86v, 93, 110v, 249, 207v, 300, 300v, 305.

periplemonie *n.* apostem in the lungs 162, 165, 170, 173v, 175, 177v, 182v.

pe(e)ris *n. pl.* Rosaceae, *Pyrus communis*, pears 49, 167, 249.

pestil *n.* pestle 174v, 274.

petrolei *n.* crude oil 76v.

**peusadanum *n.* Umbelliferae, *Peucedanum officinale*, hog's fennel 77.

phicisiens *n. pl.* physicians 181v.

pic(c)he, picch *n.* pitch 145v, 275, 275v, 298v. Cf. **colofoyne**.

pye *n.* magpie 101v.

pigami see **rw(e)**.

pike *n.* pike fish 181v. See **fysshe**.

piliol, puliol, pileol, puleol *n.* Labiatae, *Mentha pulegium*, penny-royal 68, 103, 115v, 122v, 159v, 234v, 247, 273v, 204v, 295v, 307v, 308; *p. monteyn*, **polie** = ? *Teucrium polium* 76v, 148v, 230v. See **oyl(e)**.

pillules *n. pl.* medicine made by rolling a substance into pills 54, 60, 61, 62, 68, 73, 77, 78, 123, 123v, 132-133, 148, 148v, 150, 157, 159v, 174v, 183v, 234, 201v; *p. Arabie* 50v; *p. of diacastor* 76; *cold p.* 222v.

pyment *n.* spiced and sweetened wine 200.

pimpernel *n.* Umbelliferae, *Pimpinella saxifraga*, burnet saxifrage 249, 292.

pimple, pemple *n.*, **-s** *pl.* pimple 103v, 104, 128v, 129v, 130, 140, 289, 300, 302, 303.

pyn *n.* clouding of the eye resembling a pin head 95v.

pynes *n. pl.* pine nuts from Pinaceae, *Pinus* spp., 148v, 161, 167, 183v; *pyne appil* pinecone 161v, 275.

pyntis *n. pl.* pints 141v.

pyony(e) *n.* Paeoniaceae, *Paeonia mascula*, peony 68v, 141v, 286v; *seeds of p.* 67v, 69.

pipe *n.*, **-s** *pl.* pipe 115, 119, 258v, 259v, 302, 307v.

piretre, peletre, peretre, peritori(e), peritre *n.* Urticaceae, *Parietaria diffusa*, pellitory-of-the-wall 49v, 62, 62v, 68, 69v, 73, 76v, 77, 85, 98, 105v, 124v, 131v, 136-137v, 141, 142v, 145v, etc., also 268, 308; *p. leves* 105; *clensing of p.* 148v, 162; *p. of Spayne* Compositae, *Anacyclus pyrethrum*, pellitory of Spain 117v, 239. See **oyl(e)**.

pisse *n.* urine 55v, 65v, 294v; *mere p.* watery or foamy urine, not suitable for uroscopy 61v. See **vryn**.

pisse *v.* urinate 284, 285, 287, 287v, 291v, 292; **pissiþ** *pr. 3 sg.* 285, 288, 289; **(bi)pissen** *3 pl.* 282, 289, 294, 294v, 295v, 302; **bipissid** *p. p.* 268.

pissing *vbl. n.* urination 280, 281, 282, 285, 288, 291, 291v, 294, 310.

planteyn *n.* Plantaginaceae, *Plantago major*, great plantain or waybread, or *P. lanceolata*, lesser plantain or ribwort (L *plantago*) 69v, 83, 96v, 92, 96v, 97, 107v, 129, 171, 173, 177v, 242v, 256v, 257, 258, 259, 263v, 198, 216v, 290, etc.; *iuse of p.* 82v, 87v, 90, 91, 93, 94v, 97, 127v, 143v, 146, 146v, 171, 223, 239, 240v, 245, 249, 253, 256v, 257v, etc.; *sede of p.* 109, 171, 178v, 179v, 258, 258v, 293; *p. boþe þe more and þe lasse* 290v; **rib(be)wort** *n.* ribwort (L *lanceola*) 290v, 292; *iuse of r.* 298; **weybrode** *n.* waybread (L *arnoglossa*) *iuse of w.* 140.

(em)plastir, (em)plastre *n.*, **(em)plastris** *pl.* thick or sticky medicine applied externally, plaster 49, 51v, 56v, 57, 62, 73, 73v, 81, 81v, 83, 84v, 85, 92, 99-100, 102, 104, 105v, 110v, etc.

plastre *imp.* apply a plaster 105, 110, 124v, 250v, 253, 261, 268, 287v, 292v, 304v, 306v; **(y)-plastrid** *p. p.* 51v, 83, 97, 97v, 100, 111v, 136v, 137v, 174, 272; **emplastrid** 306v.

plemeros *n.* Primulaceae, *Primula vulgaris*, primrose 98. MED **prime-rose**.

plumb *n.*, **plum(b)es** *pl.* Rosaceae, *Prunus domestica*, plum 156, 188v, 221v, 292v, 310; *black p.* 167; *kirnels of p. stones* 284v; *soure p.* 233; *swete p.* 156v. See **sirip**.

pluresi(e) *n.* apostem of the diaphragm 162v, 165-166, 167v, 170, 173v, 175v, 177v, 182v.

**pocio muscata *n.* electuary containing musk 186v.

pocion *n.* medicinal drink 68v, 293v, 307.

y-poisened *p. p.* poisoned 193.

policarie *n.* Compositae, *Pulicaria dysenterica*, fleabane 307v.

polie see **piliol**.

pol(l)ipodi(e), polipodium *n.* Polypodiaceae, *Polypodium vulgare*, polypody 76v, 137v, 261v, 262v, 209v, 293v, 307v.

****pollitricum adiantos** *n.* kind of fern 219, 283. See **feren leues, meiden-her(e)**.

pomgarnard *n.* Punicaceae, *Punica granatum*, pomegranate tree; *iuse of p.* 186; *rynde of p.* 186v; **balaustia, balaustie** *n.* 140, 145, 171, 179, 258v, 259, 275v, 298v; **psidie** *n.* 171, 258v, 259, 298v, 308v; the bark is **psidie**, the flower **balaustia**. See **wyn(e)**.

popi *n.* Papaveraceae, *Papaver rhoeas*, red poppy or *P. somniferum*, black or white poppy 84v; *p. sede* 80v, 81, 109, 157, 179v; *blacke p.* 57; *blacke p. sede* 80v; *iuse of rede p.* 93v; *rynde of p.* 124v; *white p.* 182v; *white p. seed* 152, 155v; . See **opium**.

popilion *n.* ointment made from poplar buds 57, 157v, 168, 186, 239, 245v, 197v, 209v, 282v.

pore *n.*, **po(o)ris** *pl.* opening 185, 197v, 209, 281; *p. of þe brayn* 52v; *p. in þe eris* 120; *p. of þe lyuer* 202-204v; *p. of þe nosepirles* 124; *p. of þe reines* 281; *p. of þe skynne* 74, 184v, 292v; *p. of þe spleen* 211v, 213v; *p. of þe stomake* 235, 235v, 237, 243v.

porke *n.* pork 49.

portulake see **purs(e)lane**.

pose *n.* a cold 83v, 86, 120, 120v, 121v, 122v, 124v, 147.

postem(e), postom(e), postum *n.*, **-s** *pl.* morbid gathering of undigested or badly digested humors, apostem 52, 55v, 56, 58, 61, 63, 75, 85v, 87, 100v, 104, 105v, 107, 108v, 110v, 111v, 112, 113v, 114v, 121, etc., also 144v, 145v, 146, 154, 162, 247v.

potage *n.* soup 249v, 216v, 309v.

potagre *n.* gout 54v. See **goute**.

pouse *n.* pulse 56, 61v, 106v, 142v, 143, 185.

practis *n.*, **practises, practiues** *pl.* subdivision of a chapter 74v, 103v, 105v, 120, 129, 133, 146v, 162, 221, 253v, 194, 275v, 299v, 305v. See **title, tre(a)tes**.

psidie see **pomgarnard**.

ps(c)illie, silly(e), psilly *n.* Plantaginaceae, *Plantago psyllium*, fleawort 81, 97v, 150, 223; *iuse of p.* 180; *musculage of p.* 91v, 97v, 156v, 158, 186; *seed of p.* 91v.

psilotrum þat is made to doo awey heris *n.* depilatory 89.

ptisane see **(p)tisane**.

ptisike see **(p)tisike**.

puliol see **piliol**.

purgacion *n.*, **-s** *pl.* purging 55, 56v, 60v, 62, 68, 73, 76, 77v, 78, 82, 99, 109v, 116v, 119, 119v, 121v, 128v, 129, 145, 149v, etc.

purge, purgen *v.* rid the body of something, esp. a humor 49v, 54, 55, 62, 77v, 96, 98, 143, 186, 189v, 226v, 237, 274v, 214, 218v, 276v, 277, 292; **purgeþ** *pr. 3 sg.* 54, 54v, 155v, 256, 274v, 201v; **purgen** *3 pl.* 50v, 54, 107, 112, 187v, 271v, 201, 204v, 220v; **purge** *imp.* 84, 116v, 123v, 124v, 135, 148v, 159v, 178, 187, 192, 221v, 226, 233, 239v, 244v, 256, 261v, 262, 263, 267, etc.; **(y)-purgid** *p. p.* 72v, 98v, 107, 108, 132, 136, 137v, 148, 155v, 175, 186, 227, 228-229, 232, 243, 251, 256v, 260v, etc.; **purgynge** *ppl. adj.* 204.

purs(e)lane *n.* Portulacaceae, *Portulaca oleracea*, purslane (L *portulaca*) 59v, 222, 228v, 233, 245v, 249, 266v, 208, 283, 292, 292v, 295; *iuse of p.* 178v, 198; *seed of p.* 178v, 182, 182v, 247, 197, 198, 293; **portulake** *n.* purslane (L *portulaca*) 81, 129v, 130, 134v, 179v, 228v; *iuse of p.* 57v, 156; *sede of p.* 148, 150v, 156, 171v, 177v.

quantum sufficit *adj.* as much as necessary 60v, 64v, 69v, 145v, 150v, 152, 153, 161v, 162, 171v, 173, 174, 174v, 183, 192v, 225v, 230v, 231v, 238v, 247, etc.

quartron, quarte *n.* quart 142, 299, 309v.

quibibis *n. pl.* fruit of Piperaceae, *Piper cubeba*, cubeb 54v, 64v, 131v, 132v, 141v, 226v, 241, 250.

quiter(e), quytour, qwiter *n.* purulent matter, pus 105v, 111v-113, 128v, 162v, 170, 173-174, 177, 250v, 251, 208-209, 279, 280, 280v, etc.

quitering *vbl. n.* releasing of pus 113, 114v.

quiteriþ *pr. 3 sg.* releases pus 128v.

radiche *n.* Cruciferae, *Raphanus sativus*, radish 123, 171, 174, 180v, 183, 189v, 237, 237v, 197v, 217, 283v, 284; *branchis of r.* 206; *iuse of r.* 83, 113, 114, 115, 115v, 117v, 118, 119, 119v, 189, 238, 283v; *iuse of þe rote of r.* 113, 197v; *rote of r.* 50, 161. See **oximel**.

rapis *n. pl.* Cruciferae, *Brassica napus*, turnip 237.

reche *v.* stretch 296.

rede, reed *adj.* red, esp. from blood or choler 53, 56, 61v, 72, 75v, 85v, 89v, 92v, 95v, 96, 106, 106v, 125, 133v, 143, 155, 185, 222v, 206v, 279, etc.; *brovn-r.* 75v; *derke r.* 139, 155v; *swart r.* dark red 55v, 134, 158v, 303v. See **chekenmete, ciceres, coler(e), coral, net(t)le, popi, ro(o)ses, sandris, snayl, tuc(h)ie, vynegre, wax(e), wyn(e)**.

reednes, redenes *n.* red, esp. as a symptom of sanguine or choleric illness 75, 75v, 89v, 95v, 96, 102, 103v, 116v, 126, 128, 134, 142v, 146, 165, 195, 302.

reynes[1] *n. pl.* kidneys 74v, 77, 121, 162, 238v, 264, 201, 275v-279, 280, 280v, 281v-282v, etc. See **kidney**.

reynes[2] *n. pl.* rains 53. See **watir**.

reisen(e)s, reysyns *n. pl.* dried fruit of Vitaceae, *Vitis* spp., grape 157, 166v, 167, 167v, 168v, 177, 181, 183, 183v, 231, 250v. See **grapes**.

repercussyues see **(re)percussyues**.

repercussif *adj.* (of a medicine) repelling harmful matter 89v.

reson *n.* rational faculty 52; **vnresonable** *adj.* irrational 221, 224v, 225, 226, 226v, 230.

resta bouis *n.* Leguminosae, *Ononis repens*, restharrow 257.

retentif *n.* ability or tendency of the body to retain something 254v. Cf. **expulsif**.

reubarbe, rwebarbe, reupont *n.* Polygonaceae, *Rheum* spp., rhubarb 54, 76v, 103, 182, 234, 239, 244v, 245, 247, 197, 201v, 208v, 215v; *Englisshe r.* 70v.

reule *n.* rule, guide 205.

reule *imp.* subject to a regimen of health 266v; **rulid** *p. p.* 242v.

rewme, revme *n.* mucous discharge 76, 77, 120v, 121, 122, 124, 134, 134v, 136v, 174v, 178v, 181v, 262, 276.

ribbis *n. pl.* ribs 162v, 165v, 203.

rib(be)wort see **planteyn.**

riche *adj.* rich 245v, 198v, 199.

rigge *n.* back 237v, 254, 263v, 203, 280v, 281v, 282; *r.-boon* backbone 69v, 207, 281v.

ri3t *adj.* right (side of the body), esp. with reference to diseases that are hot or of the liver 116v, 126, 166, 169, 193v, 260v, 264, 194v, 195, 196, 203-203v, 206v, 207, 277, 288v, 289v. Cf. **lift(e).**

riys, rise *n.* Gramineae, *Oryza sativa*, rice 127, 173, 249v, 258, 302.

roche *n.* roach, a type of carp 181v. See **fisshe.**

root *n.*, **rotis** *pl.* roots of plants, root vegetables 226, 238, 197v; root of hair 105; *r. of colde duretike erbis* 197. See **chache.**

roris ciriaci see **oke.

**rosata nouella *n.* electuary made from roses 186v, 252, 196v.

ro(o)ses *n. pl.* Rosaceae, *Rosa* spp., rose 48, 54, 55, 64v, 80, 81, 81v, 82v, 83v, 84v, 87v, 88, 91-92, 94v, 98v, 99v, 100v, 102, etc., also 125, 134v, 187, 193v, 204v; *r. lyues* rose petals 48; *iuse of r.* 78, 266v, 197, 215v, 282v, 283, 286, 289v, 292, 295; *rede r.* 198. See **hony, oyl(e), sirip, sugur.**

rosyn *n.* pine sap, resin 144.

ros(e)maryn, rosmary *n.* Labiatae, *Rosmarinus officinalis*, rosemary 50, 214; *floures of r.* 201, 309; **ant(h)os* *n.* 64v, 141v, 214; *croppes of a.* 200v; *floures of a.* 200v. **Anthos** most often meant the flowers of rosemary.

ruddes *n. pl.* Compositae, *Calendula officinalis*, pot marigold 51v.

rw(e), rue, rewe *n.* Rutaceae, *Ruta graveolens*, garden rue 49, 60v, 68v, 69, 70, 76v, 79v, 84v, 88v, 91, 98, 102-103, 110, 117v, 192v, 227, 233v, 234, etc., also 209, 214, 308; *iuse of r.* 62v, 73, 84v, 91, 97, 98, 102v, 113, 119v, 300v; *sede of r.* 246; ****pigami** *n.* rue seed 192v; *iuse of p.* 193. See **oyl(e).**

saf(f)ron, saffren *n.* Iridaceae, *Crocus sativus*, saffron (L *crocus*) 60, 105, 109, 150v, 160, 177, 179, 249v, 274, 201; **citre** *n.* (L *crocus*) 77v, 87v, 103, 103v, 171, 174v, 182, 225v, 230, 230v.

sa(u)ge *n.* Labiatae, *Salvia officinalis*, sage (L *salvia*) 67v, 68v-69v, 73, 84, 98, 103, 105v, 141v, 148v, 150v, 159v, 192, 246, 258, 199, 205v, 299v, 308; *iuse of s.* 142; *leues of s.* 135v; *weilde s.* prob. Compositae, *Artemisia stellerana*, dusty miller (L *abrotanum, i.e. habrotonum*) 109v.

sal(t) armoniac, s. armoniake *n.* ammonium chloride 54v, 55, 76v, 89, 105v, 141, 218v, 219. See **bo(o)le.**

saleyn leues *n. pl.* leaves of Salicaceae, *Salix* spp., willow 187, 192v, 216, 282v, 300v. See **oyl(e)**.

sal nitre see **(sal) nitre**.

salt(e) *n.* table salt, sodium chloride, either from rock salt or combined with sea salts 56v, 63, 64, 73v, 94, 112v, 127v, 137, 137v, 173, 267, 267v, 271, 272, 302v-303v, 309v; medicinal salt 54v, 160v; *s. gemme/iem* rock salt 64, 131v, 141, 237, 266v, 201v, 307v; *comyn s.* table salt 307v; *euery s.* prob. salt, sal nitre, and sal ammoniac 80, 89 (cf. 141, 307v). See **fysshe, flevme, humour, mete, watir**.

salte *adj.* salty 143, 149v, 158v, 163v.

salte *imp.* apply salt to 94; **saltid** *p. p.* 97v, 150v.

saltnes *n.* saltiness 228.

saluatelle see **veyne**.

saluitica see **veyne**.

sandeuer *n.* liquid saline substance floating on molten glass after vitrification 88v.

san(g)dragon, sandragun *n.* dried juice of Liliaceae, *Dracaena* spp., dragon's blood tree 51v, 68v, 76v, 81, 93, 96v, 97, 99, 114, 127, 127v, 135, 170, 171, 179, 179v, 240v, 242, 256v, 257v, etc.

sandris *n.* powdered wood of the trees Santalaceae, *Santalum album*, white or yellow sandalwood, or Leguminosae, *Pterocarpus santalinus*, red sanders 130v, 180, 188, 188v, 247, 249v, 204v, 208v, 283, 301v, 310; *rede s.* 132v, 140, 141v, 226v, 245, 261, 200v, 310; *pre kyndes of s.* 188v, 261, 197v, 215v, 292v; *white s.* 182, 226v, 245, 261, 198, 200v, 290v.

sangrinary(e) *n.* Cruciferae, *Capsella bursa-pastoris,* shepherd's purse 128, 257; *s. pat is clepid* **sheppardis purse** *n.* 96v, 127; *iuse of* **s. p.** 112v, 114.

sanicle *n.* Umbelliferae, *Sanicula europaea*, sanicle 69.

sansuke see **maioran**.

sape *n.* sweet vinegar made from sweet wine 142v, 143v, 156, 157, 177v, 280v. See **not(t)e, vynegre**.

sarcacol(le), sarcocol *n.* Persian gum, poss. gum ammoniac, tragacanth, or galbanum 80, 85, 87v, 88v, 91v, 93, 94v, 96v, 103v.

satiriasis *n.* involuntary penile erection 300, 301v.

sau(e)yn *n.* Cupressaceae, *Juniperus sabina*, savin 77; *branch of s.* 128; *iuse of s.* 120.

sauerey, saturey *n.* Labiatae, *Satureja* spp., savory (L *satureia*) 76v, 148v, 160, 160v, 189, 230v.

saxifrage *n.* Saxifragaceae, *Saxifraga* spp., saxifrage 283v, 284; *iuse of s.* 283v, 284. See **burnet, seed**[1].

sc. *n.* scruple, 20 grains 64v, 83v, 87v, 91v, 152, 183v, 192v, 193, 247, 201, 201v, 216, 218v.

scab(be) *n.*, **scabbis** *pl.* scab 74, 104, 194v, 203v.

scabbid *ppl. adj.* afflicted with scabs 289.

scabeous, scabious *n.* Dipsacaceae, *Scabiosa* spp., scabious 104, 129.

scales *n. pl.* scaly formations 294, 294v.

scamony(e), scamone, scamonia *n.* Convolvulaceae, *Convolvulus scammonia*, scammony 51, 54, 54v, 73v, 90, 238v, 272, 196v, 197, 198v, 287, 290, 307v.

scariole *n.* Compositae, *Lactuca serriola*, prickly lettuce 182, 222, 204v; *iuse of s.* 186, 249, 198, 205v; *seed of s.* 156.

scorpion *n.* scorpion 90v.

scotomy(e) *n.* spots before the eyes 52, 52v, 236, 195v.

sebesten *n.* Boraginaceae, *Cordia* spp., sebesten plum 181.

see *v.* see 75, 83v, 91, 99, 102, 107, 115, 117v, 143v, 158v, 180v, 280; **seeþ**[1] *pr. 3 sg.* 52v, 72, 72v, 101, 191; **seen** *pr. 3 pl.* 58v; **seest** *subj.* 185v, 256v; **see** *imp.* 299v; **(a)-seen** *p. p.* 100v, 247v, 195, 207, 214v, 296.

seed[1]**, sede** *n.*, **seedis** *pl.* seed (of a plant); *iiii colde s.* prob. seeds of melon, gourd, portulake, and citonies 208v, 216v, 282v, 293, 310; *s. of þe iiii colde herbis* 167v; *s. þat breken þe stoon* burnet or saxifrage 68. See **co(o)lde**[2]**, duretike, hote.**

seed[2]**, sede** *n.* sperm 300, 300v, 301.

seeþ[2]**, seþe** *v.* simmer, soak 69v, 141v, 144, 246, 250, 273v; **seeþ** *pr. 3 sg.* 167v; **seþen** *pr. 3 pl.* 267v; **seeþ** *imp.* 50, 55, 56v, 62v, 63v, 68, 69, 70v, 73, 81, 85, 93v, 94, 101v, 102, 103v, 108v, 109, 115, etc., also 167v; **seþing** *pr. p.* 180; **y-so(o)den, y-soode** *p. p.* 49v, 55, 56v, 69, 69v, 73v, 81v, 84-85, 92, 93v, 97, 97v, 100v, 102, 105, 105v, 107v, 108v, etc.

sege *n.* privy; *at s.* 266; *go to s.* 267v, 273v; *haue s.* 238v.

Seynt Joon Baptist *n.* John the Baptist 51v.

se(e)ke, sike *n.* ill person 55, 56v, 63v, 68v, 69, 73, 150v, 152, 161v, 162, 299v.

se(e)ke, sike *adj.* ill 53v, 64, 65, 74v, 79, 162v, 170.

sekenes, sikenes *n.*, **-is** *pl.* illness 48v, 50v, 52-53v, 55v, 56, 58-59, 60v-61v, 62v, 64v-66v, etc.

sene, seen(e), cene *n.* Leguminosae, *Cassia* spp., senna 50v, 54, 55, 56v, 64v, 68, 159v, 187, 252v, 261v, 201v, 209v, 217, 218v, 220v, 226v, 307v.

serapinum, serapionis *n.* gum from Orchidaceae, *Orchis* spp., serapine 76v, 105v, 242, 298v.

serid clooþ *n.* waxed cloth 77v.

serpentarie *n.* 238; *rote of* **dragance** *n.* 271v; both terms mean Polygonaceae, *Polygonum bistorta*, snake-root.

shar(e), sher(e), sheer *n.* groin 257v, 263, 264, 275, 280v, 282, 284, 284v, 285v, 287-288, 289, 290v, 293, 295v-296v, 297v, 300.

sharpe *adj.* strong, acute 54, 55v, 73v, 106, 114, 118, 121v, 125, 126v, 131, 132, 139, 149v, 151, 158v, 264v, 272, 202v, 206v. See **feuer.**

shaue *v.* shave 63v, 124; **(y)-shaue** *p. p.* 73, 112v; **shaue** *imp.* 56v, 299; **shauing** *vbl. n.* shaving 254-255, 261v.

shep(p)ardis ʒeerd/ʒerd(e) *n.* Dipsacaceae, *Dipsacus fullonum* ssp. *fullonum*, teasel 171v, 177v, 257; *iuse of s. ʒ.* 111v.

sheppardis purse see **sangrinary(e).**

shite *v.* move the bowels 251v, 253v, 272, 272v, 274, 275v, 296v, 307, 309; **shiteþ, sheteþ** *pr. 3 sg.* 253v, 194v; **shiting** *pr. p.* 281v, 297v.

shuldir, *n.* **shuldris** *pl.* shoulder 77v, 165, 176, 176v; s-**blade(s)** 60v, 84, 155v, 165, 176.

siclamen see **erþe appel.**

sycomour *n.*, -**is** *pl.* Moraceae, *Ficus sycomorus*, sycamore 143v; *iuse of s.* 140.

sign(e) *n.*, -**es** *pl.* diagnostic sign 55v, 60, 65v, 66v, 71v, 116v, 236, 236v, 247v, 260. See **token.**

si3t(e) *n.* sense of sight 51, 54, 71, 71v, 77v, 85v, 101, 102-103v, 230v, 201v.

siler(is), ciler *n.* Umbelliferae, *Seseli* spp., sesely 64v; *s. mo(u)nteyn* sesely 76v, 103, 230, 231v, 280, 307v, 308; **sileos** sesely 174v, 247.

silke *n.* silk; *brent s.* 64v, 220v; **syndel** 90v.

silly(e) see **ps(c)illie.**

siluer *n.* silver 193v.

symphite see **comfery(e).**

simple *adj.* (of a medicine) not compounded 79v, 155v, 189v; (of a person) not wealthy 198v; (of a disease) uncomplicated 199v, 291. See **oxymel, flux(e), riche.**

sincopis *n.* disease of the heart 72, 184, 190, 193.

syndel see **silke.**

syneuey, seneuey, cineuei *n.* Cruciferae, *Brassica nigra*, mustard 62, 62v, 69v, 73, 98, 115v, 125, 140, 141, 149v, 214; *leues of s.* 206. See **carses, oyl(e).**

syn(e)grene, sen(e)green *n.* Crassulaceae, *Sempervivum tectorum*, houseleek 50v, 81, 83, 120, 188, 292; *iuse of s.* 57, 81v, 107v, 108v, 112, 119, 119v, 127v, 188, 239, 244v, 245, 292v.

siphac, ciphac *n.* membrane lining the abdominal cavity; peritoneum 296, 296v, 297.

sirip, sirup(e), sirep *n.*, -**s** *pl.* medicinal syrup 69, 141v, 156, 156v, 161, 167, 167v, 170, 172v, 171, 173v, 177v, 180, 182v, 183, 186v, 226v, 233, 239v, 240, 245, etc., also 310v; *s. of borage* 186; *s. of fumiter* 128v; *s. of gourdes* 228v; *s. of horehoune* 222v; *s. of inubes* 157, 159, 167, 170; *s. of ysop* 160v; *s. of myntis* 240v, 252; *s. of plumes* 221v, 234v; *s. of roses* 63, 64v, 126v, 167, 182v, 226, 229, 247v, 249, 252, 261, 295, 301v; *s. of smyþþis watir* 216; *s. of spikenard* 209v; *s. of vinegir* 237v; *s. of violet* 63, 148v, 150, 152, 153, 156, 167, 180, 221v, 226, 228v, 229v, 232v, 234v, 237v, 245, 249, 196v; *s. of watir-lilies* 300v; *s. of wormod* 209v; *cold s.* 63, 221v, 226, 228v, 245, 266v, 289v; *drie s.* 181v; *hoot s.* 230v.

sisymbre *n.* Cruciferae, *Sisymbrium officinaie*, hedge mustard 69v.

skyn(ne) *n.*, -**es** *pl.* skin (of a person) 48, 61, 74, 105v, 196, 276, 305v; covering 104; peritoneum 296, 296v, 303v; *s. of þe brayn* 55v; *s. of þe herte* 184; *s. of þe stomake* 235, 236v, 237, 243v, 247v, 250v; *hare-is s.* 297; *olde lambes s.* 158; *newe weþires s.* 298v, 299. See **mawe, pore, siphac.**

skirewhites *n. pl.* Cruciferae, *Eruca sativa*, rocket 206.

skulle *n.* skull 61.

slepe, sleep *n.* sleep 48, 57, 61, 61v, 62v, 63, 66, 82v, 106v, 107v, 122, 226, 251v, 260v, 265v, 270, 195v.

slepe, sleep *v.* sleep 50v, 60, 185, 229, 248v; **slepiþ** *pr. 3 sg.* 194v, 276v; **slepen** *3 pl.* 78, 203, 203v; **slepte** *past* 67.

sloo(n) *n.* Rosaceae, *Prunus spinosa,* sloe; *iuse of s.* 80; *rinde of a s. tre* 298v. See **acacia, þorne.**

slouþe, slevþe *n.* sluggishness 65v, 66, 71v, 147v.

smalache see **marche.**

smale *n.* (of drink) weak and clear 78. See **ale, wyn(e).**

smel(le) *n.,* **-s** *pl.* odor 70, 127v, 194.

smel(le) *v.* smell 63, 68v, 74, 131, 187, 193v, 194, 300v; **smelliþ** *pr. 3 sg.* 121; **smelling** *ppl. adj.* 115v, 122v, 132, 133, 159v, 160v, 176v, 187v, 193v, 226, 226v, 270v.

smelling *vbl. n.* sense of smell 71, 120v.

smoke *n.,* **-s** *pl.* fume or smoke 51v, 52, 52v, 53v, 55v, 56v, 63, 66, 66v, 75, 98v, 106v, 119, 122, 135v, 136v, 143, 147v, 158v, 160v, etc., also 180, 228, 257v, 273, 195v, 209, 304v.

smoky *adj.* smoky 229.

snayl *n.,* **-s** *pl.* snail 93v, 145, 209; *rede s.* 94.

snes(s)e *v.* sneeze 62, 98, 113v, 117, 119, 124v, 139v; **sneseþ** *pr. 3 sg.* 121v.

snesing *vbl. n.* sneezing 234, 234v, 297v.

s(e)newis *n. pl.* nerves, sinews 64v, 70v, 71v, 138v, 140v, 185, 221, 285v, 293v, 294, 294v.

snowe *n.* snow 78v.

(y)-so(o)den see **seeþ**[2].

solatre *n.* Solanaceae, *Solanum dulcamara,* bittersweet 100, 134v, 249, 277; *iuse of s.* 57, 81, 111, 140, 145, 249, 197v, 207v, 208v, 292v, 310.

so(u)le *n.,* **-s** *pl.* spirit or mind 241; sole of the foot 56v, 187v, 245, 211.

sommer *n.* summer 163, 163v, 249v; **mydsommer** 48.

sooking beestis *n. pl.* nursing mammals 59v.

so(o)pe, soop *n.* soap 303; *blacke s.* 73v; *white s.* 73v, 104v.

sorel *n.* Polygonaceae, *Rumex* spp., sorrel (L *acedula*); *iuse of s.* 129v, 188; **sour(e)-doc** *n.* sorrel (L *acedula*) 282v, 283.

sorow(e), sorew *n.* grief 50v, 58v, 98v, 185v, 190, 190v, 269v.

souereyn(e) medicyn/remedy *n.* best medicine 72v, 240v, 274v, 275v.

sour(e)-doc see **sorel.**

soure/sorowe dowe *n.* fermented bread dough 145v, 209v, 309v. See **bred(e).**

souþerenwode *n.* Compositae, *Artemisia campestris,* southernwood 63v, 159v, 233v, 267, 272, 199.

sowne *v.* faint 66v; **y-sovned** *p. p.* 248.

(y)-sparplid *p. p.* scattered 154v, 190v.

speche *n.* power of speech 121, 231, 269v.

special *adj.* (of treatment or medicine) specific 60v, 68v, 78, 110, 114, 137, 165, 183, 186v, 189v, 262v, 268, 271, 275, 196, 197, 218v, 220.

speke *v.* speak 57, 138v, 142v, 176v; mention 126v, 127, 127v, 129, 176v, 242v; **spek** *subj.* 66v; **speking** *pr. p.* 151, 176v, 228v.

spica celtica *n.* Valerianaceae, *Valeriana celtica,* spike celtica 174.

spices *n.* species, type 204.

spicis, spicery *n. pl.* spices 79v, 132, 180, 257v, 258, 200, 201; *hote s.* 133, 138.

spike *n.* Valerianaceae, *Nardostachys jatamansi*, spikenard 62, 64v, 76v, 87v, 88v, 98v, 131v, 137, 141, 148v, 153v, 162, 178, 182, 187, 225v, 226v, 230, 246v, 250, etc.; **spikenard** *n.* spikenard 84v, 119, 233, 208v, 209v, 278v, 310. See **sirip.**

spinage *n.* Chenopodiaceae, *Spinacia oleracea*, spinach (L *spinarchia*) 59v.

spiritis *n. pl.* small bodies in the eye by which sight is accomplished 101, 102; substances or qualities contained in the heart and blood associated with bodily heat, fever, and the emotions 172, 184, 190, 190v, 191v, 193v.

spleen, splene *n.* spleen 50, 77, 95v, 126, 127v, 162, 169, 175v, 193, 131v, 201-202, 203v, 205, 210, 210v, 211v-212v, etc., also 276v, 277v, 288v, 289v, 309v. See **veyne.**

spodi(e) *n.* spodium, powder from calcination 64v, 127v, 161v, 171v, 179v, 182, 186v, 240, 245, 246v, 253, 258v, 197-198, 204v, 292v, 298v.

spon(e)ful *n.* spoonful 64, 119v, 132v, 161v, 226v, 299v, 309, 309v.

sponge of þe see *n.* marine sponge 240v.

spue *v.* vomit 53v; **spuyng** *vbl. n.* 234v. See **cast(e), volate(n).**

spume *n.* foam 262, 265, 195, 202v, 211; **s. of þe see** pumice 94.

sp(o)urge *n.* Euphorbiaceae, *Euphorbia* spp., spurge; *iuse of s.* 238; *sede of s.* 89, 90 .

squill(i)e, squillia *n.* Liliaceae, *Urginea scilla*, squill 144, 217, 219; *onyon of þe see þat is clepid in Latin s.* 50. See **oxymel.**

squynacy(e) *n.* apostem of the throat, quinsy 142v-143v, 175v, 249v.

squinantum, squinant(e), squinanti *n.* Gramineae, *Cymbopogon schoenanthus*, camel hay 55, 62, 64v, 76v, 162, 230, 230v, 246v, 250, 262v, 201, 201v, 309v.

squoyme *imp.* skim 167v.

stancrop *n.* Crassulaceae, *Sedum* spp., stonecrop; *iuse of s.* 272.

staphi(e), staphyne, staphizagre, staffie *n.* Ranunculaceae, *Delphinium staphisagria*, stavesacre 62, 68, 69v, 76v, 77, 98, 136, 137, 141.

steel *n.* steel 216.

stering *vbl. n.* starting, leaping 55v.

sticados *n.* Labiatae, *Lavandula stoechas*, French lavender 62.

stiche *n.*, **-s** *pl.* stitch in the side 156v, 264.

stille see **distille.**

stomak(e) *n.* stomach 50v, 52v, 53v, 56, 65, 66, 69v-70v, 76, 95, 101, 102v, 106, 107, 109v, 121, 122v, 130v, 131, etc., also 221; **stomakes** *poss.* 52v, 224v; **mouþe of þe s.** top of the stomach 62, 184v, 224v, 225, 233, 235-236v, 241v, 253. See **pore, skyn(ne).**

stomaticon *n.* digestive or purgative electuary 73, 251v; *colde s.* 245, 251; *grettir s.* 187v; *hoot s.* 251.

ston(e), stoon *n.*, **-s** *pl.* urinary calculus 68, 90v, 162, 275v, 280v-282v, 283v-284v, 285v, 286, 287, 288; stonelike apostem 104; stone 123v, 189v, 222v, 256v, 259, 274v, 218v, 310v; testicle 296v, 300, 300v-302, 303v, 304v; kernel 233v; *tiyl s.* 84v, 149, 192v, 240, 258, 258v, 273v. See **chiry, fysshe, magnes, plumb.**

stonied see **a-stonyen.**

storax, storace, storacis *n.* resin from Hamamelaceae, *Liquidamber orientalis,* styrax tree 64v, 76v, 122v, 123v, 137, 172v, 174v, 183v, 241, 301v.

strangury(a) *n.* difficulty in urination, strangury 162, 251, 285, 286, 289, 293; **stranguriam** 286v.

straw-beri leues *n. pl.* Rosaceae, *Fragaria vesca,* wild strawberries 307.

strictory *n.*, **-es** *pl.* constricting medicine 82, 86v, 92, 93, 96v, 135, 136, 137, 181v, 186v, 251, 252, 256v, 257, 262, 263v, 276v, 301v; *adj.* 126v, 240, 259v, 275, 293v; *s. herbs* 252, 261, 298. See **constrictif.**

stufe, st(e)we, stue *n.*, **-s** *pl.* bath or hot vapor used as medicine 77v, 84, 107v, 108, 109v, 110, 114v, 117, 119-120, 122v-123v, 129, 142, 148v, 159v, 233v, 199, etc.

stufe(n) *v.* treat with a bath or vapor 151v, 160, 246; **stuwe** *imp.* 107v; **stufen, stwid, y-stufed** *p. p.* 84, 108, 148v; **stufyng** *vbl. n.* 108, 109v.

stupefacris, stupefactiues *n. pl.* very cold medicines having a numbing effect 80v, 138.

subtilatiues, subtilitiues *n. pl.* medicines making harmful matter thinner 178v, 183.

sugur, sugyr *n.* sugar 48, 48v, 103, 140v, 141v, 156-157, 161v, 167v, 168, 171, 177v, 182v, 186v, 222v, 228v, 230v, 239v, 241, etc.; *s. of borage* 55; *s. roset* 48, 48v, 55, 63, 126v, 167, 186v, 229, 233, 252, 260v, 290, 292, 292v, 301v; *s. of violet* 48, 48v, 63, 149, 167, 187v, 229, 196v, 208v, 216v, 286.

sumac *n.* Anacardiaceae, *Rhus* spp., sumac 140, 145, 171, 258, 297.

sunne, sonne *n.* sun 48, 60, 75, 78v, 85, 91, 94v, 102, 102v, 104v, 188, 190v, 192v, 194, 309v.

superfluite(e)s *n. pl.* waste products 48.

suppository(e) *n.*, **-s** *pl.* suppository 64, 69, 73v, 192, 259, 266, 268, 268v, 273, 274, 198v, 306v.

surgery *n.* surgery 172. See **kutting, oyn(e)ment.**

swalme *n.* swelling 139, 143, 304, 304v, 305v, 308v.

swelle *v.* swell 120v, 229v; **swelliþ** *pr. 3 sg.* 85v, 126, 139, 224, 244v, 248v, 195; **swellen** *3 pl.* 72, 75v, 85v, 120v, 130v, 308; **(to)-swolle(n)** *p. p.* 55v, 133v, 139, 195, 302v, 304, 305, 305v, 308v; **swol(we), to-swolowe** *p. p.* 107, 279, 301.

swelling *vbl. n.*, **-is** *pl.* swelling 74v, 75v, 105v, 133v, 134, 135v, 139, 142v, 147, 165, 173v, 191, 231, 231v, 244v, 246, 246v, 247v, 195v, 207, etc.

swete, soot, swote *n.* a sweat 67, 82v, 108v, 184v, 185.

swete *adj.* sweet 132, 155, 156v, 193v, 225, 271, 205v, 206v. See **flevme, mete, mylke, vynegre, wyn(e)**.

swete *v.* sweat 107v, 288; **swetiþ, swete** *pr. 3 sg.* 61v, 215v; **sweting** *vbl. n.* 61v, 304v.

swetnes *n.* sweetness, esp. from the humor blood 147, 164v.

swolle, swolewe, swolowe, swollewen *v.* swallow 131v, 180v, 189v, 221v, 223v, 248; **swolwiþ** *pr. 3 sg.* 221v, 222; **swolowid** *p. p.* 223v; **swolewing** *vbl. n.* 143v, 221.

taast *v.* taste 138v; **tasting** *vbl. n.* 71.

talowe *n.* rendered fat 299; *t. of a goot bucke* 111; *boles t.* 100v; *gotis t.* 275, 298, 298v; *shepis t.* 273v, 280.

tamarindi(s) *n. pl.* Leguminosae, *Tamarindus indica*, tamarind 261v; *rynde of t.* 218v; **oxifistula** *n.* t. bark 228v.

tansey *n.* Compositae, *Chrysanthemum vulgare*, tansy 171v.

tartarum of whijt wiyn *n.* white wine dregs 140v.

temperat *adj.* tempered 63v; hot and moist 64; neither too hot nor too cold 229v, 216v, 217v; moderate 67. See **mete**.

templis *n. pl.* temples 53, 57v, 72, 81, 81v, 85v, 135, 137, 188.

tempriþ *pr. 3 sg.* temper 150; **tempre, temper** *imp.* 51v, 54, 62v, 81v, 83v, 85, 87v, 88, 91, 94, 94v, 96v, 123, 123v, 132v, 141v, 142v, 148v, 156, 171, etc.; **(y-)temp(e)rid** *p. p.* 63v, 87, 223, 253, 199v, 309v. See **distemp(e)ring**.

tenasmon *n.* painful urge to move the bowels but inability to do so 272, 274, 275, 203v.

tentis *n. pl.* small rolls 64.

terebentyne *n.* resin of Anacardiaceae, *Pistacia terebinthus*, terebinth tree 160v, 161.

theodoricon *n.* a purgative medicine 72v.

tyme *n.* Labiatae, *Thymus* spp., thyme 50, 54v, 103, 117, 159v, 247, 209v, 214, 217, 218v, 220v, 307v; *floris of t.* 84; **epityme (þat is þe flour of tyme)** 60, 76v, 159v, 187, 204v, 209v, 218v, 307v.

(p)tisane *n.* barley water 149, 150, 152v, 166v, 170v, 174v, 183v, 222v, 223v, 228v, 232v, 237, 310.

(p)tisik(e) *n.* wasting caused by loss of natural moisture, phthisis 151v, 162v, 168, 175-177, 180-182v, 185, 200v.

titimalle *n.* Euphorbiaceae, *Euphorbia paralias*, sea spurge; *iuse of t.* 238v.

title *n.*, **-s** *pl.* title, chapter 103v, 105v, 120, 129, 133, 138v, 146v, 162, 184, 221, 253v, 194, 275v, 299v, 305v. Cf. **practis**.

tittis *n. pl.* teats 130v.

token *n.*, **-es** *pl.* diagnostic or prognostic sign 52v, 53, 55v, 56, 57, 57v, 61, 61v, 65v, 66, 72, 75-76, 107, 110v, 125-126, 128, etc.; *t. of deeþ* 57v, 60, 61v, 72, 72v, 126, 172, 173v, 176v, 227v. See **sign(e)**.

toon *n. pl.* toes 191v. See **veyne**.

tooþ *n.*, **teeþ** *pl.* tooth 67, 74, 120v, 129v, 130v-137v, 138, 138v, 269v. See **ache**.

tose *imp.* pull apart 278v.

traue(i)l *n.* effort 172, 226, 227v, 215v.

traue(i)l *v.* work 241v, 216v, 288, 291, 297; **traueliþ with child** *pr. 3 sg.* 264.

trauelous *adj.* painful, difficult 165v, 265, 195v.

tre(a)tes *n.* subdivision of a chapter, treatise 74v, 150. Cf. **practis.**

triacle *n.* theriac, a medicine esp. effective against poison 251, 253, 263v, 283v, 286v, 287, 295, 295v; *t. diatesseron* 192v, 193, 267.

triafera sarasenica *n.* a cleansing medicine 197, 208v, 215v.

triasandri *n.* electuary made of three kinds of sandalwood 182v, 186v, 229, 245, 196v, 218.

trouble, trobelid *ppl. adj.* turbid 61v, 207, 288v.

trussid *ppl. adj.* wearing a truss 299v.

tuc(h)ie, thuchie, thuchia, tute *n.* natural zinc ores or zinc oxide flakes found inside smelting furnaces 88-89, 91v, 92, 94, 94v, 103v.

tunge, tonge *n.* tongue 55v, 65v, 120v, 129v, 130, 132v, 134v, 138v-142, 143, 148v, 149v, 150, 155v, etc.

turbit *n.* Convolvulaceae, *Ipomoea turpethum*, turpeth 262v.

turmentil *n.* Rosaceae, *Potentilla erecta*, tormentil 102, 249, 259, 216, 282v, 298v; *rote of t.* 299v.

turmentyne *n.* turpentine 144, 223, 238v, 219, 298v, 305.

þenke (*on*) *v.* think about 58v; **þenken** *pr. 3 pl.* 58v.

þerf *n.* tharf, unleavened bread 202v.

þick(e) *adj.* thick or viscous in consistency 53, 91v, 92v, 95, 97, 101v, 126, 127, 133v, 143v, 144, 153v, 154v, 158v, 159, 160, 163v, 170v, 176v, 225, etc.; (of the pulse) frequent 56.

þin(ne) *adj.* watery or thin 50, 53, 56, 83, 92v, 101v, 125, 154v, 158v, 163, 163v, 244, 255, 260, 262v, 195v, 196, 210v, 211-213, etc.

(nose)þirl(e), noseþril *n.*, **-s** *pl.* nostril 77, 120, 120v, 121v, 124, 124v, 126, 128, 137v, 188, 191v, 193, 193v, 269v.

þirst(e), þurste *n.* thirst 142v, 151, 155, 159, 163v, 185v, 221, 224, 227-229, 248, 251, 265v, 196, 212v, 291v.

þirstful(le), þurstful *adj.* thirsty 158v, 185v, 221v, 224, 244v, 264v, 265, 203, 206v, 211v, 293.

þistil *n.* Compositae, *Silibum marianum*, St. Mary's thistle; *seed of Oure Lady þ.* 284v.

þombe n. thumb 293. See **veyne.**

þorne *n.* **-s** *pl.* Rosaceae, *Crataegus oxyacanthoides*, white thorn; *Prunus spinosa*, sloe or black thorn 145v; *rinde of þ.* 298v; *branchis of a white þ.* 302v; *leues of a white þ.* 302v; *rinde of a blac þ.* 257. See **acacia, sloo(n).**

þou3t *n.* study , mental effort 48, 172; thought 53; mental processes 53.

þrote *n.* throat 127v, 141, 142v, 143v, 144v, 145v, 147, 154v, 155, 158v, 159, 164v, 228; **þ.-bolle** larynx 147, 149-150.

y-þrowe (*into*) *p. p.* (of an enema) propelled into 259v.

vnkynde *adj.* unnatural 48v, 179v, 251, 198. See **kyndeli.**
vryn *n.* urine 53, 56, 61v, 126, 185, 243, 250v, 251, 264v, 265, 194v-
196v, 203, 202v, 203v, 206v, 207, etc. See **child(e), pisse, watir.**

valerian *n.* Valerianaceae, *Valeriana officinalis*, valerian 69, 83.
veyne *n.*, **-s** *pl.* vein, blood vessel 72, 85v, 96, 113v, 121, 122, 125, 125v,
127, 128, 134v, 142v, 147, 155, 164v, 165, 169, 169v, 172v, 178v,
etc., also 184v, 195, 277v, 291, 301, 305v, 307v; *v. vndir þe ancle*
216, 276, 277v, 279, 282v, 283v, 301, 303v, 304, 306v; *v. of þe arme*
207v; *v. of þe arme y-callid basilica* basilic vein 155v, 185v, 205v;
v. of þe brayn cephalic vein 169; *v. vndir þe eere* 216; *v. of þe
elbowe* 84, 96v, 99; *v. in þe myddil of þe foreheed* 57; *v. of þe
guttis* 260, 202, 210; *heed v. (of þe arme)* cephalic vein 53v, 68,
72v, 77v, 96v, 99, 126v, 134, 143, 148; *herte v.* median cephalic
vein 206; *v. þat ben in þe y3e* 96v, 99; *v. þat clenseþ þe y3en and
þe heed* 99; *liuer v. (of þe arme)* basilic vein 260v, 277, 301, 302v,
306v; *v. about þe li3te* 164; **saluitica/saluatelle** salvatella 216,
218v; *splene v.* left salvatella 206; *v. on þe grete too* 143; *v. þat is
vndir þe tunge* 134v, 139v, 140v, 143, 155v; *v. of þe þombe* 96v; *v.
bitwene þe þombe and þe nexte fyngir* 70, 99.
veneson *n.* venison 49.
vertigrece, vertegrese *n.* verdigris 89, 97v, 302v.
vertu *n.* power 97, 152, 167v, 284v, 287v, 292, 310v.
verueyn *n.* Verbenaceae, *Verbena officinalis*, vervain 80, 99v, 107v,
109v, 137v, 138, 290v; *iuse of v.* 82v, 94, 94v, 97, 127v.
vyne *n.* Vitaceae, *Vitis vinifera*, grape vine 80, 97, 219; *v. leues* 187,
216, 282v; *knot of v.* 88v; *root of white v. and blacke wield v.*
Cucurbitaceae, *Bryonia dioica*, white bryony; Dioscoreaceae,
Tamus communis, black bryony 113. See **brionie, grapes.**
vynegre *n.* vinegar 49v, 50, 56v, 57, 63, 68, 73, 94, 95, 99, 104v, 109,
112v, 113, 114, 117v, 123v, 127v, 134v, 135, etc.; *rede v.* 298; *swete
v.* 142v, 156; *white v.* 197. See **sape, sirip.**
violet *n.*, **-tis** *pl.* Violaceae, *Viola* spp., violet 54, 63v, 64v, 69v, 81,
107v, 108v, 111, 124v, 129, 152, 156-157, 167-168, 177, 179v, 182v,
etc., also 193v, 222; *v. floures* 181, 187, 215v; *iuse of v.* 81v, 87v;
leues of v. 187; *sedis of v.* 197. See **oyl(e), sirip, sugur.**
visage *n.* face 56, 129, 142v, 147, 155, 155v, 164v, 192v, 194, 194v,
195v, 207.
voice, voys *n.* voice 134v, 147.
volate(n) *v.* vomit 169, 191, 235; **volatiþ** *pr. 3 sg.* 60, 235v, 265v, 194v;
volaten *3 pl.* 270; **volating** *vbl. n.* 234v. See **cast(e), spue.**
vomeþ *pr. 3 sg.* foams at the mouth 270v.

wagging *vbl. n.* remaining awake (L *vigilia*) 149v.
wake *v.* remain awake, keep a vigil 300v; **waking** *vbl. n.* 48, 49v, 50v,
55v, 63, 151, 172, 188v.

walle-notte, walis-not, walisshe-notis *n.* Juglandaceae, *Juglans regia*, walnut 249; *quantite of a w.* 173, 174, 174v.

walwort *n.* Caprifoliaceae, *Sambucus ebulus*, danewort 238; *iuse of w.* 271v.

warm(e) *adj.* neither hot nor cold 48, 48v, 51v, 56v, 57, 62, 62v, 81v, 82, 86v, 98, 107v, 115v, 117v, 136v, 145, 148v, 161v, 169v, 173, etc., also 228, 234.

watir *n.*, **-s** *pl.* water 48v, 53, 56v, 57, 58, 60v, 62, 63v, 64, 69v, 70, 78, 78v, 81, 82, 84, 86v, 90, 91v, 93v, etc., also 147, 150, 252v, 213; medicinal water 48, 55, 69, 73v, 79v, 80, 81, 81v, 82v, 83v, 84v, 87-88, 91, 92, 93v, 94, 97, 98, etc., also 152, 156v; tears 75, 75v, 102v; urine 281, 281v; *w. foules* 67v; *w. leche* 57v, 61v, 112v, 289; *fresshe w.* 260v, 273; *reyne w.* 87v, 88, 171, 240, 251, 256v, 258, 273, 290; *smypþes w.* water from a forge 99v, 216; *souffri w.* 69v; **aqua** 183, 286v. See **fysshe, salt(e)**.

watren *pr. 3 pl.* (of the eyes) water 67, 85v, 86; **watryng** *vbl. n.* 103v.

watri *adj.* watery 163, 270v, 203.

watrines *n.* watery quality 212v, 280v.

wax(e), wex(e) *n.* bees' wax 56v, 62v, 69v, 77, 77v, 111, 129v, 130v, 144, 157v, 299; *reed w.* with vermilion added 142, 287; *white w.* 146v, 157v.

web(be) *n.*, **webbis** *pl.* weblike growth over the eye 75, 87, 88, 92v, 94-95v, 99v, 103v.

weybrode see **planteyn**.

wem *n.* blemish on the eye 88, 92v.

wesaund(e), wesaunt *n.* throat 143, 146v, 221v-223.

whei *n.* whey; *gotis w.* 180v, 197, 205v.

wherte *n.*, **-s** *pl.* wart 118, 118v.

wheston *n.* whetstone 95, 105; *barbours w.* 94v.

whete *n.* Gramineae, *Triticum* spp. wheat 100v, 145v, 170v, 259v, 267, 310; *w. flour* 60. See **bred(e), bran(ne), mele**[1].

white, whiyt *adj.* white, esp. as an effect of phlegm or melancholy 53, 56, 58, 74, 75, 76, 86, 87v, 87, 89v, 92v, 95, 134, 139, 163, 163v, 174, 177, 244, 262, etc. See **bred(e), ceruse, coral, ey(e), horeho(u)ne, y3e, mete, pepir, popi, sandris, so(o)pe, vyne, wax(e), wyn(e)**.

wike, weke, woke *n.*, **-s** *pl.* week 157v, 159v, 206, 216, 218v, 283, 299.

wyn(e), wiyn *n.* wine 55, 55v, 56v, 68, 69, 70v, 73, 74, 77, 78, 80, 82v, 84-85, 89v, 92, 97, 97v, 100v, etc.; *w. drastis* wine dregs 60; *w. of Gasqwyn* 67v; *w. of pomgarnad* 89v; *rede w.* 137, 225, 258; *smale w.* 142, 183; *stronge w.* 74v, 121v, 142, 291v; *swete w.* 149, 156; *white w.* 49v, 81, 82v, 83v, 84v, 85, 89, 101v, 102v, 105, 229, 245v, 246, 251, 197, 293, 308, 309v. See **tartarum**.

w(i)ynd(e) *n.*, **-s** *pl.* flatulence or gas 102v, 106, 160, 184v, 225v, 229v-230v, 234v, 243v, 244v, 246-247, 248v, 264v-265v, 267v, 268, etc.; breeze 75, 98v, 129v, 130v, 148, 194; air 154, 194; *norþen w.* 160.

wyndi, wiyndi *adj.* flatulent 116, 116v, 245v, 268v, 220, 300. See **mete**.

wynd(i)nes, wyndenes *n.* windiness 210, 213v, 219v, 220, 296, 297.

wynter *n.* winter season 105, 160, 163, 163v, 164, 249v.

wit(t), wit(t)e *n.*, **-s** *pl.* sense, sensory perception 48, 51, 52, 52v, 55v, 56, 60v, 65v, 70v-71v, 169, 224, 227v, 248v, 264, 270v, 195v.

wode, wood *adj.* mad 224, 270; (of choler) raging 241v; *w. dog* 60; *w. hounde* 193.

wo(o)dnes *n.* madness 52, 55v, 58, 220.

wol(le) *n.* wool 108v, 116, 250v, 299; *shepis w.* 62; *vnwasshe shepis w.* 143v, 168v, 189, 266, 267v, 209, 309v.

woman *n.*, **women, wymen** *pl.* woman 51, 264, 306; *company of w.* 48, 67v, 172; *medling with w.* 291. See **mylke**.

worde *n.*, **-s** *pl.* word 59, 310v.

worme *n.*, **-s** *pl.* parasitic worm 104, 105, 105v, 114v-116, 133, 134, 135v, 136, 184v, 253, 264v, 265v, 268v-270v, etc., also 217; snake 193.

worm(w)od(e), wermod *n.* Compositae, *Artemisia absinthium*, wormwood 49, 54, 63v, 67v, 69, 77, 84, 107v, 109v, 110, 117, 129, 142, 172v, 226v, 227, 233, 241, 250, 258v, etc.; *w. sede* 271; *iuse of w.* 62v, 102v, 115, 115v, 117v, 119v, 130, 132v, 233v, 234, 271, 272, 208-209. See **sirip**.

worte *n.*, **-is** *pl.* wort, decoction of malt 271, 277, 278.

wound(e) *n.*, **-is** *pl.* wound 100v, 129v, 145v, 177-179, 181, 181v, 223, 223v, 260, 280, 280v, 289, 305.

wowes *n. pl.* walls 56.

wraþ(þe), wreeþ *n.* anger 49v, 55v, 67v, 172, 297v. See **angir**.

ȝeer, ȝere *n.* year 59v, 87, 120, 160, 214v, 306.

ȝeere see **(e)ere**.

ȝelew(e), ȝelow, ȝelov *adj.* yellow, esp. as an effect of melancholy 71v, 126, 164, 177, 255v, 194v, 202v, 212v, 276v, 306; *swarte ȝ.* deep yellow 139, 158v, 160, 174, 244, 244v, 203v, 210v, 211, 276v, 281, 294v; *ȝ. yvel(e)* jaundice 95v, 182, 182v, 202v-204, 216v.

ȝelew(e)nes *n.* yellowness, esp. as an effect of melancholy 53, 61v, 134; *swart ȝ.* deep yellowness 134.

ȝerde, ȝeerd *n.* penis 101v, 284-285, 288, 290v, 294v, 296, 300, 300v, 301v-303; stick 265v, 309.

zedeware, zedwale, zedoare, zeduare, zedwarie *n.* Zingiberaceae, *Curcuma* spp., zedoary 54v, 76v, 187, 193, 230, 200v, 220v.

ziloaloes see **lignum al(l)oes**.

zilobalsamum *n.* wood of Burseraceae, *Balsamodendron opobalsamum*, balsam of Gilead 182, 225v, 230v, 251, 201. See caropbalsamum, opobalsamum

zilocassia see **cassie**.

zinziber Alexandrium *n.* electuary made of ginger 252.

zosking *vbl. n.* hiccup 221v, 231v, 232, 233-234v.

zoskiþ *pr. 3 sg.* hiccups 232v.

Alphabetical List of Plants by Genus

(See above pp. xlix-l)

Modern Plant Name	Name in Glossary
Acacia senegal	gum arabike
*Achillea millefolium	mylefoyle
Acorus calamus	calamus aromaticus
*Adiantum capillus-veneris	meiden-her
*Aegopodium podagraria	ameos
*Agrimonia eupatoria	egrimoyn
*Ajuga chamaepitys	camapiteos
*Ajuga reptans	myddel comfery
Allium ampeloprasum	erbe þat is like leek
*Allium cepa	onyon
*Allium porrum	leke
*Allium sativum	garlik
*Allium ursinum	affodille
Aloe spp.	aloes
Aloe perryi	aloes cicotryn
Aloe vera	aloes epatike
*Alpina officinarum	galengal
*Althaea officinalis	holy-hock, bismalue
*Amaracus dictamnus	ditteny, ditandre
Amomum cardamomum	amomum
*Amomum melegueta	greyne
*Anacyclus pyrethrum	piretre of Spayne
*Anagallis arvensis	chekenmete ...flour
*Anchusa officinalis	langdebef
*Anethum graveolens	anet
*Anthriscus cerefolium	cerfoil

*Apium graveolens	marche, smalache
Aquilaria agallocha	lignum aloes
*Aquilegia vulgaris	columbine
*Arctium lappa	berdane
*Aristolochia spp.	aristologia
*Aristolochia clematitis	long aristologie
*Aristolochia rotunda	aristologia rotunda
*Artemisia absinthium	wormod
*Artemisia campestris	souþerenwode
Artemisia stellerana	weilde sage
*Artemisia vulgaris	mugwort
*Arum maculatum	aaron
Asarum europaeum	asarum
Astragalus spp.	dragagant
*Atriplex spp.	arage
*Avena spp.	otis

Balsamodendron spp.	bdellie
*Balsamodendron myrrha	mirre
Balsamodendron opobalsamum	carpobalsamum
	opobalsamum
	zilobalsamum
*Bellis perennis	daies-i3e
*Berberis vulgaris	b rberis
*Beta spp.	betis
*Betonica officinalis	betayn
Betula spp.	birche
*Borago officinalis	borage
Boswellia spp.	olibanum
*Brassica spp.	caul
Brassica napus	rapis
Brassica nigra	syneuey
*Brassica oleracea	wilde caul
Brassica rapa	neep
Bryonia dioica	brionie, gorde, white vyne

*Calamintha officinalis	calamynt
*Calendula officinalis	ruddes
*Cannabis sativa	hempe
Capparis spinosa	caparis
*Capsella bursa-pastoris	sangrinary, sheppardis purse
*Carum carvi	carewey
Cassia spp.	sene
Cassia fistula	cassia fistula
Castanea sativa	chesteyn
*Centaurium erythraea	centori
Ceratonia siliqua	carabe

Ceterach officinarum   ceterake
*Chamaemelum nobile   camomil
*Chelidonium majus   celidon
*Chenopodium bonus-henricus   mercury
*Chrysanthemum balsamita   cost
*Chrysanthemum leucanthemum   oxi3e
*Chrysanthemum vulgare   tansey
*Cicer arietinum   ciceres
Cichorium intybus   cicori
Cinnamomum camphora   camphor
Cinnamomum cassia   cassie, zilocassie
Cinnamomum zeylancium   canel
Cistus spp.   lapdanum
Citrullus colocynthis   collaquindida
Citrus medica   citernes
Colchicum autumnale   hermodactalis
*Conium maculatum   hemloc
Convolvulus scammonia   scamony
Cordia spp.   sebesten
*Coriandrum sativum   coliandre
Corylus avellana   hasil, note
Crataegus oxyacanthoides   þorne
*Crocus sativus   safron, citre
Cucumis melo   melone
Cucumis sativus   cucumer
*Cuminum cyminum   comyn
Curcuma spp.   zedeware
*Cuscuta epithymum   cuscute
Cyclamen neapolitanum   erþe appel, siclamen
Cydonia oblonga   citonie
Cymbopogon schoenanthus   squinantum
*Cynoglossum officinale   houndistonge
Cyperus longus   ciperi
Cytinus hypocistis   ypoquistidos

*Daphne laureola   lauriole, alipiados, coconidie
*Daucus carota   dauke
*Delphinium staphisagria   staphi
Dipsacus fullonum ssp. fullonum sheperdis 3eerd
Dorema ammoniacum   amoniac
Dracaena spp.   sandragon

Ecballium elaterium   electarie
Elettaria cardamomum   cardamomum
*Eruca sativa   skirewhites
*Euphorbia spp.   spurge
Euphorbia paralias   titimalle

Euphorbia resinifera	euforbe
Euphorbia uralensis	esula
*Euphrasia officinalis	eufrace

*The botanical family Filicales	feren leues, pollitricum
Fagus sylvatica	beche
Ferula spp.	ase
Ferula galbaniflua	galbanum
Ficus carica	fyge
Ficus sycomorus	sycomour
*Filipendula vulgaris	filipendula
*Foeniculum vulgare	fenel
*Fragaria vesca	straw-beri leues
Fraxinus excelsior	assh
*Fumaria officinalis	fumiter

*Gentiana lutea	gencian
*Geum urbanum	auence
Glaucium flavum	memyth
*Glechoma hederaceae	hayhoue
*Glycyrrhiza spp.	liquoris
*Gnaphalium uliginosum	filago
Gossypium spp.	coton

*Hedera helix	yue
*Helleborus niger	eleborus niger
*Hordeum distichon	barliche
*Hyoscyamus niger	henbane
*Hypericum androsaemum	ypericon
*Hyssopus officinalis	ysop

*Inula helenium	horshel, elena campana
Ipomoea turpethum	turbit
*Iris spp.	accorun, yreos

Juglans regia	walle-notte
Juniperus communis	iuniper
*Juniperus sabina	sauyn

The botanical family Lauraceae	folii
*Lactuca sativa	letuse
Lactuca serriola	scariole
*Lactuca virosa	endyue
*Lamium purpureum	reed netle

Laurus nobilis	lorer
*Lavandula officinalis	lauendre
Lavandula stoechas	sticados
Lens spp.	lentes
*Lepidium sativum	carses, 3erde carses
*Levisticum officinale	louage
*Linum spp.	lynseed
Liquidamber orientalis	storax
*Lithospermum officinale	gromel, milum solis
	palma Christi
Lolium temulentum	nigel
*Lonicera spp.	licium
*Lupinus albus	lupynes
*Malus spp.	appil
*Malva sylvestris	hock, malue
*Mandragora officinalis	mandrake
Marchantia polymorpha	lyuer-worte
*Marjorana hortensis	maioran, sansuke
*Marrubium vulgare	horehone
*Melilotus officinalis	mellilot
*Melissa officinalis	bawme, melisse
*Mentha spp.	mynt
Mentha longifolia	mentastre
*Mentha pulegium	piliol
Morus spp.	mylbery, mores
*Myristica fragrans	notemyg, macis
Myrtus communis	mirtille, mirte
*The botanical family	lily
Nymphaeaceae	
Nardostachys jatamansi	spike, spikenard
*Nepeta cataria	nepte
Nigella damascena	gith
Ocimum spp.	basilicon, ozmi
*Ononis repens	resta bouis
Opoponax chironium	opoponac
*Orchis spp.	serapinum
*Origanum vulgare	origanum
Oryza sativa	riys
*Paeonia mascula	pyony
*Papaver rhoeas	rede popi
*Papaver somniferum	blacke/white popi

*Parietaria diffusa	piretre
*Pastinaca sativa	pasnep
*Petroselinum spp.	parseli
*Peucedanum officinale	peusadanum
Phoenix dactylifera	datis
Phyllanthus emblica	(mirabolanis) emblici
*Phyllitis scolopendrium	hertistonge
*Pimpinella anisum	anyse
*Pimpinella saxifraga	pimpernel
Pinus spp.	pynes
Piper cubeba	quibibis
*Piper nigrum	pepir
Pistacia lentiscus	mastik
Pistacia terebinthus	terebentyne
*Pisum sativum	pees
*Plantago lanceolata	planteyn þe lasse, ribwort
*Plantago major	planteyn (þe more), weybrode
*Plantago psyllium	psillie
*Polygonum aviculare	corigiole
*Polygonum bistorta	serpentarie, dragance
*Polypodium vulgare	polipodi
Polyporus officinalis	agarike
*Portulaca oleracea	purslane, portulake
Potentilla erecta	turmentil
*Potentilla reptans	pentafilon
*Primula veris	herbe of þe palesy
*Primula vulgaris	plemeros
*Prunus amygdalus	almondis
Prunus avium	chiry
Prunus domestica	plumb
Prunus domestica ssp. insititia	damasenes
Prunus spinosa	acacia, sloo, blac þorne
Pterocarpus santalinus	sandris
*Pulicaria dysenterica	policarie
Punica granatum	pomgarnard, balauste, psidie
Pyrus communis	peris

Quercus spp.	oke

*Ranunculus lingua	lanceola þat groweþ in watir
*Ranunculus sceleratus	apium ranarum
*Raphanus sativus	radiche
Rheum spp.	reubarbe
Rhus spp.	sumac
*Rorippa nasturtium-aquaticum	watir-carses
*Rosa spp.	roses
*Rosmarinus officinalis	rosmaryn, antos

*Rubia tinctorum   madir
Rubus caesius   breris þat growen in þe fildis
*Rumex spp.   sorel, sour-doc
*Ruta graveolens   rw, pigami

Salix spp.   saleyn leues
Salvia horminoides   centrum-galli, gallitricum
*Salvia officinalis   sage
*Sambucus ebulus   walwort
Sambucus nigra   elern
*Sanguisorba officinalis burnet
*Sanicula europaea   sanicle
Santalum album   sandris
*Sarothamnus scoparius   brome
*Satureja spp.   sauerey
*Saxifraga spp.   saxifrage
*Scabiosa spp.   scabeous
*Sedum spp.   stancrop
*Sedum telephium   orpyn
Semecarpus anacardium   anacardi
*Sempervivum tectorum   syngrene
*Senecio vulgaris   groundswili
Seseli spp.   siler (mounteyn)
Silibum marianum   þistil
*Sinapis alba   mustard
Sinapis arvensis   carloke
*Sisymbrium officinale   sisymbre
*Smyrnium olusatrum   macedo
*Solanum dulcamara   solatre
*Solanum nigrum   morel
*Spinacia oleracea   spinage
*Stellaria media   chekenmete, oculus Christi
*Symphytum officinale   comfery, symphite
Syzygium aromaticum   clowes

Tamarindus indica   tamarindi, oxifistula
*Tamus communis   blacke wield vyne
Terminalia chebula   (mirabolanis) kebulis
Terminalia citrina   mirabolani citri, m. indi
Teucrium chamaedrys   camedreos
*Teucrium polium   piliol monteyn, polie
*Thymus spp.   tyme
*Trifolium pratense   iii-leuyd gras
*Trigonella foenum-graecum   femygreke
Triticum spp.   whete

*Ulex europaeus	gorst
Ulmus glabra	elme
*Umbilicus rupestris	penyworte
*Urginea scilla	squille
*Urtica spp.	netle
Valeriana celtica	spica celtica
*Valeriana officinalis	valerian
Verbascum thapsus	moleyn
Verbena officinalis	verueyn
Vicia faba	bean
*Vicia orobus	orobus
*Viola spp.	violet
Vitex agnus-castus	agnus castus
Vitis spp.	reisens
*Vitis vinifera	grapes, vyne
Zingiber officinale	gynger
Zizyphus jujuba	inubes

Bibliography

Ariès, Philippe. *The Hour of Our Death*. Translated by Helen Weaver. New York: Knopf, 1981.

Arnaldus de Villanova. *Arnaldi de Villanova Opera medica omnia II: Aphorismi de gradibus*. Edited by Michael R. McVaugh. Granada-Barcelona: Seminarium historiae medicae Granatensis, 1975.

Articella. Lyons, 1519.

Bacon, Roger. *The Opus Majus of Roger Bacon*. Vol. 2. Edited by J. H. Bridges. London, 1900.

Bacon, Roger. *De retardatione accidentium senectutis cum aliis opusculis de rebus medicinalibus*. Edited by A. G. Little and E. Withington. Brit. Soc. Franciscan Studies 14 (1928).

Bailey, L. H. *Manual of Cultivated Plants*. Revised. New York: Macmillan, 1977.

Bartholomaeus Anglicus. *On the Properties of Things: John Trevisa's Translation of* Bartholomaeus Anglicus De proprietatibus rerum: *A Critical Text*. Edited by M. C. Seymour et al. 3 vols. Oxford: Clarendon Press, 1975-1988.

Bateson, Mary, ed. *Borough Customs*. Vol. 2. Selden Society 21 (1906).

Beaujouan, Guy. "Manuscrits médicaux du moyen âge conservés en Espagne." *Mélanges de la casa de Velazquez* 8 (1972): 161-221.

Beck, R. Theodore. *The Cutting Edge: Early History of the Surgeons of London*. London: Lund Humphries, 1974.

Bennett, H. S. *Chaucer and the Fifteenth Century*. 1947. Revised. Oxford: Clarendon Press, 1970.

Bennett, H. S. "Medicine," "Translations and Translators," "Trial List of Translations into English Printed between 1475-1569." In *English Books and Readers, 1475-1557*. 2d ed. Cambridge: Cambridge University Press, 1970.

Bennett, H. S. "Science and Information in English Writings of the Fifteenth Century." *Modern Language Review* 39 (1944): 1-8.

Bernardus de Gordonio. *Practica seu Lilium medicinae.* Naples, 1480.

Bierbaumer, Peter. *Der botanische Wortschatz des Altenglischen.* Teil 3: *Der botanische Wortschatz in altenglischen Glossen.* Frankfurt a. M.: Peter Lang, 1979.

Bloch, H. *Monte Cassino in the Middle Ages.* 3 vols. Cambridge: Harvard University Press, 1986.

Boase, T. S. R. *Death in the Middle Ages: Mortality, Judgment and Remembrance.* London: Thames and Hudson, 1972.

Briquet, C. M. *Les filigranes: Dictionnaire historique des marques du papier.* Edited by Allan Stevenson. 4 vols. Amsterdam: Paper Publications Society, 1968.

Brodin, G|sta, ed. *Agnus Castus: A Middle English Herbal.* Cambridge: Harvard University Press, 1950.

Carlin, Martha. "Medieval English Hospitals." In *The Hospital in History,* edited by Lindsay Granshaw and Roy Porter, pp. 21-39. London: Routledge, 1989.

Carlin, Martha. "The Medieval Hospital of St. Thomas the Martyr in Southwark." *Soc. Social Hist. Medicine Bull.* 37 (1985): 19-23.

Catalogue of Additions to the Manuscripts in the British Museum in the Years 1876-1881. Reprint. London, 1968.

Chaucer, Geoffrey. *Works.* 2d ed. Edited by F. N. Robinson. Boston: Houghton Mifflin Co., 1957.

Clapham, A. R.; Tutin, T. G.; and Warburg, E. F. *Flora of the British Isles.* 2d ed. Cambridge: Cambridge University Press, 1962.

Cockayne, Thomas Oswald, ed. *Leechdoms, Wortcunning and Starcraft of Early England.* 1864-66. 3 vols. Rev. ed. London: Holland Press, 1961.

Constantine the African. *Opera.* Basel, 1536.

Cook, Harold J. *The Decline of the Old Medical Regime in Stuart London.* Ithaca: Cornell University Press, 1986.

D'Alverny, Marie-Thérèse. "Translations and Translators." In *Renaissance and Renewal in the Twelfth Century,* edited by Robert L. Benson and Giles Constable, with Carol D. Lanham, pp. 421-62. Cambridge: Harvard University Press, 1982.

Davis, Norman, ed. *Paston Letters and Papers of the Fifteenth Century.* 2 vols. Oxford: Clarendon Press, 1971.

Dawson, Warren R., ed. *A Leechbook or Collection of Medical Recipes of the Fifteenth Century.* London: Macmillan, 1934.

Demaitre, Luke. *Doctor Bernard de Gordon: Professor and Practitioner.* Toronto: Pontifical Institute of Mediaeval Studies, 1980.

Demaitre, Luke. "Scholasticism in Compendia of Practical Medicine, 1250-1450." *Manuscripta* 20 (1976): 81-95.

Dictionary of Medieval Latin from British Sources. Edited by R. E. Latham. London: Oxford University Press, 1975-1986.

Dictionary of Scientific Biography. 16 vols. Edited by Charles Coulston Gillispie. New York: Scribner, 1970-1980.

Diverres, P., ed. *Le plus ancien texte des Meddygon Myddveu*. Paris, 1913.

Dobson, Jessie, and Walker, R. Milnes. *Barbers and Barber-Surgeons of London: A History of the Barbers' and Barber-Surgeons' Companies*. Oxford: Blackwell Scientific Publications, 1979.

Eisner, Sigmund, ed. *The Kalendarium of Nicholas of Lynn*. Athens: University of Georgia Press, 1980.

Finucane, R. C. "Sacred Corpse, Profane Carrion: Social Ideas and Death Rituals in the Later Middle Ages." In *Mirrors of Mortality: Studies in the Social History of Death*, edited by Joachim Whaley, pp. 40-60. New York: St. Martin's Press, 1981.

Fischer, Hermann. *Mittelalterliche Pflanzenkunde*. 1929. Reprint. Munich: Münchner Druke, 1967.

Fisher, John H. "Chancery and the Emergence of Standard Written English in the Fifteenth Century." *Speculum* 52 (1977): 870-99.

Fisher, John H. "Chancery Standard and Modern Written English." *Jour. Soc. of Archivists* 6 (1978-79): 136-44.

Flower, C. T., ed. *Introduction to the Curia Regis Rolls, 1199-1230*. Selden Society 62 (1944).

Furnivall, F. J., ed. *The Book of Quinte Essence*. 1866. Reprint. EETS 16 (1965).

Garrett, Robert M., ed. "A Middle English Rimed Medical Treatise." *Anglia* 34 (1911): 163-93.

Getz, Faye Marie. "Charity, Translation, and the Language of Medical Learning in Medieval England." *Bull. Hist. Medicine* 64 (1990): 1-17.

Getz, Faye Marie. "Gilbertus Anglicus Anglicized." *Medical History* 26 (1982): 436-42.

Getz, Faye Marie. "John Mirfield and the *Breviarium Bartholomei*: The Medical Writings of a Clerk at St. Bartholomew's Hospital in the Later Fourteenth Century." *Soc. Social Hist. Medicine Bull.* 37 (1985): 24-26.

Gilbertus Anglicus. *Compendium medicine*. Lyons: J. Saccon for V. de Portonariis, 1510.

Grant, Edward, ed. *A Source Book in Medieval Science*. Cambridge: Harvard University Press, 1974.

Green, Monica. "Women's Medical Practice and Health Care in Medieval Europe." *Signs* 14 (1989): 434-73.

Grieve, Maud. *A Modern Herbal*. 2 vols. in 1. 1931. Reprint. Edited by C. F. Leyel. New York: Penguin, 1978.

Gross, Charles, ed. *Select Cases from the Coroners' Rolls, A.D. 1265-1413*. Selden Society 9 (1896).

Guy de Chauliac. *The Cyrurgie of Guy de Chauliac*. Edited by Margaret S. Ogden. EETS 265 (1971).

Hallaert, M. R. "The *'Sekenesse of Wymmen'*: A Middle English Treatise on Diseases of Women." *Scripta* 8 (1982).

Hammond, Eleanor Prescott, ed. *English Verse between Chaucer and Surrey*. 1927. Reprint. New York: Octagon Books, 1965.

Handerson, Henry E. *Gilbertus Anglicus: Medicine of the Thirteenth Century*. Cleveland, Ohio, 1918.

Hanna, Ralph. *A Handlist of Manuscripts Containing Middle English Prose in the Henry E. Huntington Library. Index of Middle English Prose, Handlist I*. Cambridge: D. S. Brewer, 1984.

Hargreaves, Henry. "Some Problems in Indexing Middle English Recipes." In *Middle English Prose: Essays on Bibliographical Problems*, edited by A. S. G. Edwards and Derek Pearsall, pp. 91-113. New York: Garland, 1981.

Hartley, Percival Horton-Smith, and Aldridge, Harold Richard. *Johannes de Mirfeld of St. Bartholomew's, Smithfield: His Life and Works*. Cambridge: Cambridge University Press, 1936.

Hatcher, John. *Plague, Population and the English Economy, 1348-1530*. London: Macmillan, 1977.

Heinrich, Fritz, ed. *Ein mittelenglisches Medizinbuch*. Halle, 1896.

Henslow, George, ed. *Medical Works of the Fourteenth Century*. 1899. Reprint. New York: Burt Franklin, 1972.

Hippocratic Writings. Edited by G. E. R. Lloyd. London: Penguin Books, 1978.

Hunt, Tony. *Plant Names of Medieval England*. Cambridge: Brewer, 1989.

Hunt, Tony. *Popular Medicine in Thirteenth-Century England*. Cambridge: Brewer, 1990.

James, M. R. *The Western Manuscripts in the Library of Trinity College, Cambridge*. Vol. 2. Cambridge, 1902.

Jenks, Stuart. "Astrometeorology in the Middle Ages." *Isis* 74 (1983): 185-210.

John of Arderne. *Treatises of Fistula in Ano*. 1910. Edited by D'Arcy Power. Reprint. EETS 139 (1968).

Jones, Ida B., "Halfod 16: A Mediaeval Welsh Medical Treatise." *Etudes celtiques* 7, fasc. 2 (1955): 270-399.

Jones, Peter Murray. "British Library MS Sloane 76: A Translator's Holograph." In *Medieval Book Production: Assessing the Evidence*, edited by Linda L. Brownrigg, pp. 21-39. Los Altos Hills, Calif.: Red Gull Press, 1990.

Jones, Peter Murray. "Four Middle English Translations of John of Arderne." In *Latin and Vernacular: Studies in Late Medieval Manuscripts*, edited by Alastair Minnis, pp. 61-89. Woodbridge: D. S. Brewer, 1989.

Jones, Peter Murray. *Medieval Medical Miniatures*. London: British Library, 1984.

Jones, Peter Murray. "'*Sicut hic dipingitur . . .*': John of Arderne and English Medical Illustration in the 14th and 15th Centuries." In *Die Kunst und das Studium der Natur vom 14. zum 16. Jahrhundert*, edited by Wolfram Prinz and Andreas Beyer, pp. 103-26, 379-92. Weinheim, 1987.

Kealey, Edward J. "England's Earliest Women Doctors." *Jour. Hist. Medicine* 40 (1985): 473-77.

Keil, Gundolf. *Die urognostische Praxis in vor- und frühsalernitanischer Zeit.* Freiburg: Institut für Geschichte der Medizin, 1970.

Ker, N. R. *Medieval Manuscripts in British Libraries.* Vol. 1. Oxford: Clarendon Press, 1969.

Kingsford, C. L. ed. *The Stonor Letters and Papers, 1290-1483.* 2 vols. Camden 3d ser. 29-30 (1919).

Kristeller, Paul Oskar. "Bartholomaeus, Musandinus, and Maurus of Salerno and Other Early Commentators of the 'Articella,' with a Tentative List of Texts and Manuscripts." *Italia medioevale e umanistica* 19 (1976): 57-87.

Kristeller, Paul Oskar. *Studi sulla Scuola medica salernitana.* Naples: Istituto Italiano per gli Studi Filosofici, 1986.

Lanfrank's Science of Surgery. 1894. Edited by Robert von Fleischhacker. Reprint. EETS 102 (1973).

Maitland, F. W., ed. *Select Pleas of the Crown.* Vol. I: *A.D. 1200-1225.* Selden Society 1 (1888).

Manzalaoui, M. A., ed. *Secretum Secretorum: Nine English Versions.* EETS 276 (1977).

Marcellus of Bordeaux. *Marcelli de medicamentis liber.* Edited by Max Niedermann and Eduard Leichtenhan. 2d ed. Corpus medicorum Latinorum 5 (1968).

Matthews, Leslie G. *History of Pharmacy in Britain.* London: Wellcome Institute, 1962.

Matthews, Leslie G. *The Royal Apothecaries.* London: Wellcome Institute, 1967.

Matthews, William, ed. *Later Middle English Prose.* London: Peter Owen, 1962.

Mesue. *Opera quae extant omnia.* Venice, 1562.

Middle English Dictionary. Edited by Hans Kurath et al. In fascicules. Ann Arbor: University of Michigan Press, 1956-.

Moorat, S. A. J. *Catalogue of Western Manuscripts on Medicine and Science in the Wellcome Historical Medical Library.* Volume I: *MSS Written before 1650 A.D.* London: Wellcome Institute, 1962.

Mowat, J. L. G., ed. *Alphita.* Oxford: Anecdota Oxoniensia, Mediaeval and Modern Series, 1887.

Mowat, J. L. G., ed. *Sinonoma Bartholomei.* Oxford: Anecdota Oxoniensia, Mediaeval and Modern Series, 1882.

Müller, Gottfried, ed. *Aus mittelenglischen Medizintexten.* Leipzig, 1929.

Müller, Irmgard. *Die pflanzlichen Heilmittel bei Hildegard von Bingen.* Salzburg: Otto Müller Verlag, 1982.

Mustain, James K. "A Rural Medical Practitioner in Fifteenth-Century England." *Bull. Hist. Medicine* 46 (1972): 469-76.

Norri, Juhani. *Compound Plant-Names in Fifteenth-Century English.* Turku: Publications of the Department of English, 1988.

Norri, Juhani. "Notes on the Study of English Medical Vocabulary from the Historical Point of View." *Neophilologica Fennica* 45 (1987): 335-50.

Norri, Juhani. "Premodification and Postmodification as a Means of Term-Formation in Middle English Medical Prose." *Neuphilologische Mitteilungen* 90 (1989): 147-61.

Ogden, Margaret, ed. *Liber de diversis medicinis*. Revised. EETS 207 (1969).

Parkes, Malcolm B. "The Influence of the Concepts of *Ordinatio* and *Compitatio* on the Development of the Book." In *Medieval Learning and Literature: Essays Presented to Richard William Hunt*, edited by J. J. G. Alexander and M. T. Gibson, pp. 115-41. Oxford: Clarendon Press, 1976.

[Partridge, John]. *The Treasurie of Hidden Secrets . . . Practised by Men of Great Knowledge*. London, 1627.

Payne, Joseph Frank. "English Medicine in the Anglo-Norman Period." *British Medical Jour.* 2 (1904): 1281-84.

Penso, Giuseppe, ed. *Index plantarum medicinalium totius mundi eorum synonymorum*. Milan: O. E. M. F., 1983.

Pollard, Graham. "Describing Medieval Bookbindings." In *Medieval Learning and Literature: Essays Presented to Richard William Hunt*, edited by J. J. G. Alexander and M. T. Gibson, pp. 50-65. Oxford: Clarendon Press, 1976.

Power, Eileen. "Some Women Practitioners of Medicine in the Middle Ages." *Proc. Roy. Soc. Medicine* 15 (1921-1922): 20-23.

Rawcliffe, Carole. "The Hospitals of Later Medieval London." *Medical History* 28 (1984): 1-21.

Rawcliffe, Carole. "Medicine and Medical Practice in Later Medieval London." *Guildhall Studies in London History* 5 (1981): 13-25.

Rawcliffe, Carole. "The Profits of Practice: The Wealth and Status of Medical Men in Later Medieval England." *Soc. Hist. Medicine* 1 (1988): 61-78.

Richardson, Malcolm. "Henry V, the English Chancery, and Chancery English." *Speculum* 55 (1980): 720-50.

Riley, Henry T., ed. *Memorials of London and London Life*. London, 1868.

Robbins, Rossell Hope. "Medical Manuscripts in Middle English." *Speculum* 45 (1970): 393-415.

Rowland, Beryl, ed. *Medieval Woman's Guide to Health*. Kent, Ohio: Kent State University Press, 1981.

Rufinus. *The Herbal of Rufinus*. Edited by Lynn Thorndike. Chicago: University of Chicago Press, 1946.

Schöffler, Herbert, ed. *Mittelenglischen Medizinliteratur*. Halle, 1919.

Shaaber, M. A. *Check-list of Works of British Authors Printed Abroad, in Languages Other than English, to 1641*. New York: Bibliographical Society, 1975.

Sharpe, Reginald, ed. *Calendar of Coroners' Rolls of the City of London, A.D. 1300-1378*. London, 1913.

Sharpe, Reginald, ed. *Calendar of Letter-books Preserved among the Archives of the Corporation of the City of London* [to 1497]. 11 vols. London, 1899-1912.

Slack, Paul. "Mirrors of Health and Treasures of Poor Men: The Uses of the Vernacular Medical Literature of Tudor England." In *Health, Medicine and Mortality in the Sixteenth Century*, edited by Charles Webster, pp. 237-73. Cambridge: Cambridge University Press, 1979.

Stannard, Jerry. "Botanical Data and Late Mediaeval 'Rezeptliteratur.'" In *Fachprosa-Studien: Beiträge zur mittelalterlichen Wissenschafts- und Geistesgeschichte*, edited by Gundolf Keil et al., pp. 371-95. Berlin: Erich Schmidt Verlag, 1982.

Stannard, Jerry. "Rezeptliteratur as Fachliteratur." In *Studies on Medieval Fachliteratur*, edited by William Eamon. *Scripta* 6 (Brussels, 1982): 59-63.

Steinschneider, Moritz. *Die hebraeischen Uebersetzungen des Mittelalters*. Reprint. Graz: Akademische Druk-und-Verlagsanstalt, 1956.

Talbot, Charles. *Medicine in Medieval England*. London: Oldbourne, 1967.

Talbot, C. H., and Hammond, E. A. *The Medical Practitioners in Medieval England: A Biographical Register*. London: Wellcome Institute, 1965.

Theodoric of Lucca. *The Surgery of Theodoric*. 2 vols. Edited by Eldridge Campbell and James Colton. New York: Appleton-Century-Crofts, 1955 and 1960.

Thomas, A. H., ed. *Calendar of Early Mayor's Court Rolls*. Cambridge, 1924.

Thomas, A. H., ed. *Calendar of Select Pleas and Memoranda of the City of London Preserved . . . at Guildhall . . . 1413-1437*. Cambridge, 1943.

Thomson, George. *A Letter Sent to Mr Henry Stubbe*. London, 1672.

Thorndike, Lynn, and Kibre, Pearl. *A Catalogue of Incipits of Mediaeval Scientific Writings in Latin*. Rev. and aug. New York: Mediaeval Academy of America, 1963.

Thrupp, Sylvia. *The Merchant Class of Medieval London*. Ann Arbor: University of Michigan Press, 1962.

Trease, G. E., and Hodson, J. H. "The Inventory of John Hexham, a Fifteenth-Century Apothecary." *Medical History* 9 (1965): 76-81.

Tristram, Philippa. *Figures of Life and Death in Medieval English Literature*. London: P. Elke, 1976.

Voigts, Linda Ehrsam. "Editing Middle English Medical Texts: Needs and Issues." In *Editing Texts in the History of Science and Medicine*, edited by Trevor H. Levere, pp. 39-68. New York: Garland, 1982.

Voigts, Linda Ehrsam. "Medical Prose." In *Middle English Prose: A Critical Guide to Major Authors and Genres*, edited by A. S. G. Edwards, pp. 315-35. New Brunswick: Rutgers University Press, 1984.

Voigts, Linda Ehrsam. "Scientific and Medical Books." In *Book Production and Publishing in Britain, 1375-1475*, edited by

Jeremy Griffiths and Derek Pearsall, pp. 345-402. Cambridge: Cambridge University Press, 1989.

Voigts, Linda Ehrsam. "The 'Sloane Group': Related Scientific and Medical Manuscripts from the Fifteenth Century in the Sloane Collection." *British Library Journal* 16 (1990): 26-57.

Voigts, Linda E., and McVaugh, Michael R., eds. "A Latin Technical Phlebotomy and Its Middle English Translation." *Trans. American Philos. Soc.* 74, 2 (1984).

Walton, Michael. "The Advisory Jury and Malpractice in 15th Century London: The Case of William Forest." *Jour. Hist. Medicine* 40 (1985): 78-82.

Walton, Michael. "Stinking Air, Corrupt Water, and the English Sweat." *Jour. Hist. Medicine* 36 (1981): 67-68.

Walton, Michael. "Thomas Forestier and the *False Lechys* of London." *Jour. Hist. Medicine* 37 (1982): 71-73.

Way, A. "Bill of Medicines Furnished for the Use of Edward I. 34 and 35 Edw. I, 1306-7." *Archaeological Journal* 14 (1857): 267-71.

Webster, Charles. "Thomas Linacre and the Founding of a College of Physicians." In *Essays on the Life and Work of Thomas Linacre, c. 1460-1524*, edited by Francis Maddison, Margaret Pelling, and Charles Webster, pp. 198-222. Oxford: Clarendon Press, 1977.

Welborn, Mary Catherine. "The Errors of the Doctors according to Friar Roger Bacon of the Minor Order." *Isis* 18 (1932): 26-62.

Whittaker, W. J., ed. *The Mirror of Justices*. Selden Society 7 (1895).

Whittet, T. D. "The Apothecaries in Provincial Gilds." *Medical History* 8 (1964): 245-73.

Wickersheimer, Ernest. *Dictionnaire biographique des médecins en France au moyen âge*. 1936. Reprint. Geneva: Librairie Droz, 1979.

Williams, John, ed. *The Physicians of Myddfai*. London, 1861.

Workman, S. K. *Fifteenth-Century Translation as an Influence on English Prose*. Princeton: Princeton University Press, 1940.

Wylie, J. A., and Collier, L. H. "The English Sweating Sickness (Sudor Anglicus): A Reappraisal." *Jour. Hist. Medicine* 36 (1981): 425-45.

Young, John. *Catalogue of the Manuscripts in the Library of the Hunterian Museum in the University of Glasgow*. Glasgow, 1908.

Young, Sidney, ed. *The Annals of the Barber-Surgeons of London*. London, 1890.

Zimmermann, Volker. *Rezeption und Rolle der Heilkunde in landessprachigen handschriftlichen Kompendien des Spätmittelalters*. Stuttgart: Franz Steiner Verlag, 1986.

Wisconsin Publications in the History of Science and Medicine